www.voltaicplasma.com

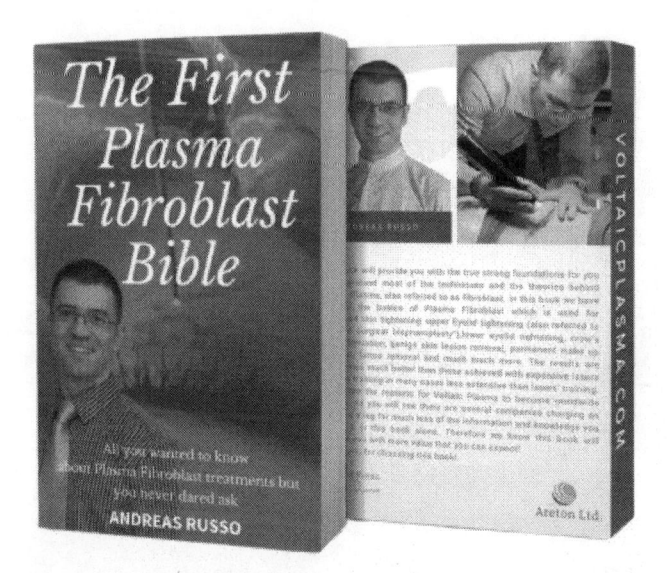

Author: Andreas Russo

Table of Content

1.0 Voltaic arc, sometimes referred to as Plasma or Fibroblast, what is it? 20

2.0 A Bit of History and context about Plasma or "Fibroblast" 22

3.0 Voltaic Arc in Aesthetics, Electrofulguration and Electrodessication 23

4.0 Familiarize with the use of electrical arc 27

    4.1 Exercise on How to generate the electric Arc or Spark 29

    4.2 Practice of the Spot Mode or Spot Operation 29

    4.3 Practice of the Spot Mode or Spot Operation 30

5.0 Fibroblast and skin tightening 31

    5.1 What to expect from Fibroblast skin tightening treatments 31

    5.2 The basics priniciple of skin tightening by using Electrofulguration (Plasma) 31

    5.3 Methods to accomplish skin tightening using electrical arcing 32

    5.4 Spot mode or spot operation 32

    5.5 Spray mode in skin tightening 33

    5.6 Spot mode treatment intensity 34

6.0 The basic principles of plasma skin tightening, why does it work? 35

7.0 The physics of Fibroblast 36

    7.1 Distance between the spots and treatment intensity 37

    7.2 Arc duration and treatment intensity 41

8.0 Introduction to Upper Eyelid Tightening 42

    8.1 Alternatives to electrical arcing for eyelid tightening (or plasma) 43

    8.2 Advantages and disadvantages of eyelid tightening in general 43

    8.3 Eyelid tightening by using aesthetic lasers 44

    8.4 Overview of eyelid tightening with electrical arcing equipment 46

    8.5 With Eyelid tightening using the appropriate plasma (or arc generating) device: 48

    8.6 Patch testing.. 49

    8.7 Before applying the numbing product 49

    8.8 Use of numbing products before the treatments 49

8.9 How to perform upper eyelid tightening	53
8.10 Treatment intensity advantages and disadvantages	54
8.11 Minor Bleeding	54
8.12 The Carbon Residues	55
8.13 Immediate apparent skin contraction during eyelid tightening	56
8.14 Swelling and downtime	57
8.15 How to reduce swelling and downtime	58
8.16 Scabbing proces	60
8.17 Pink skin	61
8.18 When can the client use make-up?	61
8.19 Broad spectrum sun screen	62
8.20 When to repeat the treatment	63
8.21 Long term adverse reactions to the plasma eyelid tightening treatments	63
8.22 Claims of non surgical blepharoplasty	65
8.23 Further advice	66
9.0 How to perform plasma upper eyelid tightening for the first time	67
9.1 Preface	67
9.2 How to carry out your first plasma upper eyelid tightening procedure	68
9.3 Medium intensity	69
9.4 High intensity treatments	69
9.5 Rarely high-intensity treatments can lead to some of the medium-term adverse effects	71
9.6 Conclusions	72
10.0 Long-term healing after plasma upper eyelid lift high-intensity treatments	72
10.1 Overview	73
10.2 What is the long-term healing process anyway?	73
10.3 Redness after localised plasma skin tightening	76
10.4 What does the long-term healing feel like	76
10.5 Plasma upper eyelid lift tightening remodeling during the long-term healing period	77
11.0 Upper Eyelid Tightening AferCare	81
11.1 Swelling	81

11.2 Healing Progression 82

11.3 AfterCare at Home 83

12.0 Plasma Upper Eyelid Healing Process Case Study 84

12.1 Introduction 85

12.2 Difference between the healing after upper eyelid tightening and other plasma localised skin tightening treatments elsewhere on the body 86

12.3 Upper plasma eyelid tightening healing process overview................................... 87

12.4 Pain 88

12.5 Comparison of three swelling cases... 89

12.6 Day one after the procedure 90

12.7 Day two after the procedure 91

12.8 Day three after the procedure 91

12.9 Day four after the procedure 92

12.10 Day Five after the procedure 93

12.11 Day six after the procedure 93

12.12 Swelling of the lower eyelid (or eyebag swelling) following upper eyelid lift 94

12.13 Plasma upper eyelid lift healing process table 95

12.13 Conclusions 96

13. Crow's feet attenuation 96

13.1 Botox and periorbital lines attenuation using plasma 97

13.2 How to perform crow's feet attenuation using plasma 97

14.0 MiniFacelift 99

15.0 Jowl Line 100

16.0 Atrophic Scar Attenuation 101

16.1 Scars can come in different shapes and forms, in this section we will discuss the most common type of scars.. 101

16.2 Types of atrophic scars, "ice pick", "box scars" and "rolling scars"........................ 102

16.3 Atrophic scar removal and attenuation treatments 107

16.4 Ice pick scars removal 109

16.5 Box scars removal 112

16.6 Minor skin grafting or punch grafting (floating) 113

16.7 Punch, discard and close 115

16.8 Subcision 116

16.9 Atrophic scar removal treatments conclusions 117

16.10 Atrophic scar attenuation treatments 118

16.11 Laser resurfacing for acne scar attenuation 120

16.12 Voltaic arcing atrophic scar attenuation treatment (plasma) 121

16.13 Micro needling atrophic scar attenuation treatment 124

16.14 Cosmetic peels atrophic scar attenuation treatment 125

16.15 How to treat atrophic scars in practical cases 125

17.0 Smoker lines attenuation 126

17.1 Introduction to perioral lines 127

17.2 The options to reduce the appearance of perioral lines 128

17.3 Laser resurfacing 129

17.4 Micro-needling 130

17.5 Peels 130

17.6 Microdermabrasion 131

17.7 Smoker lines attenuation using electrical arcing (plasma) resurfacing and tightening 131

17.8 Protocol for perioral lines attenuation using our electrical arcing devices 135

17.9 Manage perioral lines after the permanent attenuation treatments 136

18.0 Brown Spots 136

18.1 How to remove Superficial Brown Spots using Voltaic arc 136

19.0 Moles and skin lesions removal, make sure they are benign first 137

20.0 Moles and skin lesions removal 140

20.1 Manual excision using a conventional scalpel 140

20.2 Mole removal using laser 141

20.3 Mole removal with voltaic arc or voltaic plasma 142

20.4 The techniques generally used for benign mole removal is the spray operation 143

20.5 Summary 145

21. Seborrheic Keratoses 146

22.0 Syringoma 147

- 22.1 How to remove Syringoma using electrical arcing 147
- 22.2 Syringoma Recurrence 148
- 23.0 Xanthelasma 148
- 24.0 SkinTags Removal using Fibroblast 149
- 25.0 Keloids 150
  - 25.1 How and why does a Scar Form? 150
  - 25.2 Keloids and the fundamental difference from hypertrophic scars 152
  - 25.3 Keloid removal treatments 153
  - 25.4 Steroids injections (or intralesional corticosteroid injections) 154
  - 25.5 Main types of combined ablative treatments 154
  - 25.6 Types of combined ablative methods 157
  - 25.7 Home Treatments 158
  - 25.8 Conclusions 160
- 26.0 Tattoos 161
  - 26.1 What is tattoo and an overview of its physiology 162
  - 26.2 Main risk during healing: inflammatory skin infections 164
  - 26.3 Tattoo inflammatory infections symptoms 166
  - 26.4 Introduction to the stages of the tattooing process 168
  - 26.5 Stage one: healing of the open wound. Soon after the tattoo has just been made .. 169
  - 26.6 Stage two: scabbing, peeling and itching 171
  - 26.7 Stage Three 172
  - 26.8 After-care during the healing recovery period 172
  - 26.9 Adverse reactions 174
  - 26.10 Cancer scare due to pigments toxicity 174
  - 26.11 Viral and bacterial infections 175
  - 26.12 Keloids 176
  - 26.13 Allergic Reactions 177
  - 26.14 Granulomas and lymphnodes issues 178
  - 26.15 Mri errors due to tattoos 179
- 27.0 Tattoo Removal 180

27.1 Legislation on tattooing and tattoo removal procedures at european level 181

27.2 Physiological progressive fading of permanent tattoos and the impact of tanning on their brightness 182

27.3 Tattoo resilience and estimating the tattoo fading sessions required 184

27.4 Why is having a tattoo done perceived to be less risky than having it removed? 187

27.5 Tattoo removal techniques introduction, the challenges 188

27.6 Laser tattoo fading 189

27.7 Tattoo fading using plasma, or thermal abrasion with or without osmosis 189

27.8 Tattoo surgical excision 190

27.9 Tattoo fading using osmosis or salation in general 193

27.10 Tattoo fading using chemical peels 197

27.11 Tattoo fading using intense pulsed light (IPL) 198

27.12 Tattoo fading using cryotherapy 199

27.13 Tattoo removal by replacement 200

27.14 Discomfort and Pain 202

27.15 Frosting, (during laser tattoo fading) 202

27.16 Minor bleeding 203

27.17 Immediate redness and minor swelling 203

27.18 Blistering 204

27.19 Scabbing 204

27.20 Itching 205

27.21 Swelling and infections 205

27.22 Permanent and semi-permanent adverse reactions 207

27.23 Permanent adverse reactions 207

27.24 Scarring 207

27.25 Hyper-pigmentation 208

27.26 Hypopigmentation 209

27.27 Conclusions 210

28.0 Laser Tattoo Removal 210

28.1 Why are lasers so popular in tattoo fading treatments 210

28.2 An overview of laser's physics and basic principles of operation in aesthetics 211

28.3 Visually appreciating the ablation effects of the q-switched laser 215

28.4 Varying the timing of the light emission without frosting effects 216

28.5 The physics of laser tattoo removal 217

28.6 Q-Switching Lasers 221

28.7 Laser colour sensitivity 223

28.8 Introduction to tattoo fading treatments transient adverse reactions 228

28.9 Pain during the laser treatment 229

28.10 Bleeding 230

28.11 Discomfort, blistering and normal skin reactions throughout the healing process .. 231

28.12 The number of laser treatments required and the kirby-desai scale 235

28.13 Realstic results of laser tattoo fading 239

28.14 Hypo-pigmentation examples 243

28.15 Real Example 245

29.0 Electrical Thermabrasion tattoo fading 246

29.1 Tattoo Removal with Electrical Thermabrasion (Fibroblast) without osmosis 246

29.2 Plasma or Fibroblast for Tattoo Removal with Osmosis 247

29.3 The importance of Salation or Osmosis when using fibroblasting for tattoo removal 248

29.4 Why using electrical arcing for skin resurfacing before Salabration (or Osmosis)? . 251

29.5 Intensity of the treatment when using Fibroblasting before osmosis 252

29.6 Adverse reactions to Tattoo removal by applying electrical thermal abrasion with osmosis 254

29.7 About the results. How many treatments are required to remove a tattoo? 255

29.8 How much of an area can be treated at a time? 256

29.9 Multicolour tattoos 257

29.10 Tattoo Removal Aftercare 257

29.11 Healing time 258

30.0 Tattoo removal with and without osmosis 258

31.0 Permanent make-up removal 261

31.1 Our Electrical Arcing Device Removal Protocol 261

- 32.0 Pre Treatment 262
  - 32.1 Client's prerequisites to be eligible for the treatment 262
  - 32.2 Before applying the numbing product 263
  - 32.3 Patch testing 263
  - 32.4 Use of numbing products before the treatments 265
  - 32.5 Medical topical numbing product 267
- 33.0 Aftercare 268
  - 33.1 After Care Main Points 269
  - 33.2 Antiseptic, Benzalkonium Chloride Solutions 270
  - 33.3 Optional Soothing Treatment 271
- 34.0 Hot and Cold Plasma 272
  - 34.1 What is "hot plasma" ? 274
  - 34.2 What are carrier gasses in Plasma? 275
  - 34.3 What is "cold plasma"? 276
- 35.0 Electrical Arcing and the European New MDD in 2020 277
  - 35.1 Introduction 277
  - 35.2 Plasma or arcing devices for aesthetic purposes and the new european legislation on medical devices 278
- 36.0 The principle of exclusion in legislation 278
  - 36.1 Why the word "High Intensity"? Because all objects radiate electromagnetic radiations 279
- 37.0 Why does the legislation refer to as "High Intensity Electromagnetic Radiation" (HIER) and not only "Electromagnetic Radiation" ? 281
  - 37.1 are High Intensity Electromagnetic Radiation (HIER) devices as defined by the new legislation? 282
  - 37.2 Plasma (or Electrical Arcing) Devices for aesthetic purposes are not equipment emitting High Intensity Electromagnetic Radiation 283
- Annex I 287

About the author

Andreas Russo started working on Electrical Plasma also referred to as "fibroblast" in 2013. It has been a long journey and the main bulk of this book is taken from the online training platform voltaicplasma.com which Andreas Russo has worked on for a number of years now. Andreas Russo has produced the most successful training videos on the use of plasma devices and has travelled the world over to teach several professionals on the correct use of these devices. VoltaicPlasma.com at the time of writing of this book is being visited by over 100 worldwide visitors daily and the number keeps growing due to the accuracy of the online training and the detailed degree of information you can find only in this website. It is the best online training platform and resource to effectively learn how to use electrical arcing for aesthetic purposes. And one of the most amazing things is that it is mostly free. It blows away any other paid for training programme on plasma fibroblast and it is free of charge. While others charge you thousands of dollars or Pounds for one day training this platform is for most part free and it delivers an immense amount of value which the other courses will not live up to even 10% of the value of the free course we have available on our website. Andreas Russo started creating Voltaicplasma.com in 2015 out of the frustration of having several professionals being over charged for information which should have been free of charge in the first place. Today we are proud of disrupting the market place and making this knowledge ubiquitous and available at your fingertips.

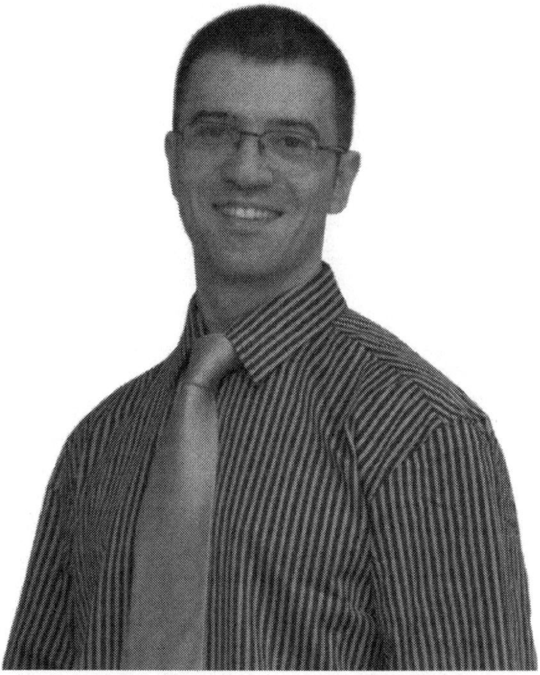

Illustration 1: Andreas Russo

Foreword

We acknowledge all the people who have undergone the several treatments we have carried out throughout the world over all these years. Most of them have already been published on our Youtube channel and you can view them all on demand free of charge.

This book and the free online training on VoltaicPlasma.com would not have been possible without them and the support from all our previous customers.

The mission of this book is to provide you with an oversight of the market place in "plasma" or "fibroblast". This has now become the norm in several clinics the world over due to the several applications this technique has.

Several people are still attempting to sell the training plus the device for 2000 to 4000 dollars however this is becoming more and more complicated in order to sustain provided the enormous resources the internet has on offer. This is why since 2015 we keep releasing all the training we have provided the world over for free.

It is simply not possible to compete with the speed and "intelligence" provided online for free. The era of the local "gurus" selling their secrets on plasma treatments and techniques are gone as there is no real secret any more in the sphere of plasma. We have almost revealed all in our open and free training platform voltaicplasma.com.

Since 2013 when I started in plasma, designing the beautyteck I had the vision of free online training. This is because this is the only future, there is not going to be space for highly priced courses. If you have ever been sold one of these courses you will have experienced the classic, once in a lifetime opportunity to join our "……whatever name…. family". You are sold a lifestyle which you are not going to have. And guess what you are not going to be part of any family. Then if you want to learn you will eventually find our videos and our website.

The people who study and do not impulse buy have access to the best training for free and they are wise in their investment in equipment. Not needing to spend this capital will allow you to invest more where it is really needed for your business. Anyway even if you have invested 2000 or 3000 USD to "allow you" to perform these treatment come to us to learn the real stuff for free.

We have worked on the VoltaicPlasma.com website for several years now to allow to learn the real stuff. Not the hipe you get from the other places where they over charge you.

www.voltaicplasma.com   Author: Andreas Russo

What is the market place like and where is it going to go?

In 2014 Plexr attemped to enter the UK maket and some other markets. This was so much fun to watch. They were selling their three devices in a box for 10000 to 15000 pound depending who you talked to. They managed to sell some, just over 50 in a couple of years. That was it.

More and more devices entered the market place and they were all better than the Plexr and less expensive. Up until 2017 when an internal partnership inside the italian company broke up, soon Plexr was literally pushed out of the UK market due to a very highly competitive market place where more and more devices where available and the knowledge of the techniques have become accessible to everyone thanks to our videos.

Now we see a similar trend, there are still companies out there selling the training with some devices but the price is constantly dropping.

This is thanks to two factors:

1 Internet

2 Cheap devices accessible from the internet.

The mission of this book is to allow you to access in book format and audio format the most important principles of Plasma or also referred to as "fibroblast". The knowledge is now commonplace. The devices are too. We foresee this market being literally commoditised and training companies trying hard selling these same techniques forced out of the market because of this knowledge which you have at your fingertips, or at your earpieces thanks to this book and all the information we placed in voltaicplasma.com

We foresee the only training academy to survive in the future being our website voltaicplasma.com This is because there is no other way. Online training is the only way and it was my vision to create a completely free online training platform wich is attracting more and more visitors over time. At the time of writing this book the daily visitors of Voltaicplasma.com is over 100, everyday people are taking our online testst and getting our certificates online.

If by anychance our website is down we get notified pretty much within one hour over an email or some other means. This is done by people completely unknown to us.

Why Did I have the vision of Voltaicplasma.com?

I was fed up of seeing people being sold very expensive overpriced programmes and devices. It was outrageous to me that in this day and age people were spending precious capital (sometimes over 5000 USD) for a two day training course including the device.

I knew that the person spelling out the secret in the open would take it all. And this is what it is happening due to two factors:

1. More people are sold these devices
2. They require real training and support

The claim I am about to make it quite bold, but I believe it is true. The best training and support on the use of this type of devices is only currently available on Voltaicplasma.com. If you do not believe me please try us, we are free. You have nothing to lose other than the time that it takes to learn and if you want to compare you can compare us with other paid for courses you will eventually come to our website to learn what you need to learn anyhow. Simply because this is the best and most comprehensive way to learn the correct use of professional plasma devices.

At the beginning of our journey with Plasma some devices were sold for 20K GBP. Then it went down to 15K then to 10K, after a while to 5K and downward. Also I have seen several companies come stay for a while in the market to then disappear. And the cycle continues. Every time I see another marketing stunt on the various social platforms advertising these courses I know it is short lived. Consequently our voltaicplasma.com website is gaining more and more visitors as companies are advertising. This is because as they advertise we gain more and more exposure as we are the only crazy ones giving it all away. And I mean it we are giving it away. We give away for nothing so much knowledge that we got several people getting in touch with us simply because they could not learn enough from the expensive courses done by others.

Why Plasma has become ubiquitous in aesthetics?

The plasma revolution this is how we refer to it. Within a very short period of time it is being adopted the world over and very fast. Why is that?

www.voltaicplasma.com   Author: Andreas Russo

There are several reasons for that:

- The number of applications in aesthetics, One device can perform so many different aesthetic treatments it is unreal. It beats most lasers in several applications, including tattoo removal. This simple technology is a real game changer. There are so many applications that it is not possible to cover them into detail just in one book and not even Voltaicplasma.com. Some people even claim to teach you everything within one day course.
- The ease of learning the techniques. Although the applications are almost infinite the most important ones are relatively easy to teach and learn.
- The fact that most devices are not very expensive. The requirements for this tyoe of device are so little thant they are not where near as expensive as their nearest competitors: the lasers. And as we will see in this book in many cases plasma beats lasers by miles.
- Lack of legislation to regulate the use of these devices in most countries. This is happening so fast that no legislator has had time to react to this revolution and plasma is now available in most parts of the world. Only in a few countries it was claimed that these are medical procedures and not aesthetic procedure therefore requiring regulation.

Limitations of this book

Before you embark in reading this book please note that a picture is worth a thousand words, a video a thousand pictures. Unfortunately there is no way we can include the videos in this book. But if you want to learn all the tricks and secrets of the "plasma job" which peple do not tell you about, then go to voltaicplasma.com where most of the videos are stored and you can learn at your own pace accessing the videos and the online training material. There are also online tests, downloadable certificates and several other electronic resources.

Unfortunately the writing word on a book is not as interactive as we have made our online training platform with all the online tests and loads of free learning tools. So after you have read this book, if you are serious about learning how to use plasma fibroblast for aesthetic treatments go to voltaicplasma.com and start your course, most of it is free.

Unfortunately we will not be adding the huge number of case studies we have published in Voltaicplasma.com, this is a matter of timing. We want to finish this book as soon as possible so that you can have it and use it. However you can access all the case studies whenever you like on our voltaicplasma.com website. The case studies will generally show you the before, healing porgression pictures as well as the afters. But this is not all!! In the case studies you can also watch how the treatment was carried out in detail. So once you have finished with this book go and have a good look

www.voltaicplasma.com   Author: Andreas Russo

at the case studies we have. We are one of the very few if not the only ones who have taken the bother to build real case studies.

Voltaicplasma.com was created in order to democratise the learning necessary in order to become familiar and ultimately an expert in this field.

Why did we build so many case studies and made them in videos?

Let me tell you a story which is going to be an eye opener. When I started this business I was competing with unscrupulous established companies, especially one which I will not mention. They where charging an arm and a leg for their device and their training. It was a true rip off and this was the main reason for me to start in this business. I wanted to be the disruptor, and indeed I was.

The competitors felt so threatened by me that tried anything including bribery to put me out of business. I was very inexperienced and I did not know how they could have possibly put me out of business. It was impossible in my head, because after all the market was with me as I was pumping out so much valuable information for free, and on top of it our devices were much cheaper and better.

One of the strategies they used was to claim that our devices were dangerous and according to them all sorts of strange things would happen to people who had the treatment performed by our devices. Anonymous blogs appeared claiming that our devices were fake, dangerous and the public was at serious risk.

I remember really well receiving a comment on one of our videos with the clear threat that our devices were dangerous and they would have been recalled.

I was terrorised and baffled, how can you recall our devices form the market? Impossible I thought, but I was still troubled. One day in May or June 2014 we had an employee form the MHRA (Medicine and Healthcare Authority) knocking on our door. I was not in but my girlfriend answered the door and the gentleman asked a number of questions also some amongst which were not pertinent at all.

It was as if this MHRA employee was getting out of his way to try and find my weak spot. He would ask questions like "is this house an HMO?", hoping that I would be running the house as an HMO without a license of course. Also he would ask other questions which were not that pertinent either, but clearly aimed at trying to find ways to see where I could have made a mistake. I was terrorised, simply because all I was doing was building the business but I did not study the law and I had no clue where I could have fallen foul of the law. I simply did not have a clue.

www.voltaicplasma.com   Author: Andreas Russo

Because the way this alleged HMRA employee behaved he was suspicious to me, I believed he was not really an MHRA employee, this is because public servants never behaved the way this gentleman did. This gentleman seemed very keen to dig as much as possible also asking some questions that felt like trick questions. It was very suspicious. Never a police officer or any other public officer was ever so keen...So I checked, called the MHRA main phone number and there certainly was a gentleman under the name given to me.

My mistake was to have marketed the device as a medical device with medical applications. Later when I had time to study the law and consult with all the public bodies it turned out not to be a problem whatsoever, because it could have been resolved very quickly and easily. But at the time since I did not have a clue of the legislation and how it was interpreted and implemented I was caught off guard.

When a device is marketed as medical it must have a medical CE mark. Obtaining a medical CE mark is an expensive and lengthy process in many ways and for several reasons, which I was about to learn very very quickly. Basicly the MHRA employee after having established that the device did not have a medical CE mark insisted that my company had to recall all devices in Europe. He cleverly first asked where they were sold and the name of the distributors, and then he ordered my company recalled all devices "to safeguard public health", such bunch of bollocks!! This was dejavue, because a few weeks earlier I received another message on one of our videos exactly stating that all devices would have been recalled from each distributor. This message came from the competitor.

It was now clear, the MHRA employee was as if was working directly under the orders of my competitor and he was determined indeed. He insisted that if I did not recall all devices I would have faced prosecutions and several fines. Although I found the legal way to get out of his remit, simply by stating in a phone call to the MHRA employee in question, that we would rewrite the manual to remove all medical claims and therefore the device would not require a medical CE certification but a simple CE declaration of conformity which is essentially a self certification. This was not good for this MHRA employee. This was confirming that the gentleman was infact working for the competition not only the MHRA. Well he was working for the MHRA but very likely with a bonus form the completion should I go down.

I lost sleep, I felt into a deep depression and I did not know what to do. It was a real nightmare. It felt so bad that I wanted to sleep all the time in order to forget what was going on. For the first time in my life I fell into a deep depression. I did not have the strengths to react. I was trying to find the way to get the CE medical mark but it took too long, in the region of 6 months to a year if I was lucky and I was still been forced to recall all devices by this MHRA employee.

I kept thinking and trying to find a solution, but there was no convincing of the MHRA employee, little by little it appeared clearer and clearer that the strategy of making the device non medical was the right one. I suspected that devices without a medical purpose and only aesthetic purposes did not fall into the Medical legislation remit, this was the key I needed to get out of trouble. I learned this because I was constantly trying to find a solution even during my depression. What I did was making several enquiries with the notified bodies those companies who issue the CE medical mark.

www.voltaicplasma.com   Author: Andreas Russo

When I was explaining the main uses of the device they said that it was not a medical device. This was strange, how was it possible that I had notified bodies saying that the main uses of the device I was marketing like tattoo removal, moles removal, skin tightening etc (also "non surgical blepharoplasty") were non medical while the MHRA employee was so adamant that it was a medical device and it was so dangerous? It was becoming clearer and clearer, the circumstantial evidence was ever in my face. The employee had vested interests! I called the MHRA asking if a device for tattoo removal was a medical device and some nice gentleman form the MHRA said it was not medical. I immediately asked for his email address and I asked the same question, this time in writing and he replied in writing. I had the evidence now, in writing, that even the MHRA said that tattoo removal devices are not medical devices.

So I knew I did not have a way out, the employee wanted his bonus from my competitor and I did make a few legal mistakes. But in hindsight not that big. I did not know how the law worked and I also hired a couple of lawyers who charged me in the region of 2500 pounds for consultation but they did know less than me. A complete waste of money and time, completely useless. I believed at the time that if I fought I would have lost more as I did not have a clue about legislation and I did not have any financial resources to whether the storm. The competitor did know what they were doing and they were doing it well, they destroyed me without them even needing to sue me. They were very smart. They decided to kill my business and they managed it, without even doing it themselves (directly).

I was at a huge disadvantage. Given the situation what I decided to do was the following: since I was operating under a limited company. The company did not have anything and it was new, all the distributors might as well have sued my company and it would have not mattered at all. I could have started afresh very soon once the storm was over. But I needed to get the MHRA employee to get his bonus and have the competitors believe that they won. I needed to rest and start afresh without those mistakes.

So I decided to play dead. When the deadline to recall all the devices imposed by the MHRA employee came, he sent me another email reminding me of the documents I needed to fill in order to fulfil the recall. I just could not fill these documents. I hated it. I would not do it.

So what I did was simply replying to the HMRA employee saying that as far as we were concerned the device was now only a tattoo removal device and the manual was changed accordingly and passed onto all the customers, hence not his remit any more. I also mentioned that a tattoo removal device by the admission of the MHRA itself is not a medical device and I also mentioned in the email that it was not the MHRA trying to force me to recall the devices, but it was him! After this email I am sure he knew I knew about his bonus. He also knew I knew he could not prosecute me that easily. But of course he wanted his bonus from the competition so what he did the following week was extraordinary. He flew to Slovenia to meet with one of my distributors, maybe to investigate or something else. Basically the MHRA employee found out that it was true that the MHRA itself confirmed in writing that a tattoo removal device is not medical and it does not require a medical CE. He knew I had a great line of defence.

www.voltaicplasma.com   Author: Andreas Russo

At that point he stopped travelling because he realised that a prosecution would not have stacked up in any way at all. So he decided to write to each single medical body enforcement agency of each European country to enforce the so called recall that way. Basically each distributor received a call from each agency intimating them to send the devices back otherwise prosecution would have ensued. One by one each distributor called me, it was one of the worst summers in my life the summer of 2014, but it taught me a very important lesson. By September the so called recall was done on paper only I refunded my largest distributor and everything was quiet once again, At that point I started feeling better in October 2014. I spent the whole summer up until October in Sicily. At the end of October given that I have had the peace I required I felt much better, I started jogging once again and I went back to the UK. I hid in Scotland, I did not want any attention from anyone while I was rebuilding the business.

In October I decided to restart. Now I would restart keeping the law in mind first not the sales and marketing. One of the first things I did was going back through my history and see what other mistakes I could have made that the competitor could have used once again. I went into great detail and whatever I could have found I made sure it was legal and in order. I checked and double checked because I knew that all I had to do to be successful was to survive the next attack. But I was determined to know the law better than the law enforcement officers themselves. I said to myself, "before I sell anything I must triple check and have the hard evidence that it is 200% legal". And so I did. One of the things I did during the summer of 2014 was to stop selling all products out of caution. I even thought for a second to stop letting my properties, in fear that my competitors tried to get a tenant of their team inside some of my properties. So I became paranoid and became very careful with selecting tenants. And guess what? During that period the enquires made by italians to trying to live in my houses was at a record high. I said to my girlfriend: "no matter what, do not get any Italian to move into my house". Such a coincidence....so many Italians were interested in renting my properties without even viewing them....

Going back to October 2014, I wanted quiet and peace. So I went to Scotland were nobody knew I had a place to stay. One of the things I did was to study the law in cosmetics as I was able to sell the XanthRemover online and this product alone was a winner. I called the council and asked to speak to the officer from trading standards to check out on my XanthRemover. I knew selling was easy but I had to put the legality of my products to the test first because I know what was coming later.

The trading standards officer from Renfrewshire council was very nice on the phone and very helpful and he suggested meeting in person. Such a contrast from our friend supposedly working for the MHRA... The trading standards officer came to meet me in the room I was staying and made all the suggestions as what was required for compliance. I took note during the meeting and I sent all the documents he requested. All good, green light on the XanthRemover! One source of income was restored, I had money coming in again!!!

Now it was the turn of the plasma device. I had to bullet proof its CE mark!! So what I did again called trading standard but now in Nottingham, because by the time I was working on the plasma device legalities I had aleary moved back to Nottingham. Once again the officers from trading standards were very helpful and they wanted to meet with me and they did in my house in Nottingham. Like the officer in Scotland they were very helpful and they later told me that the competent body for the plasma device was the HSE (the Health and Safety Executive). By that time I had already studied the interpretation of the relevant legislation, I know exactly how the MHRA could enforce and realised that the only way they could enforce anything was through real prosecutions which are not easy to carry out successfully. I knew exactly how a competent authority could have legally challenged the CE mark and realised that it required prosecution and even that was not easy.

To make it simple if a device is a medical device the only valid CE mark can only be affixed after a notified body issues the declaration of conformity. If the declaration of conformity is not issued by a notified body then the CE mark is simply not valid and the device is not safe from a legal stand point. However when a device becomes aesthetic then the CE declaration of conformity can be written by the legal manufacturer and it is backed up by something called the "technical file". The only thing a competent authority can do to challenge the validity of a CE mark of an aesthetic device is to ask for the technical file. If the competent authority deems that the technical file is not "good enough" than it can decide to start prosecution and the outcome is not certain especially if the manufacturer defends the case in court. Because of this it is extremely rare that a competent authority brings forward prosecution because it can loose it wasting loads of time and money.

In case of a medical device instead if the CE mark is not issued by the notified body the prosecution is successful by default there is no way to defend it.

Now going back to the plasma device, what I did was to send the technical file to the HSE, of course without the HSE even asking for it. Then I gave notice to the HSE in writing saying, if you would like to challenge our technical file please do so within one month time. If you do not, then I will place it on the market. Please note that the technical file was very complete and very good for a one man operation. I did this in March and April 2015 and in August I started marketing on the internet again. In this way basically my CE mark for the BeautyTeck was bullet proof.

Guess what? This work paid off because they came for me again in April 2016 but they failed this time and did it miserably.

So what does this story have to do with the insane number of case studies we have? Very simple, one of the claims made by the competitors and the haters was that that our plasma device was dangerous and ineffective. Basically a con... Since nobody was really publishing any proof of anything at all in terms of the effectiveness of their device, all I had to do was film the procedures and publish the results including the procedure itself. So I started taking loads of before pictures, the videos were easy as I was used to video every procedure and collecting the pictures from the healing progression and the final results.

Because of this today we have the vastest collection of true results where you can see the before pictures, the entire video of the procedure, the healing progression and the final results. I tell you the competition in 2016 did not know how to attack me any more. Since their last CE mark attach was not successful all they could do was saying that we were "cheap". By the way, today that italian competitor does hardly sell anything in the UK at all, pretty much dead in our market. So now you know why I am so passionate about our case studies which you can watch and study from our website.

www.voltaicplasma.com   Author: Andreas Russo

1.0: Voltaic arc, sometimes referred to as Plasma or Fibroblast, what is it?

It is simpler than many people busy selling you stuff make it out to be.

People who are interested in selling you stuff, have also the vested interest in making something simple appear difficult. Fibroblast or Plasma in essence is an electrical spark or electrical arc, nothing more nothing less. It is not as if selling you stuff is bad, it is instead that the selling methods used are sometimes confusing on purpose. In this section you will hopefully understand what plasma or electrical arcing devices are is in simple terms.

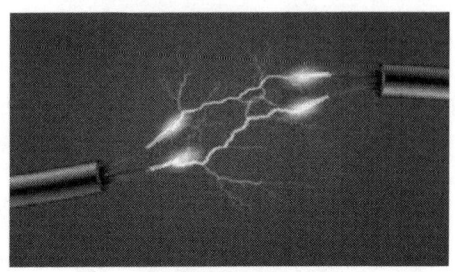

Illustration 2: Voltaic Arc

Watch Our Youtube Video

Electrical insulators, when subjected to a high enough voltage undergo an electrical breakdown. When Electrical Breakdown occurs the electric current starts flowing through the insulator and what was the insulator then becomes an electricity conducting substance during the electrical breakdown.

In other words, Voltaic arc, plasma or "fibroblast" is the electrical discharge which occurs in the insulating substance during an electrical breakdown, and this happens at a specific voltage and specific conditions in an insulator.

The electrical spark can take place in an electrical insulator (be it plastic, SF6, mineral oil, and even air or a vacuum). A dramatic electrical arc, with which we are all familiar with, is lightening, where the insulator is the air.

This natural phenomenon of arcing, sparking or "fibroblast" was first scientifically described by Sir Humphry Davy, in an 1801 paper published in William Nicholson's Journal of Natural Philosophy, Chemistry, and the Arts.

Today this natural phenomenon is very well understood and has a vast variety of applications. Many technologies using plasma have been developed over the last 200 years to help us in everyday life.

Let us look at some of the applications of electric arcs, they are used in:

- Welding, for industrial applications
- Industrial cutting, for manufacturing
- Electric or Plasma arc furnaces, for melting

www.voltaicplasma.com   Author: Andreas Russo

- Electrical discharge machining (EDM), also referred to as spark machining, spark eroding, burning, die sinking, wire burning or wire erosion, is a manufacturing process whereby a desired shape is obtained using electrical sparks.

- Arcing is also used in modern domestic and industrial light bulbs, Spotlights, Theater lighting, metal halite lamps, high-frequency lamps and many other types of light bulbs.

- Spark plugs are used in the internal combustion engines of vehicles to initiate the combustion of the fuel in a timed fashion.

- Arcing is used in movie projectors.

- Electrical Arcing devices have been used extensively for timed detonators (in controlled demolition).

- They are used to ignite our gas in domestic hobs.

- Electrical arcing is being studied for Electrically powered spacecraft propulsion.

- In Medicine electrical arcing has been in use since early 1900 for electrocoagulation, destruction of tumors and more...

- In Aesthetics electrical arcing is used for tattoo removal, skin tightening, benign mole removal etc.

All those applications and more, take advantage of the simple and well-known phenomenon of electric arcing.

The few applications we have seen are those in which the properties of electrical arcs have been harnessed to our advantage.

Sometimes, voltaic arcs are not desired physical phenomena. In electric circuit breakers, entire technologies have been developed thanks to the requirement to control and extinguish the arc. Electrical arcs are also unwanted and suppressed in electrical motors, and in oil filled powered transformers, in which a spark (or arc) could have catastrophic consequences and even cause explosions.

So we have seen, how plasma or voltaic arc have been used for many years and has many different applications in everyday life and it is applied in a vast variety of modern technologies, machines, and various devices.

If you would like to read more about voltaic arcs Click Here.

If you would like to watch some interesting videos on plasma or voltaic arcing Click Here

www.voltaicplasma.com   Author: Andreas Russo

2.0 A Bit of History and context about Plasma or "Fibroblast"

Since there is a lot of sales jargon over electrical arcing in aesthetics and medicine with some people self proclaiming themselves as the creators or inventors of this "new technology" we are providing you with some valuable context and history about plasma or "fibroblast". As we will see this is not a new technology it is just that you happen not to have seen it before in the context you are seeing it now.

Electrical arcs are used in many aspects of our lives. They are sometimes referred to as plasma or "fibroblast" for marketing purposes.

Devices generating an electrical arc have been used in the operating theaters since the early 20th century. The first electrosurgical unit, also known as the Bovie Generator, is credited to William T. Bovie while he was working at Harvard University. The first use of an electrosurgical generator in an operating theater was on October 1, 1926, at the Peter Bent Brigham Hospital in Boston, Massachusetts, in the USA.

The first operation is believed to have been performed by Dr. Harvey Cushing an American neurosurgeon. Ever since, due to its versatility, the use of electrofulguration or electrodesiccation have expanded worldwide. Later thanks to the increasing availability of voltaic arc generators, the practice has extended to aesthetic uses.

The voltage used by surgical and aesthetic equipment ranges between the 500–10,000 Volts peak-to-peak and are capable of injecting high currents through the body and through its surface, depending on how they are used. So, how is it possible that these sparks, at times injecting high currents, can travel through our bodies without causing any harm?

We have all experienced mild electric shock by an accidental contact with a live wire in our houses, and we know the unpleasant it can be. So how is the same electrical power used safely?

If we were to use the same peak to peak voltage of 50Hz as found in domestic supply, we would experience an electric shock. The magic is in the operational frequency of the device. The frequency output generated by these devices starts from 50 KHz (note this is 50,000Hz not 50Hz). This higher frequency avoids the undesired electromuscular stimulation, which in turn avoids electric shocks. Because of this principle, electrical surgical devices have high currents at high voltage (therefore high power) and can thus be put through the human body without any harm either to the internal organs or nervous system. Remember that the first electro-surgical unit was used by a neurosurgeon, and this provides an idea of the level of confidence and inherent safety of such devices. Thanks to this, these devices have been in widespread use in the medical and aesthetic world since the 1930s.

Today the use of voltaic arcs in medicine include:

- Electrocoagulation, meaning coagulating blood vessels which require the blood flow to be stopped (hemostasis).
- The destruction of soft tissues – including but not limited to removal of tumors (ablation).
- The cutting of a variety of tissues in the operating theatre;

Additionally, in aesthetics electrical arcs with high-frequency currents have applications in:

- Skin tightening
- The removal of benign moles and benign skin lesions
- Tattoo removal
- Red vein cauterization and much more

3.0 Voltaic Arc in Aesthetics, Electrofulguration and Electrodessication

The difference between Electroctrodessication and Electrofulguration.

"Plasma" or "Fibroblast" is also the same as electrofulguration, something which has been very well known in medicine for a long time. In this section we will explore and explain the difference between the two so that you can even have a better context of what plasma actually is for in aesthetic applications.

<u>**As we have seen**</u>, medium and high frequency AC currents have been in use since the 1930s. This led to the development of monopolar and bipolar radio frequency currents with diverse applications in aesthetics.

In this page we will focus our attention on two particular methods used in aesthetics:

- Electrofulguration (the same principle used in electro-coagulation for medical use) and
- Electrodessication

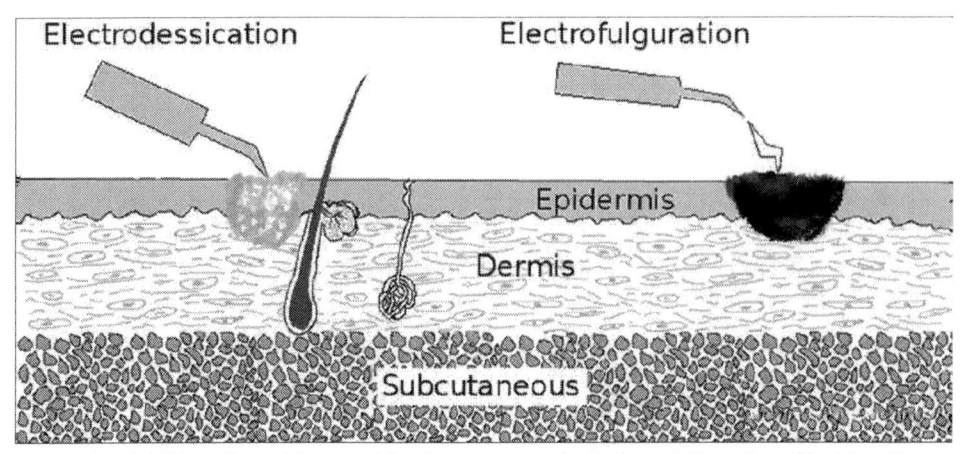

Illustration 3: This will provide you with a better context for understanding what "fibroblast " is in reality.

In the Illustration 3, we can clearly see the difference between Electrodesiccation on the left and Electrofulguration on the right. There are many devices on the marketplace which operate in one or both modes. The effects of electrofulguration are very superficial compared with the carbonization effects of electrodesiccation (also known as dehydration, ablation or sublimation). Electrofulguration occurs when the electrical arc takes place between the tit of the device and the skin. Electrodessicaiton occurs when the tip of the device touches the skin and the electrical energy is applied onto the skin by the tip of the device itself.

Effects produced by electrodesiccation are seen in the right hand side picture, the dehydration effects spread much deeper than Electrofulguration. For this reason electrofulguration (Plasma or Fibroblast) is used for superficial skin treatments in aesthetics as it provides a greater degree of accuracy than electrodesiccation. The difference in equipment operation between electrofulguration and electrodesiccation mode is very well-known as they have been used for many years for dermatological applications.

Watch Our Youtube Video on What is Plasma ?

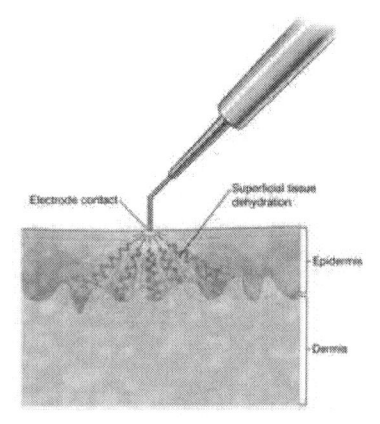

Illustration 4: Effects produced by electrodesiccation

www.voltaicplasma.com   Author: Andreas Russo

So, what is the difference in configuration of these devices which allows either electrofulguration or electrodesiccation?

The answer is: the operating frequency and the power levels are usually the same or similar in both configurations. In Electrofulguration the voltage level is usually higher than when the equipment is set at Electrodessication mode. Also the other difference between the two types of configurations is the way that current flows through the body. Also the difference stands on the fact that in electrodesiccation the electrode is either in direct contact with the skin or even inserted inside the skin (for permanent epilation).

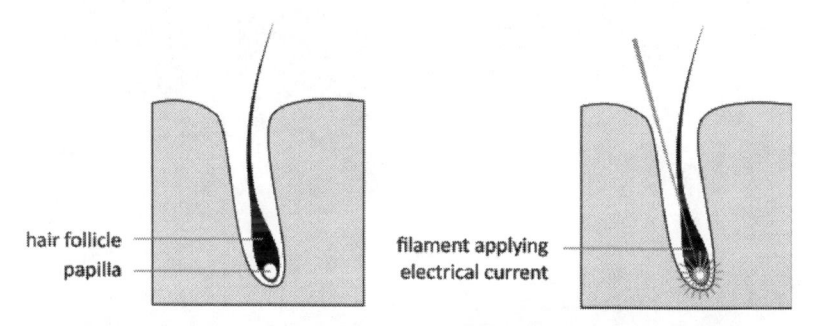

Illustration 5: Permanent epilation by using electrodessication with a return pad.

Electrofulguration Configuration

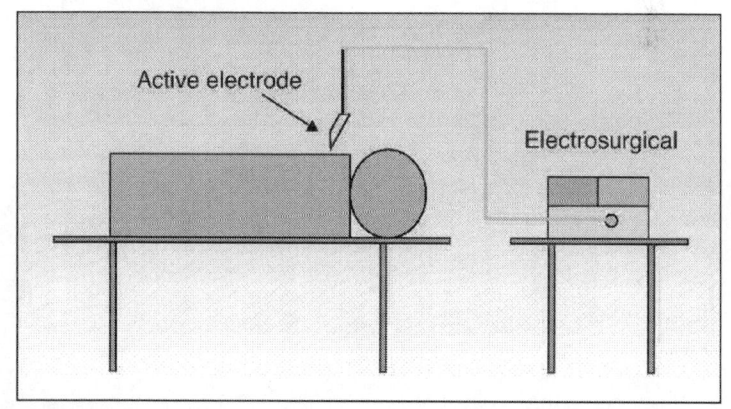

Illustration 6: In Fulguration Configuration, the electrode does not touch the skin or tissue and once the spark occurs the current flows from the tip of the electrode down to earth following the path of least resistance.

When the equipment is set up in electrofulguration mode the electricity flows from the tip of the electrode through the body (which at medium/high frequency reacts as a Faraday cage) down to earth, and a return pad is not usually needed. Because the current flows superficially to earth, the result is a very superficial carbonization of the superficial part of the skin (epidermis), lesion or benign mole.

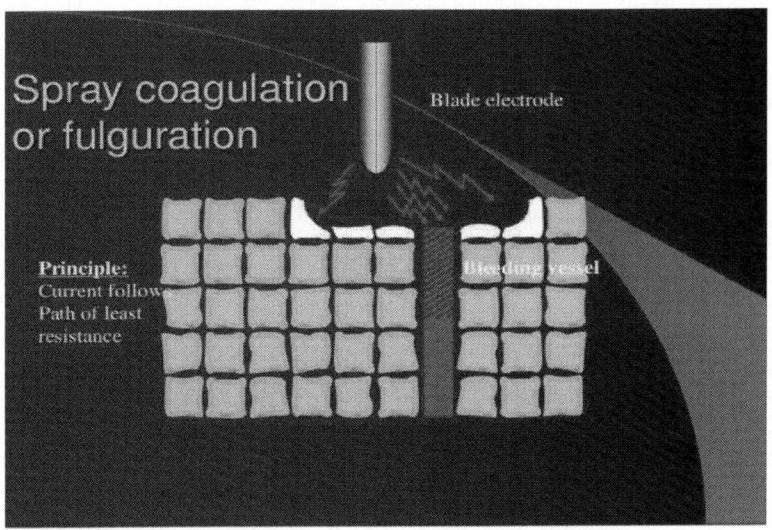

Illustration 7: Electrofulguration to stop minor bleeding, used in medicine is usually referred to as electrocoagulation.

Due to this superficial carbonization effects and precision, electrofulguration has been also used for many years in order to stop minor bleeding in medical applications, during surgery. In Electrodesiccation a return pad is used in order to close the current flow back into the equipment. In this case, the current flows from the needle/electrode, through the body, into the return pad in a loop fashion (as seen right hand).

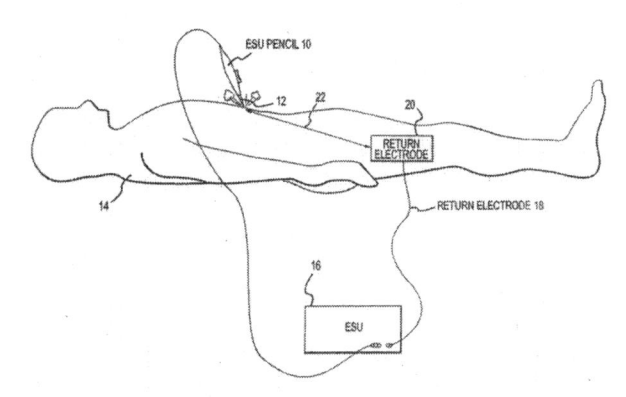

Illustration 8: In Electrodessication configuration a return pad is applied to close the current flow back to the equipment as shown in the figure.

www.voltaicplasma.com   Author: Andreas Russo

As a result of this electric current closed path, the dehydration effects are far more effective and the ablation effects spread much deeper into the skin than the electrofulguration mode (in which the current simply flows to earth). Because the dehydration effects of electrodesiccation penetrate deeper into the skin, in aesthetics electrodesiccation configurations are mainly used for red vein coagulation/removal and permanent epilation. This is because when the return pad is in use, the current flows deeper inside the dermis and this is the configuration normally used for the cauterization of small thread veins or for permanent epilation (permanent hair removal).

So to recap, when the equipment is required to function in electrofulguration mode the return pad is not needed and the voltage of the tip of the device is increased in order for the spark to be generated.

On the other hand in Electrodesiccation the voltage of the tip of the device is decreased and the return pad applied on the patient (subject).

Because of its higher degree of precision in tissue carbonisation, electrofulguration (plasma or Fibroblast) is used in aesthetics for:

- ◆ Benign moles and benign skin lesions removal in general.
- ◆ Tattoo removal.
- ◆ Permanent Makeup removal.
- ◆ Rownspots removal.
- ◆ Skin tightening ...,and more besides.

The uses of ElectroDesication (When the Equipment configured with a return pad) are usually:

- ◆ Permanent epilation or permanent hair removal.
- ◆ Red vein coagulation for aesthetic reasons.
- ◆ Benign skin lesions removal in General.

4.0 Familiarize with the use of electrical arc

Learn the basic principles of electrical arcing, so that, with enough practice, you will gain the confidence you require to then start to apply these basic principles for aesthetic purposes. Please do not take this information lightly, this is because in the past, several companies charged sometimes thousands of US dollars for you to go though this type of exercise and now you can do it on your own accord without spending a penny. This is one of the first exercises all those expensive companies will have you to go through. So pay special attention and replicate it in your own time. Watch our youtube video on this topic.

www.voltaicplasma.com   Author: Andreas Russo

Explanation VIDEO Transcript

How to familiarize with the operation and immediate effects of AC electrical arc generators for aesthetic purposes. In this example we will show you this exercise using "hot plasma", which is to say electrical arcing in air and not in argon which we refer to as "cold plasma".

Since the use of electrical arcs sometimes seems quite daunting at the very beginning, this video will guide you through the basics in the operation of Voltaic arc for aesthetic applications. So the main purpose of the experiments you are about to watch is for you to learn the basic principles, so that, with enough practice, you will gain the confidence you require to then start to apply these basic principles for aesthetic purposes. For convenience, the test subjects are usually: chicken wings, beef steaks and chicken legs, found at any local butcher.

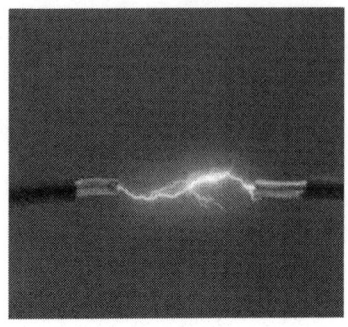

Illustration 9: Electric Arc

As you will see in <u>our youtube video the carbonisation effects of AC electrical arcing</u> (or also referred to as plasma) are dependent on three main factors:

- ✓ How long the arc has been applied for at any point
- ✓ The power output of the specific device you are using
- ✓ When the voltaic arc is applied in spray mode, the speed of movement of the electrode while the arc takes place.
- ✓ The output frequency at the tip of the device.

In the video we will show you the basics of the <u>"spot operation" and the "Spray operation</u>". These two modalities of operation are the two fundamental ways of using, voltaic arc for aesthetic purposes.

For the purposes of the type of device we are using in this demonstration, and ease of operation, if you are right-handed, grab the device as if it is a large pen in this way. This way if you are left-handed.

Position the bottom of your palm on a stable hard surface, be it the forehead of your client or any other hard and stable surface available on your client's body. This will allow you the maximum degree of control of operation by simply moving your wrist in this way. Often, during the first attempt on using an electrical arc generator, people tend to touch the skin (or surface) with the tip of the electrode. As you can see, at very low power, this has no or very little effect on the test meat or the skin. The best way to practice and learn how to generate the arc with this particular device is to increase the power setting of the device and slowly moving the tip of the electrode closer to the surface until the arc takes place. This exercise will help you familiarise with the way voltaic arcs are initiated.

www.voltaicplasma.com   Author: Andreas Russo

With this portable device, operated at minimum power, there is very little effect if the tip of the electrode touches the working surface or skin. Generally, in order to generate the arc, the electrode has to be kept at a minimum distance from the skin before the arc takes place. With this battery operated device, when set at very low power and the electrode touches the skin or any particular surface, the arc extinguishes and there will be little effects on the skin or the soft tissue (ie mole or benign skin lesion).

4.1 Exercise on How to generate the electric Arc or Spark

For the sake of this exercise, set the equipment power setting at a high enough level so that it is easy for you to generate the arc. Then slowly decrease the distance between the tip of the electrode and the surface. While you are slowly decreasing the distance, at a certain point the spark will take place (see the Paschen Law). In order to extinguish the arc simply increase the distance again. You will notice that the higher the power setting of the device the wider the minimum distance required to generate the arc, conversely the lower the power setting the closer the tip of the electrode needs to be in order to start generating the spark.

The following experiment is meant for you to understand why (with this particular portable device) it is recommended to place your other hand on the client's body while you are applying the AC voltaic arc. With this particular battery-powered device, in this experiment, set the output power at maximum level. Start trying to generate the arc but keep the other hand away from the meat. Now as the arc is generated touch the meat with the other hand. Notice how the arc increases in power as you touch the meat with the other hand, conversely the power is much lower when you do not touch the meat with the other hand. This is because when you touch the meat with the other hand the high frequency current has an extra low resistance path to earth which decreases the overall resistance it encounters therefore increasing the power of the arc and hence the carbonisation effects.

4.2 Practice of the Spot Mode or Spot Operation

This mode of operation is mainly used for skin tightening for aesthetic purposes.

Now that we have practiced the fundamental exercise which allows to generate voltaic arcs, we can start practicing the simplest of the methods used in aesthetics. The "spot operation". This type of operation is normally used for skin tightening. Please note that other methods are also suitable for the same applications, however, the spot operation is generally very effective and easy to use for skin tightening purposes. Because this is only an exercise, in order to familiarize with this technique set the equipment at any given power level which allows you ease of operation. In this video we have used the highest possible power setting to demonstrate this principle. When you will be applying the "spot mode" or "spot operation" for aesthetic purposes, the power levels will generally be far lower.

www.voltaicplasma.com   Author: Andreas Russo

First of all apply very short bursts in different areas as shown here. Stop and look at the effects on the chicken skin. As you will see, the effects on the chicken skin are hardly noticeable.

Then move to another area and apply the arc for approximately one second, two seconds, three seconds, six seconds and finally ten seconds. Observe the effects. So now as you can see, the longer you keep the arc on, the more the carbonation effects at each spot. So the longer the arc is applied the larger and deeper the effects of the voltaic arc. So with this exercise we have learned how the carbonation or ablation effects are directly dependent on the duration of the exposure to the arc.

4.3 Practice of the Spot Mode or Spot Operation

This mode of operation is preferred in aesthetics for:
- Thermabrasion, for tattoo removal
- Brown and age spots removal
- Mild thermapeeling for localised skin tightening
- Benign moles and Benign skin lesions removal and more

For ease of this exercise, the first time you practice the spray mode operation, set the equipment at maximum power and as soon as the spark is generated while keeping the electrode at constant distance from the surface of the chicken skin (or meat) make a sweeping movement while keeping the arc on. The power will be set high only for this exercise to allow you ease of practice. As you gain confidence at high power levels, then practice at lower power levels, down to the minimum setting. Normally the power levels used for aesthetic treatments, with exception for mole removal, by using voltaic arc are very low.

In this last exercise you will see that by increasing or decreasing the speed of the sweeping movement the carbonisation effects vary, even if the power setting of the equipment remains unchanged. What you will notice, is that the higher your sweeping speed, the more superficial the carbonisation effects, whereas as the sweeping speed decreases the carbonisation effects penetrate deeper into the skin of the chicken or meat surface.

In order to later move to utilising voltaic arcs for aesthetic applications, practice on your own by using all the different power levels and spend some time practicing and having fun drawing whatever you wish on the meat.

As you have seen in this video the effects produced by the electric arc are directly related to the way the equipment is used and the arc applied. In aesthetic treatments, the final results will be dependent on the way you perform each procedure. Therefore, if you purchased a voltaic arc generator for aesthetic purposes, the best advice is to start practicing as shown in this video. Practise makes it perfect and there is nothing called as too much practice. So repeat all these exercises on your own and have fun.

www.voltaicplasma.com   Author: Andreas Russo

5.0 Fibroblast and skin tightening

5.1 What to expect from Fibroblast skin tightening treatments

Skin tightening using voltaic arcing also referred to as PLASMA, produces mild appreciable cumulative improvements in the appearance of fine lines and also reduces the appearance of sagging skin. Although it has been heavily advertised as the substitute to surgery, Voltaic Arcing or "fibroblast" is not the substitute for cosmetic surgery. The only known way to achieve dramatic results is through the use of cosmetic surgery.

5.2 The basics priniciple of skin tightening by using Electrofulguration (Plasma)

Young, elastic skin depends on the number of structural proteins such as collagen and elastin. These proteins help your skin resist temporary changes such as stretching, folding, or wrinkling. As we age, our bodies produce less of these structural proteins, making our skin more prone to show signs of ageing, such as fine lines and wrinkles.

A mild superficial controlled burn by using AC voltaic arcs, DC voltaic arcs or Lasers induces a skin tightening effect which helps the skin restore more of its natural elasticity. This occurs because localized heat stimulates the skin's regenerative response, resulting in firmer, tighter skin between the wrinkles and hence the reduction in the appearance of wrinkles and fine lines. Similar results are also possible by using other skin rejuvenation methods, like AHAs (alpha hydroxy acid) based cosmetic peels, however the use of voltaic arc or cosmetic lasers are generally more selective because it can be applied exactly where required, therefore inducing the skin tightening exactly were your client needs it, with a higher degree of precision. We refer to this type of skin tightening as "**localised skin tightening**" or "**targeted skin tightening**"

Generally, *Localised Skin Tightening* **can be accomplished by using:**
- Lasers devices,
- Electrical arcing devices.

The basic principle used by all these types of devices is the same, which is the targeted delivery of heat into the skin. When this is done the skin tends to respond by generating new collagen which results in tighter and firmer skin.

5.3 Methods to accomplish skin tightening using electrical arcing

Skin tightening using electrical arcing (or also referred to as Plasma) can be accomplished in two main ways:

- Using the spot mode or spot operation.
- Using the spray operation.

Both methods deliver the required heat into the skin needed to cause a very localized skin tightening. This localized skin tightening, in turn, reduces the appearance of saggy skin and fine lines. In particular, the fine lines are improved by the pulling effect of the skin tightening effect applied between the lines.

5.4 Spot mode or spot operation

The spot mode is the preferred method to apply skin tightening by using electrical arcing, on various parts of the face. It is the preferred method because it delivers consistent and repeatable results and it is very easy to learn especially for beginners.

The spot mode is used extensively for:

- → Upper Eyelid tightening.
- → Lower Eyelid tightening
- → Crow's feet attenuation (Periorbital lines attenuation)
- → MiniFacelifts
- → Smoker lines attenuation. (Perioral lines attenuation)
- → **Atrophic Scars attenuation including acne and chicken pox scar attenuation.**

In Illustration 10 below, we can see how the intention is to feather out the treatment as we move away from the wrinkles. In other words, the spots are applied in a more tight fashion where the wrinkles are deeper, closer to the eye. As we move away from the eye then the distancing of the spots is increased.

You will also note that, in case of fine lines, the wrinkles tend to disappear while are you applying the spots. This is not a permanent effect. This is a normal immediate reaction of the skin to the dehydration effects of the superficial carbonization caused by the electrical arcing (also referred to as plasma).

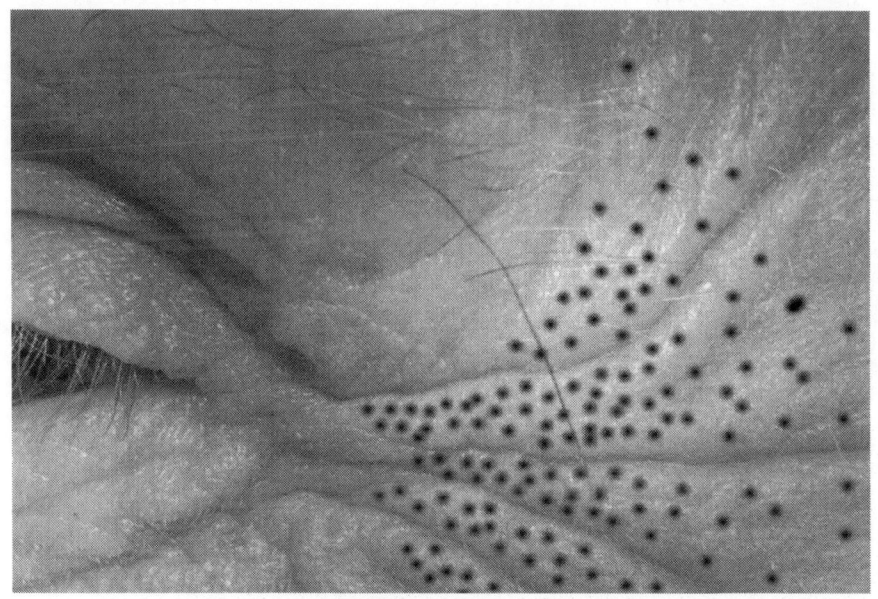

Illustration 10: Spot Mode

Watch our youtube video   Watch our youtube video

The spot mode is carried out in the following way:

- By applying short bursts between the wrinkles and not inside the wrinkles' folds. Applying the spots inside the wrinkles could worsen the appearance of fine lines instead of improving them.
- The bursts must be placed randomly, without forming lines or patterns of any type. Applying the spots randomly ensures the most uniform skin pulling effects.

5.5 Spray mode in skin tightening

The spray mode is not normally used for skin tightening, instead, it is commonly used for:

- Tattoo Removal.
- Permanent Make-Up Removal.
- Moles Removal, including Xanthelasma, Seborrheic Keratosis, Syringoma Removal and most of the other benign lesions and hypertrophic skin imperfections removed for aesthetic reasons.
- Skin resurfacing to improve the appearance of hypertrophic scars.

www.voltaicplasma.com   Author: Andreas Russo

However, after several numbers of treatments, when the users gain plenty of confidence with the use of electrical arcing for skin tightening, some prefer to move to the spray operation.

In some cases, this is also the natural way to increase the treatment intensity while using the spot mode. As we will see later on, one of the ways to increase the treatment intensity is decreasing the distance between the spots.

5.6 Spot mode treatment intensity

When using the *"spot-mode"* or *"Spot Operation"* the treatment intensity is dependant on a number of factors, the power setting on the device is only one of them.

Namely, the overall intensity of skin tightening treatments using Electrical arcing is dependant on:

1. **duration of the arc.** The longer the arc is applied at each point, during the spot operation, the higher the intensity of the skin tightening treatment. Conversely the shorter the duration of the arc the milder the intensity of the treatment. Remember that, in any case, excessive exposure to any voltaic arc at any intensity can result in injury.
2. **power level.** The higher the device power setting the higher the intensity of the treatment.
3. **the distance between the spots.** The shorter the distance between the spots the higher the treatment intensity. Conversely, as the distance between each spot is increased the treatment intensity is reduced.
4. **the area covered.** The wider the overall area covered the higher the overall intensity of the treatment.

Therefore the intensity of the treatment in the spot mode or spot operation is determined by four main factors and not only the power setting of the device itself.

However, said all the above it is important to mention that a high-intensity treatment does not necessarily lead to proportional improvements. In other words, the degree of improvement is not directly proportional to the intensity of the treatment.

If for example, over the course of a treatment the duration of the arc at each point is approximately a quarter of a second and this leads to an improvement of approximately say 4, if we increase only the duration by doubling it, by keeping all the other parameters the same (like power level, area covered and distance between carbonisation spots), the improvement will not necessarily be double because we have doubled the duration of the arc at each spot.

More generally, doubling the overall intensity of the treatment, does not necessarily lead to an improvement which may be twice as good, it will only be slightly better. Therefore, *even after you have gained enough confidence,* it is generally advisable to conduct milder treatments than you would otherwise consider possible.

6.0 The basic principles of plasma skin tightening, why does it work?

In this section we will explain the basics as why and how plasma skin tightening works for skin tightening and the physics that lead to its efficacy in skin tightening.

This is a very important section becasue plasma skin tightening has applications in:

- Upper Eyelid tightening also referred to "Non Surgical Blepharoplasty"
- Lower Eyelid Tightening
- Crow's Feet Attenuation
- Neck lift
- and several more....

First of all, plasma skin tightening should not be referred to as skin shortening. This is because the physics of the procedure itself does not allow the skin to shorten as advertised by, several marketers. Skin shortening is only currently possible by using surgery. It is understandable how the desire for short term earnings from marketing hypes, can appeal many companies the world over.

The way Fibroblast plasma works in terms of skin tightening is relatively simple and more simple than several marketers would like you to believe. Here you will see how simple it is and it is not rocket science.

Plasma skin tightening is based on the phenomenon of skin contraction after burns. As we know (and if you do not you can verify this information very easily on the internet) after burns the skin contracts. As you should know plasma or "fibroblast" causes a controlled small burn into the skin. It is controlled because otherwise, the burn would cause a scar in the area where you applied the treatment. Hence the burn has to be calibrated well so that the effects of skin tightening of the burn take place but there is no scarring at the end of the treatment.

In severe cases of deep burns, the skin contraction is so severe that skin grafting becomes necessary

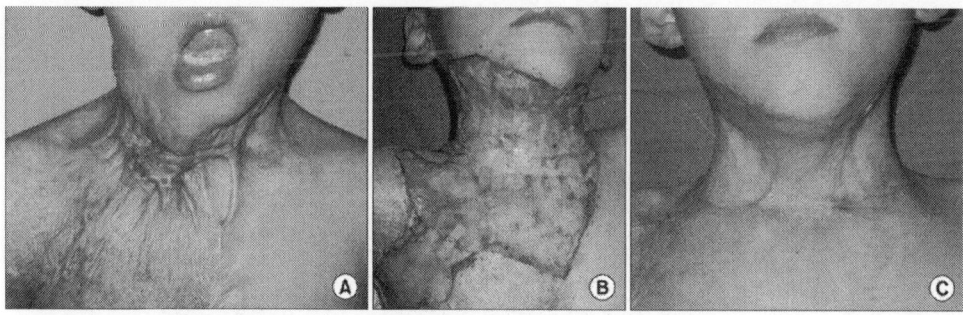

Illustration 11: (A) the skin contraction is so strong that it literally pulls down the mouth from one side. (B) immediately after the skin grafting operation. (C) After the area has healed from the skin grafting surgery.

In the above image (illustration 11) we can see on A how the skin contraction causes the pulling of the mouth. On the right (c) we can see how after skin grafting the pulling effect is gone. This is because the natural effect of skin burning is the contraction of the skin itself. It could not be simpler.

With "fibroblast" all we are doing is inflicting a controlled skin burn. This is all. But we have to be careful not to cause any scarring. This is why plasma skin tightening works so well that some marketers have referred to it as skin shortening. But as you can see from our several case studies we have published this is not shortening but it is tightening. This is because in order to cause a shortening you would need to cause a burn so deep that a scar would be in most cases inevitable.

7.0 The physics of Fibroblast

All we are doing with the magic word "fibroblast" or "plasma" is injecting heat into the skin by simply using a small electrical spark. This is the most simplistic way to explain it. Some sparks may be different to others depending on the circuitry of each device and the frequency at the output of the device. What we mean by frequency is not power level but it is actual frequency. If you want to learn the definition of frequency this is simply the period inverted or 1/T, where T is the period. You do not need to even understand what the period is but to make it simple at the output of these devices you have a sinewave which has a certain frequency.

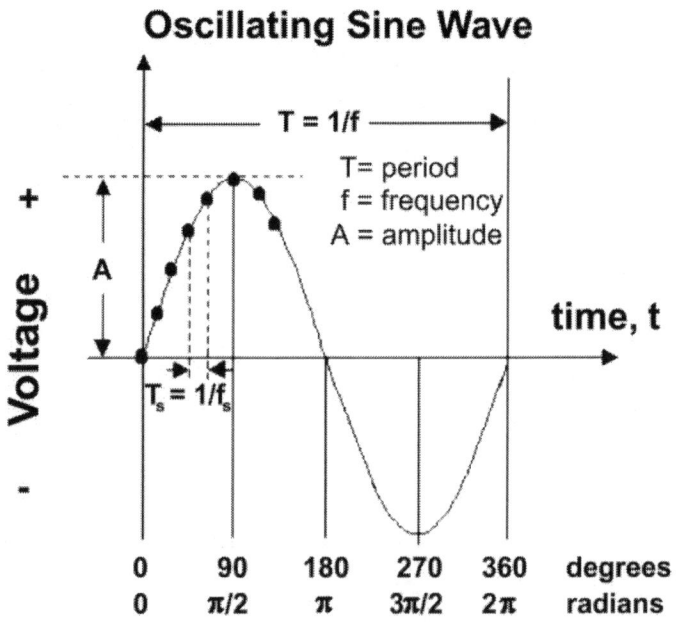

Illustration 12: Frequency

In the Illustration 12, If you examine the output of one of these plasma devices on the market they pretty much have a certain output frequency. The output at the tip of their electrode is an oscillating Sine Wave similar to the one you see in the picture above. Depending on the frequency and the circuitry of the devices the effect on the skin may vary in terms of how deep the burn penetrates inside the skin and its effects on the skin.

7.1 Distance between the spots and treatment intensity

The spot operation is the fundamental technique used in plasma skin tightening.

Below you can see the classic spot mode or spot operation applied between the wrinkles as it should. Never apply the spots inside the wrinkles.

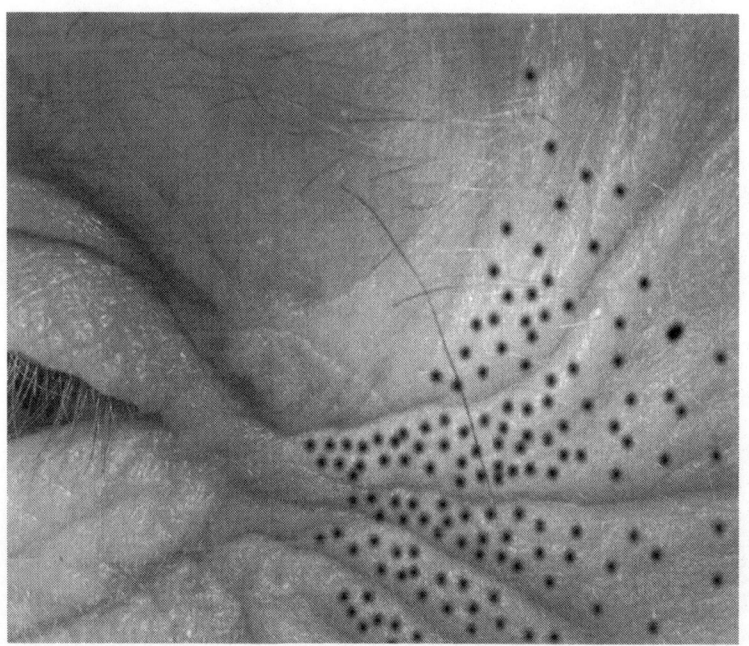

Illustration 13: classic spot mode or spot operation applied

Now we assume that the spark which the device we are using is producing an injury in the right way not to leave any scar. In the picture we can see the illustration of an electrical arc onto the skin. **As you can see in the picture on the right** the spark produces a carbonisation of the epidermis.

Also besides the carbonisation of the skin, given the high temperature at the point of contact between the skin and the arc, there is heat propagation into the skin.

One of the claims made by heavy weight marketers in the early 2010s (who have now disappeared from the UK market) was that their device had magic power of only delivering heat on to the carbonised area without affecting other areas of the dermis beneath it. These claims, although made with financial motivated scientific rigor, was of course revealed to be false. This is yet another reminder that any so called "Scientific Studies" or "Papers" will demonstrate whatever the company will want you to believe.

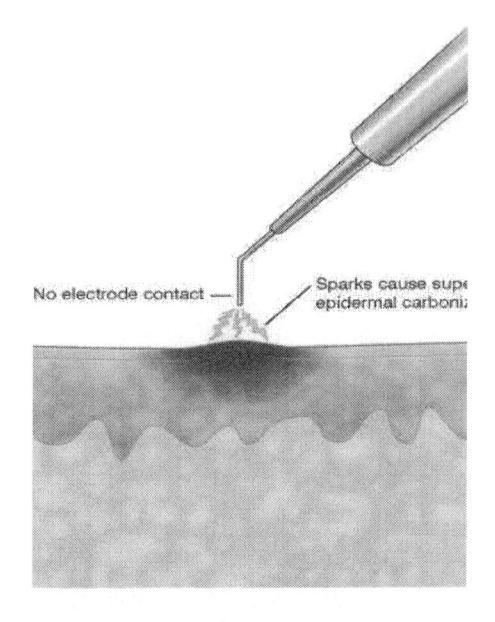

Illustration 14: As you can see in the picture above the spark produces a carbonisation of the epidermis

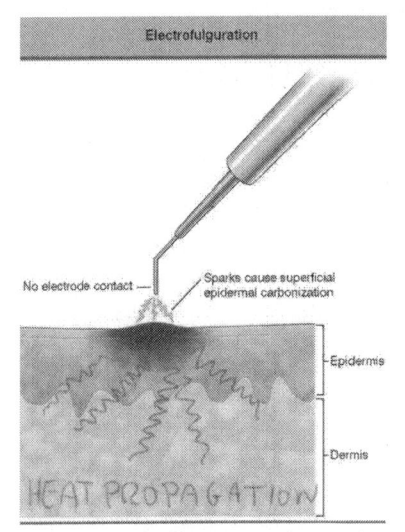

Illustration 15: This picture depicts the heat propagation caused by the electrical arc.

So if you are a doctor obsessed with scientific "papers based evidence" please note that the results of any scientific paper will demonstrate whatever the company who funds the study wants you to believe. This is especially true if there is a brand name in the so called "scientific paper" or "study". This is simply because doctors want to have scientific evidence and all the marketing companies have to do to sell you a device at a high price is to produce the so called "scientific evidence" which always demonstrates whatever the original manufacturer wants you to believe. Over the years we have seen plenty of claims made by maketers of supposedly "unique" features which then disappeared from the horizon.

Author: Andreas Russo

In the figure below we simply show the temperature distribution in the skin when an electrical arc is applied onto the skin.

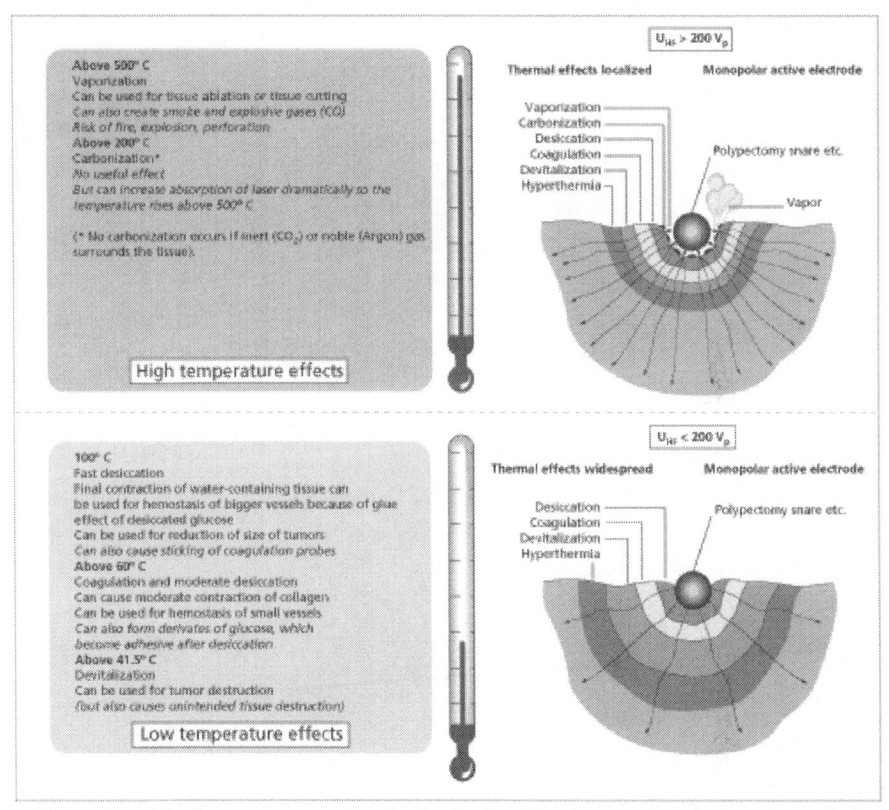

Illustration 16: the temperature distribution in the skin when an electrical arc is applied onto the skin

The carbonisation effect on the skin due to electrical arcing is a very well known phenomenon, it is nothing new. It is also known that electrical arcing produces different gradients of temperatures from the carbonisation surface (different temperature distribution as shown in the above figure) and hence irradiates heat into the skin.

In the picture below (Illustration 17) we have the representation of two separate sparks side by side at a certain distance between one another. This is to explain the heat propagation inside the skin from two carbonisation sources.

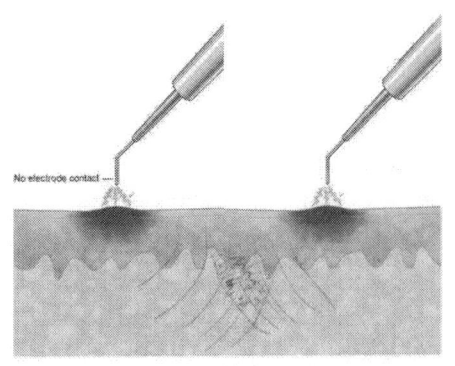

Illustration 17: we have the representation of two separate sparks side by side at a certain distance between one another. This is to explain the heat propagation inside the skin from two carbonisation sources.

Point X the total heat felt by that point is the sum of the heat emanated by source 1 on the left and also source 2 on the right. Therefore the total heat at the poit x is x1+x2.

Illustration 18: if we place the arc 1 and arc 2 closer together the heat felt at point x

As a consequence if we place the arc 1 and arc 2 closer together the heat felt at point x will be higher of course. Conversely if we increase the distance between the two arcs 1 and 2 at point x the heat will be lower, of course.

This is why the **distance between the spots** is so important in determining the intensity of the treatment. The closer the spots are together the higher the intensity of the treatment because the higher the quantity of heat injected into the skin. Conversely the further apart the spots are the less intense the treatment. This is why the distance between the spots is a major determining factor of the treatment intensity using electrical arcing.

7.2 Arc duration and treatment intensity

Also the duration of the arc is a fundamental factor in the intensity of the aesthetic treatment using the spot operation.

Lets assume for talk sake, that the left most picture depicts the arc been operated on the skin for half a second. In the middle picture for 1 second and in the right most picture for 3 seconds. Obviously the longer the arc is applied onto the skin for the higher the ablation effect and more heat is injected into the skin. As seen in the left most picture the carbonisation and the ablation of the skin is very shallow compared to the ablation of the carbonisation while the arc is applied for longer.

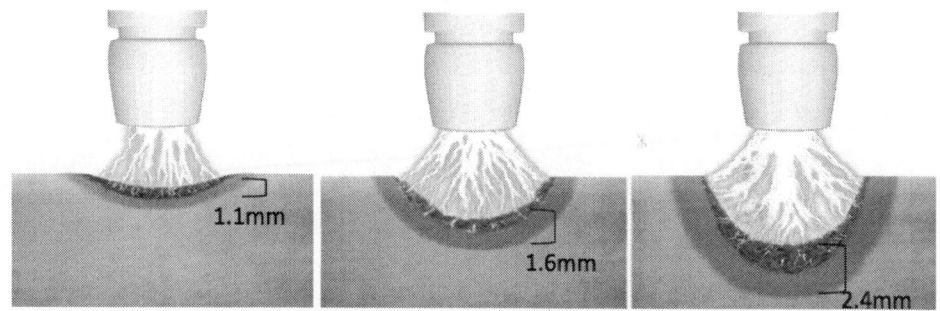

Illustration 19: in the middle picture for 1 second and in the right most picture for 3 seconds

Hence also the longer you apply the arc, while keeping the power of the device the same, the deeper the ablation and also the deeper the heat penetrates into the skin. As you have seen in the section how to get familiarised with electrical arcing device the longer you keep the arc on the deeper the ablation and also the deeper the heat penetrates into the skin.

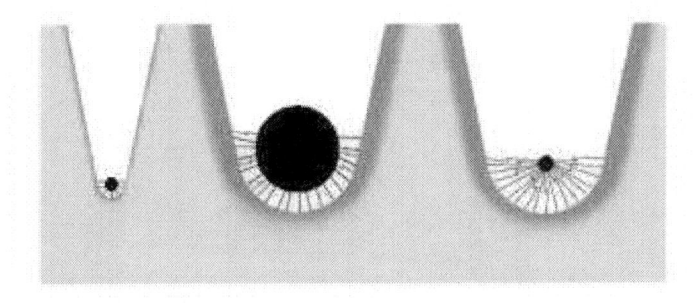

Illustration 20: In conclusion the longer the duration of the arc the higher the intensity of the treatment due to the higher amount of heat injected into the skin.

8.0 Introduction to Upper Eyelid Tightening

One of the applications of plasma skin tightening is upper eyelid tightening. Eyelid tightening using Plasma or Electrical Arcing is becoming more and more popular around the world because:

- it is cost effective,
- it leads to very good appreciable predictable results,
- the results are cumulative, this means that you build upon the improvements already achieved after previous treatments,
- it is generally very easy to carry out, and
- it is also every easy to learn

<u>Localised Skin Tightening</u> using AC Electrical arcing, also referred to as plasma, is applied for upper eyelid tightening with very good cumulative results. Therefore after a few sessions with AC Electrical arcing, your client will enjoy a substantial more youthful look by improving the appearance of saggy and heavy looking eyelids.

Upper eyelid tightening has been so successful the world over that this treatment has been sold to doctors by several companies and to patients by doctors as **"non surgical blepharoplasty"**. This is because of the, sometimes, very good short term results which the treatment can produce.

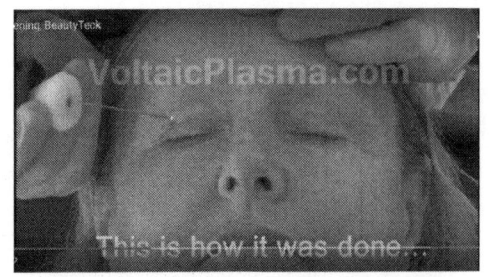

Illustration 22: <u>Watch our youtube video on Eyelid tightening</u>

www.voltaicplasma.com

Author: Andreas Russo

8.1 Alternatives to electrical arcing for eyelid tightening (or plasma)

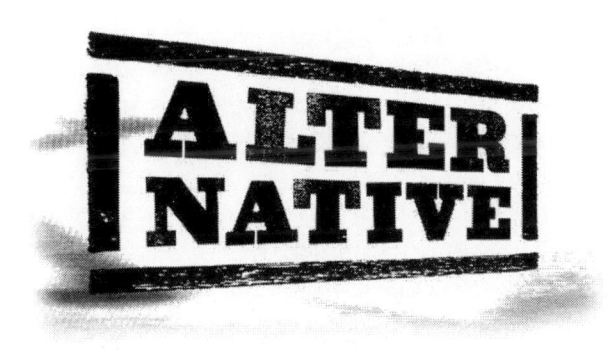

Electrical arcing or Plasma is only one of the several methods used for eyelid tightening. Similar <u>Skin Tightening Effects</u> are accomplished with use of cosmetic lasers (mainly CO_2 lasers) and also some electrocautery units properly configured. Generally the power level required for this type of aesthetic treatments is very low. Additionally similar results can be accomplished with certain specialised cosmetic peels.

To summarise, similar eyelid skin tightening effects can be also performed by using:

- Cosmetic Lasers (Mainly CO_2)– There are many different devices available on the market which can be set-up at the right wavelengths in order to carry out these types of cosmetic treatments. (Consult the manufacturer's recommendations).
- Specialised chemical peels. (ie Glycolic and or Mandelic peels made in special formulations)
- Specialised radio frequency equipment functioning in electrofulguration mode. Clear protocols are in place, results are consistent and repeatable (Consult the manufacturer's recommendations).

8.2 Advantages and disadvantages of eyelid tightening in general

The following are the advantages and disadvantages of eyelid tightening using CO_2 lasers, electrical arcing and specialised cosmetic peels. Please note that although the clients can generally resume their normal activities after this type of aesthetic treatment the *perceived* downtime of eyelid tightening procedures can be similar to surgery, especially if the treatment intensity is high. This is because of the swelling which usually follows one to two days after this type of aesthetic treatment.

Advantages over conventional surgery:

- These techniques require only topical anaesthetic (i.e. numbing products like Emla) and are very easy to perform. With exception of the use of cosmetic peels which do not require it.

- The skin recovery process lasts normally between 3 to 10 days after every session, depending on the **treatment intensity**, and other factors including the method or product used.
- Of course bleeding during and after these aesthetic procedures do not usually occur. It can occur with certain CO2 lasers and electrical arcing devices if the power level is set over a certain threshold or if the electrical arcing is applied for longer than a certain period of time during the spot operation, then some minor bleeding can occur.
- The risks of infection are very low compared with surgery.
- No general risks associated with surgery as these are non surgical easy aesthetic procedures.
- No incisions are performed and therefore no scarring is usually left.
- These procedures are extremely easy to learn and can be carried out by any trained beautician.
- The clients are able to resume their normal activities immediately after every session, provided that this does not increase the risks of infections (however a certain after-care has to be followed until complete recovery).

Disadvantages versus conventional surgery:

- Eyelid skin tightening brings about minor cumulative improvements in the appearance of saggy eyelids. If the amount of skin to be tightened is considerable in order to achieve the desired results, surgery is the best and most effective method.
- The results of eyelid tightening are not comparable to blepharoplasty and should not be proposed as an alternative to surgery. This is because dramatic results can only be achieved using surgery.
- Fat cannot be removed by using any skin tightening method.
- More than one session, sometimes several, may be required to achieve the desired results, depending on the amount of skin droopiness and the overall intensity of the treatment.
- If the amount of lose skin is significant, surgery may be the best option for those who desire dramatic changes. This is also because there is a perceived downtime due to swelling, therefore it is not advisable to attempt several treatments to achieve dramatic cumulative results while exposing the client to several swelling episodes, if a simple blepharoplasty can achieve the desired results in one session only.

8.3 Eyelid tightening by using aesthetic lasers

As we have discussed electrical arcing is not the only effective method used to achieve eyelid tightening. Some conventional surgical lasers or cosmetic lasers (often CO2 lasers) can be set up to carry out eyelid tightening by using standard skin tightening techniques. When using lasers to carry out this type of cosmetic procedure, the client should wear intra ocular laser eye-shields, for protection. In the video below you can see an example of eyelid tightening carried out using an aesthetic laser.

Page 45

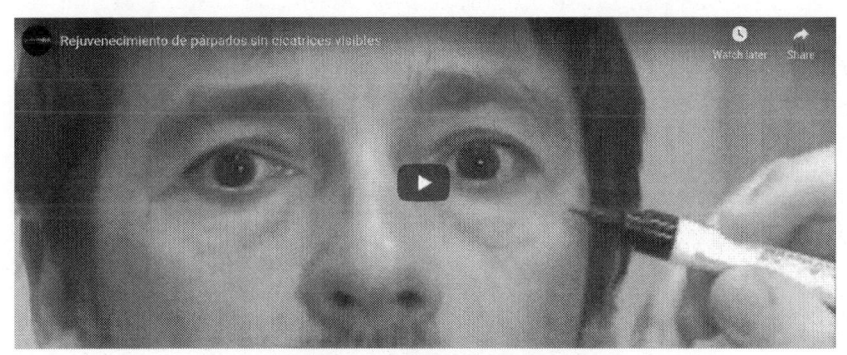

Illustration 23: Click Here to Watch Video

The laser is used on the orbital and periorbital area superficially in order to cause mild non harmful burns. This has to be done carefully, because if not set properly, the device could damage the dermis causing permanent scarring to the client.

Immediately after each session the area will appear full of tiny burns caused by the laser. The area treated will recover a week after undergoing the session with the skin tightening laser.

With a skin tightening lasers, a typical treatment ablates 11-33% of the skin, removing the old or damaged collagen which contributes to laxity. The heat generated in the tissue also helps the surrounding skin tightening, stimulating further collagen remodelling and reducing the skin area (Skin Tightening).

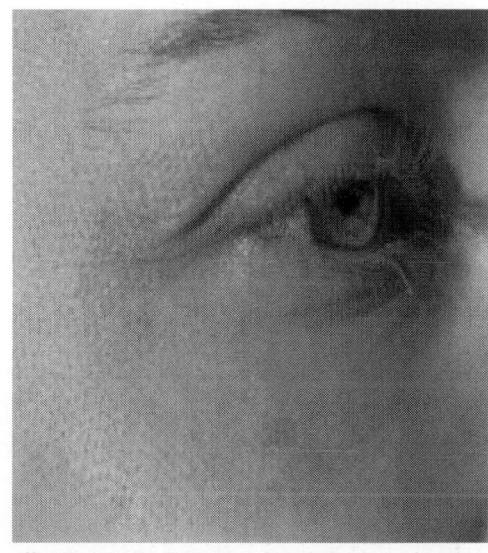

Illustration 24: Example of immediate results after co2 laser skin tightening on the periorbital area.

For most people with moderate wrinkles or hooding, 4-5 treatments will result in satisfactory results. For those with very early signs of 'crow's feet' and fine lines, 2-3 sessions can help as a maintenance type of aesthetic treatment to slow signs of ageing.

www.voltaicplasma.com   Author: Andreas Russo

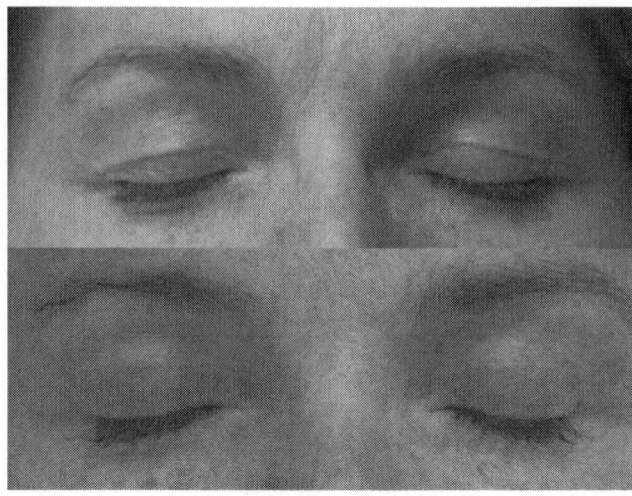

Illustration 24: Typical results after a number of laser skin tightening treatments.

8.4 Overview of eyelid tightening with electrical arcing equipment

Electrofulguration equipment or AC voltaic arcing specialised equipment are widely used throughout the world for Eyelid tightening.

In the picture right hand we see the result of the BeautyTeck being used to perform a single session of Eyelid Tightening. Eye protection during this type of procedure is not required like in laser treatments. The use of topical numbing products is recommended for the comfort of the client and ease the treatment. Each session usually lasts between 5 to 15 minutes at most, depending on the area to be treated.

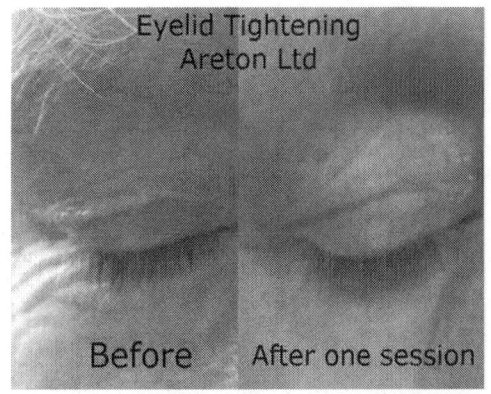

Illustration 25: Results after only one high intensity treatment with the BeautyTeck. Please, click on the picture to watch how the treatment was carried out.

Also, AC electrical arcing can be used to tighten the skin around the eye resulting in the attenuation of peri-orbital wrinkles, this can be done during the same session of eyelid tightening if required. It is important to avoid reapplying the arc on the area already treated until the area has recovered properly (usually after 4 to 6 weeks).

Additionally, although in many cases it is possible to achieve the desired results within few sessions (2 to 3), it is preferable to split the treatment into multiple sessions instead (3 to 5). This is because spreading the treatment allows the aesthetic practitioner to have more control over the outcome of the procedure. This is done by varying the intensity of the treatment. Also, during the skin recovery period, some areas could tighten more than others, therefore it is advisable to perform at least two sessions on every client, even in those cases where the desired results can be achieved within one session only.

Usually, during the first session the experienced beauty practitioner will normally cover a wide area of the upper eyelid in order to achieve the best possible results. The subsequent sessions can be used to fine tune and correct any imperfections or unevenness left after the first or previous sessions. In certain cases, due to particularly high client's pain threshold, the whole eyelid tightening procedure can be carried out without the use of any topical numbing product. However the use of an appropriate numbing cream is always advisable to make sure the client is at ease during the treatment. No medication of any kind shall be applied neither by the beautician nor by the client, other than appropriate antiseptic products to reduce the likelihood of infections during the recovery period. At home the client should only wash and rinse the whole face as usual, dry with a clean cotton cloth, being careful to gently pat and not rub the treated area. No make-up nor other creams should be worn before the area treated with the plasma device has recovered completely. During every session the beauty therapist must always take precautions to minimise any unexpected sudden movements of the client.

In certain cases, due to particularly high client's pain threshold, the whole eyelid tightening procedure can be carried out without the use of any topical numbing product. However the use of an appropriate numbing cream is always advisable to makethe client at ease during the treatment.

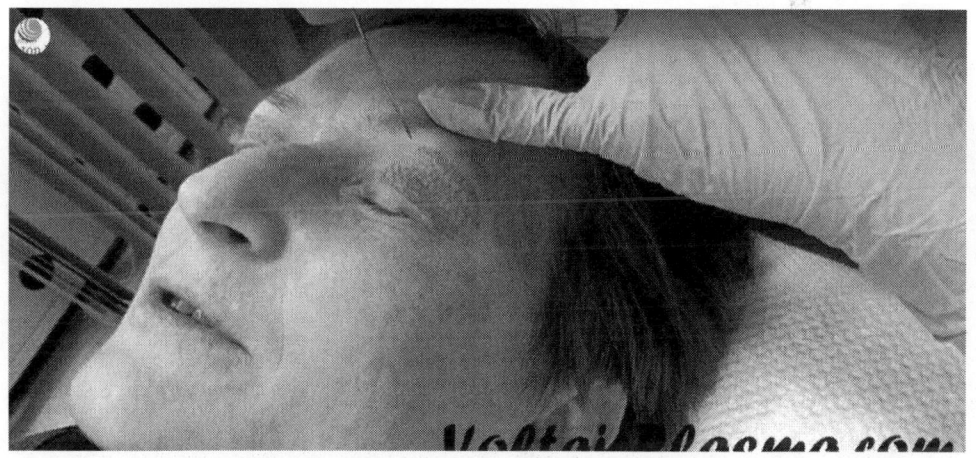

Illustration 26: Eyelid tightening using the appropriate plasma (or arc generating) device.

www.voltaicplasma.com   Author: Andreas Russo

8.5 With Eyelid tightening using the appropriate plasma (or arc generating) device:

- After a number of treatments, the results of eyelid tightening may resemble those of a Blepharoplasty. However Eyelid tightening will not bring about the same diagrammatic results only achievable with surgery.
- Eyelid tightening can be performed by appropriately trained beauticians, as well as doctors, dermatologists and plastic surgeons as sedation is not required, the procedure is very easy to learn and risks to the client are remote.
- Eyelid tightening with the appropriate plasma device has the added advantage that even minor corrections can be made in a virtually risk free and cost-effective way.
- Each correction made to the client is long lasting.
- No scarring has ever been reported using the appropriate plasma device properly.
- Each session can last 15 minutes at most. It will last longer depending if the user covers a particularly large area.
- Topical anaesthetic is not strictly necessary, but the use of an appropriate numbing product is always advisable for the comfort of the client.
- The client can always resume their activities immediately after each session.
- It is recommended that the desired results are achieved in more than one session, especially if the area to be tightened is extensive.
- The costs associated with eyelid tightening are reduced by over 60% to 70% compared with conventional surgical procedures.
- Increased business due to many clients being in fear of surgery or higher costs of traditional surgery. This enable more clients to opt for this type of treatment as it is only minor.

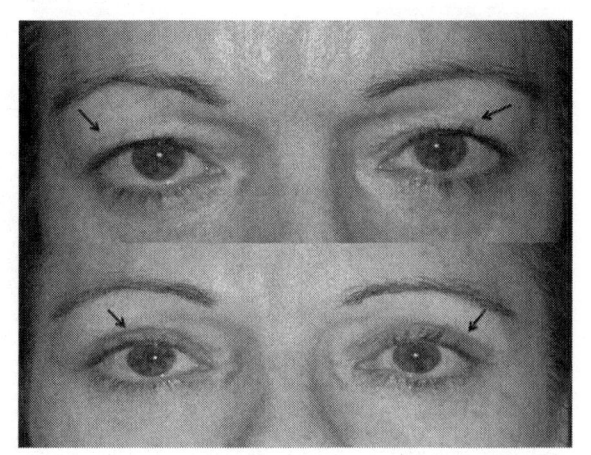

Illustration 27: Minor improvement in the appearance of saggy eyelids.

What to tell the client before the treatment:

- **WAIT** until all the scabs have fallen off. Although clients can resume their activities immediately after each session, they will not look their best during the healing process which lasts up to 7 to 10 days in normal circumstances.
- The area treated **MUST NOT** be covered with any type of make-up, mascara, creams or any other product, until the area has fully healed. Wash gently with soap twice a day. Any other treatment or wearing of any type of make-up could result in unnecessary infections and undesired effects.
- The treatment could be uncomfortable to the client, therefore numbing products shall be used for ease of treatment and comfort reasons during the eyelid tightening procedure.
- Swelling one to three days after the cosmetic treatment is normal and to be expected. It is always better make the client aware of this at consultation stage.
- Eyelid tightening brings about cumulative minor improvements of the appearance of saggy or droopy eyelids. Do not promise the dramatic results which can only be accomplished with surgery.

8.6 Patch testing

Patch testing should always be performed before starting a full eyelid tightening treatment. Patch testing is important so that you can demonstrate that if the after-care is performed correctly the skin will recover well and there are no adverse reactions to this aesthetic treatment.

The patch testing for eyelid tightening has to be performed at the same treatment intensity you intend to carry out the treatment. For example if you would like to use the equipment at a certain power setting, with the spots at a certain distance (say 1 mm apart) and the arc duration a quarter of a second (instantaneous bursts), perform this the treatment at the intensity you intend to carry out the treatment and perform it on a small area behind the ear.

8.7 Before applying the numbing product

Remove all make up thoroughly by using normal make up removal procedures. Remove all make-up from the face. Once you have removed all make-up, apply an appropriate non flammable antiseptic on a clean cotton pad and gently rub the area you are going to treat with the electrical arcing device (The upper eyelids). At that point you can apply the appropriate numbing product on the upper eyelids.

8.8 Use of numbing products before the treatments

Eyelid tightening is not the only aesthetic treatment when the use of numbing products is recommended. Tattooing, laser tattoo removal, lasers skin tightening, moles removal procedures and several other aesthetic treatments require the use of some numbing products to put the client at ease during the aesthetic treatment.

Like with most other aesthetic treatments, it is possible to perform eyelid tightening using electrical arcing without applying any numbing products. However most clients have a low pain threshold, therefore if the area is not numbed properly, eyelid tightening can become a very unpleasant experience for both to the client and the beauty therapist. The unpleasantness of the treatment, may prevent the client from undergoing further sessions due to the discomfort caused by the previous treatment. Also, when the client has an unpleasant experience, it becomes much harder for the beauty therapist, to perform the treatment correctly. This is all easily resolved by using the appropriate numbing product correctly before beginning the treatment.

A very common topical numbing product available on the market, in most parts of Europe, including the **UK is EMLA. (EMLA is available in 5% formulations from most chemists in the UK)**. This is a product which can be purchased and used without a medical prescription. Because of this, EMLA is also the preferred numbing product used by tattoo artists for tattooing and performing body piercings.

EMLA is used by applying the cream on the eyelids and covering the cream with a normal cling film. The same that can be purchased from any supermarket. The cling film is applied in order to cause an *occlusion effect* which will amplify the effects of the numbing ingredients of the EMLA numbing cream. The area is then left to rest for approximately 40 to 45 minutes in order to achieve the desired numbing effects.

Unfortunately, although available without prescription form any chemist in the UK, the EMLA formulation requires a relative long wait in order to become effective and it is not generally very effective if a cling film is not applied on top of the cream. If you attempt to start the aesthetic treatment before the 40 minutes the area will likely not be numb enough, in order to carry out the aesthetic treatment in ease and comfort. Additionally the topical effects of the EMLA formulation end within 5 to 10 minutes from the time the cling film is removed and the EMLA residues are wiped off. Therefore

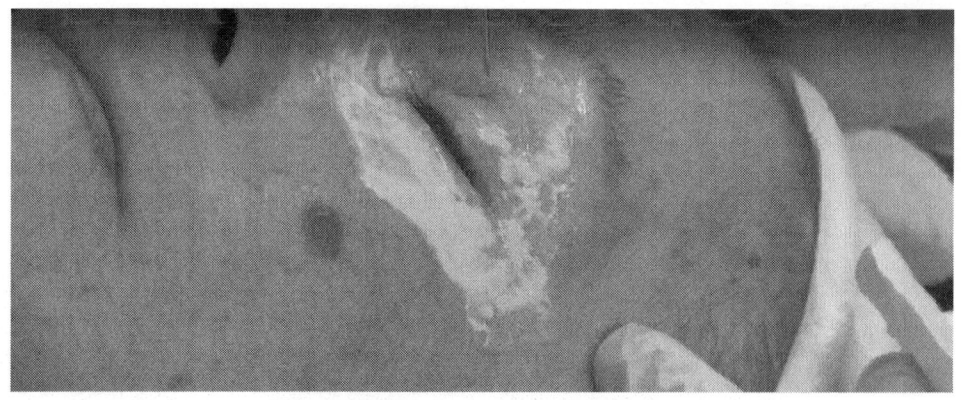

Illustration 28: Numbing cream example

the window of time while you can perform the treatment in comfort is relatively brief. Given that the use of numbing products are heavily regulated, EMLA is the main product available over the counter in the UK. Some Medical practitioners can be authorised to use other numbing products. The formulation that has been used extensively and successfully by medical practitioners who use electrical arcing devices for aesthetic purposes is a topical custom formulated product.

Formulation active ingredients are: lidocaine 20%, prilocaine 5%, tetracaine 5%.

This topical product is either made in a gel or cream formulation. In European countries like Italy and Spain this is made by most local chemists who also have an internal licensed laboratory to manufacture these types of products. In Europe, this type of topical formulation can only be made under medical prescription *(therefore under the sole responsibility of the medical practitioner who orders the product).*

Due to current regulations, this is a product which can be used by medical practitioners only or under their direct supervision. The main advantage of using this type of formulation is that the desired numbing effects are achieved almost immediately and are so good that the client will only feel a tickling sensation when the electrical arc is applied. The area where this formulation is applied becomes numb within 5 to 10 minute after the application. Please note that these types of products are not meant to be completely absorbed, therefore all you have to do is to apply the cream or gel, on the area you intend to treat and leave the product to do its job. With this formulation, there will be no need to apply a cling film because the product itself will be strong enough to achieve the desired numbing effects.

Whenever you start the treatment on the client remember to remove the topical anaesthetic on a small area. The common mistake made by beginners is to remove all the numbing product at once. For example if the topical anaesthetic has been placed on both upper eyelids, the untrained beginner usually removes the cream on both eyelids before starting the treatment. The min problem is that the effect of most topical numbing products do not last long (in case of EMLA only 5 to 10 minutes at most). Therefore the effect of the topical anaesthetic could start to fade before the end of the treatment making the procedure cumbersome.

In the video below you can see an example of the spot mode operation during of a high intensity treatment (the spots are deliberately applied very tightly in order to carry out a high in intensity treatment). As you can see the topical numbing product is only removed on one upper eyelid and in stages, while it is left on the lower eyelid which is going to be treated as soon as the upper eyelid treatment is over. In the video a custom numbing product is applied, there is no need for occlusion with cling film. The video is fast forwarded.

Page 52

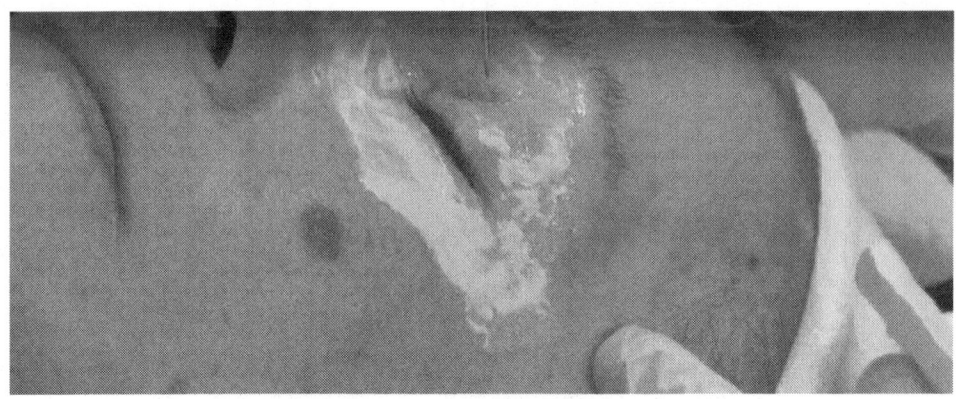

Illustration 29: [Click here to watch video](#)

Therefore is is advisable to remove any type of topical numbing product in small patches while you carry out the electrical arcing treatment. This will ensure that the area you will be treating is still numb, ensuring maximum comfort to your client and ease of operation to the beauty therapist.

In the video you can see an example of lower eyelid tightening. The treatment was performed by a trainee. As you can see the topical numbing product is still applied on the upper eyelid. In this way the upper eyelid will still be numb when the beauty therapist will perform eyelid tightening (Custom numbing product applied, no need for occlusion with cling film).

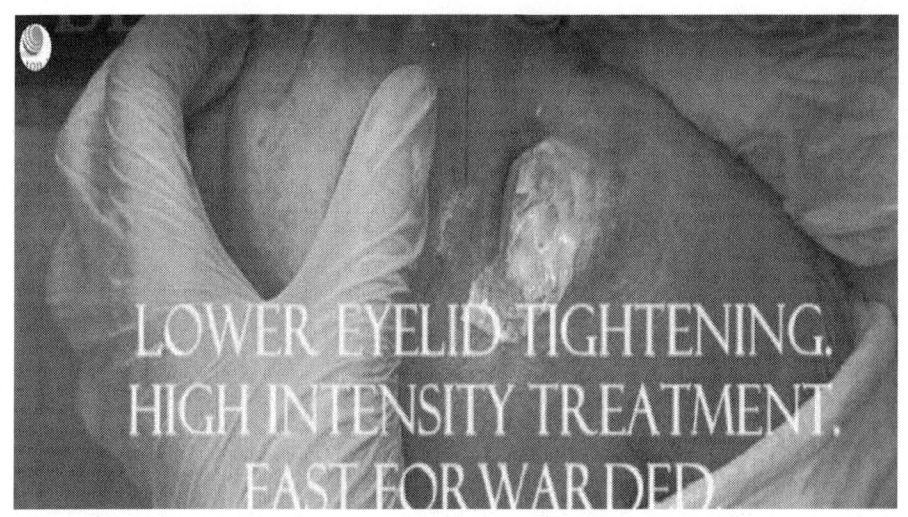

Illustration 30: For eyelid tightening and similar skin tightening procedures, using electrical arcing, the use of local injectable anaesthetics must be avoided even if the beauty practitioner is authorised to use them. [Watch our video](#)

www.voltaicplasma.com   Author: Andreas Russo

8.9 How to perform upper eyelid tightening

The preferred method of performing eyelid tightening is the **spot mode or spot operation**. This is because, the spot mode or spot operation, is very easy to learn and leads to consistent and predictable results.

The spots should be applied randomly without forming any straight line or particular recognisable pattern. One method commonly used to ensure that the spots are applied randomly is to try and apply the voltaic spots in a zigzag fashion. The distance between each spot varies according to the intensity of the treatment of the specific treatment. This varies between 3 to 4 mm apart for very mild intensity treatment to a very dense spot application which resemble the immediate result of the spray operation. A smoke evacuator should be used to get rid of the fumes caused by the cosmetic treatment.

In the video below you can see an example of overall high intensity treatment. The treatment begins as a low intensity treatment but then the intensity of the treatment is increased by applying more voltaic spots. The treatment was carried out by a trainee under supervision.

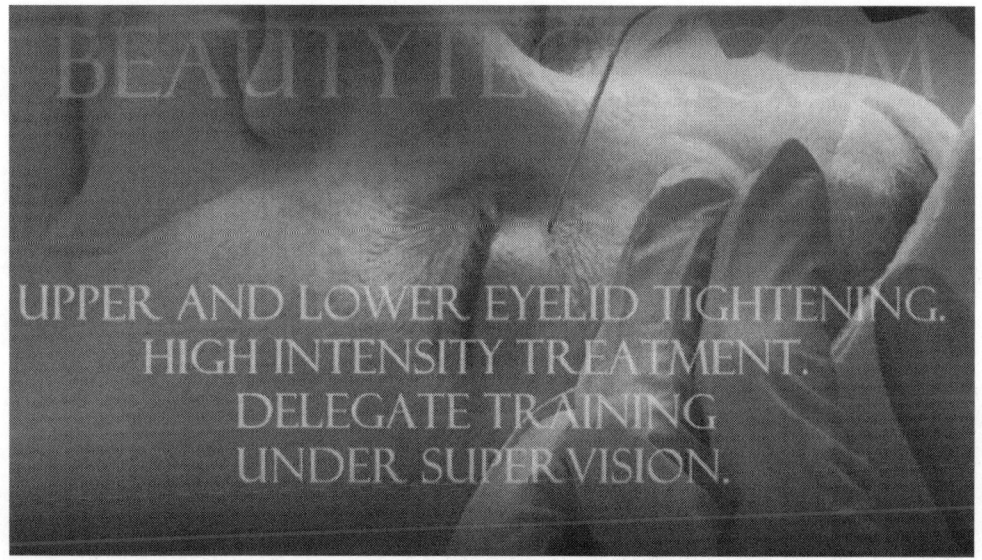

Illustration 31: Click here to watch video

As we can see in the video above upper eyelid tightening, lower eyelid tightening and crow's feet attenuation can be all incorporated within one session. However this is not advisable in most cases because the overall intensity is increased dramatically. This causes dramatic swelling events and a certain level of discomfort which can be easily avoided by simply spitting the treatment in various different sessions, each dedicated to the particular area to be treated. For example one for the upper eyelids, one for the lower eyelids and another for crow's feet attenuation.

www.voltaicplasma.com   Author: Andreas Russo

Please avoid performing high intensity treatments in any case as this can lead to protracted inflammations and various adverse reactions including skin laxity. Therefore always opt for low/medium intensity treatments.

8.10 Treatment intensity advantages and disadvantages

In general the degree of tightening (skin shrinkage) achieved is related to the skin tightening treatment intensity using electrical arcing. As we have seen, in skin tightening, the intensity of the treatment is related to a number of factors and not only the power setting of the device itself. (Click Here to revise this section).

The higher the intensity of the treatment:

- The better the eyelid tightening results once the area has recovered. Therefore the less treatments will be required in order to accomplish the desired results.
- The more the swelling and blistering after the treatment.
- The more the discomfort levels after the treatment.
- The longer it will take for the swelling and blistering to subside.
- The longer the downtime.
- The higher the likelihood of undesired effects.

Conversely the lower the intensity of the treatment:

- The milder the eyelid tightening results. The less the eyelids will tighten
- The less the swelling or blistering after the treatment.
- The less the discomfort levels after the treatment.
- The less time it will take for the swelling and blistering to subside
- The shorter the downtime
- The lower the likelihood of undesired reactions.

8.11 Minor Bleeding

Minor bleeding is a rare occurrence when using AC electrical arcing devices for this type of application. Additionally minor bleeding also occurs after the use of lasers for similar skin tightening applications including laser tattoo removal.

Bleeding occurrence is particularly rare especially if the intensity of the treatment is very mild. The likelihood of minor bleeding increases as the arc duration increases, the power setting of the device increases or both. Please note that minor bleeding is not an indication that the treatment has not been carried out correctly as this can occur despite of the type of device used, technique or intensity of the treatment itself.

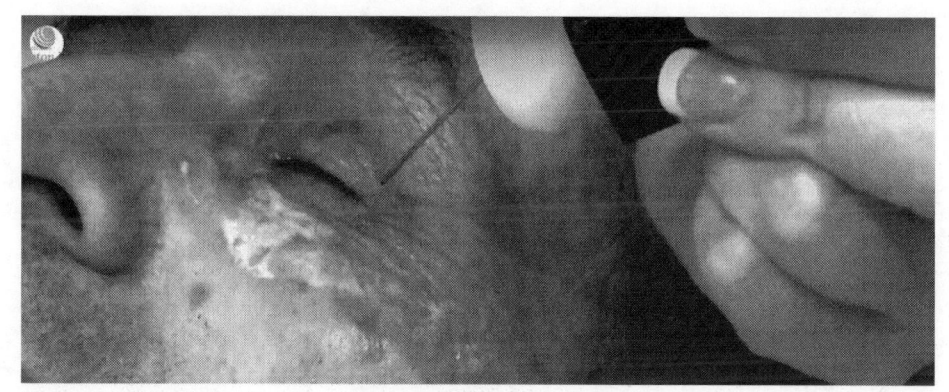

Illustration 32: Please do not be tempted to perform high intensity treatments in order to achieve dramatic results within one session. Most of the times, doing so does not lead to those dramatic results only possible with surgery.

However some degree of minor bleeding can occur even at very low intensity treatments in those cases where fine blood vessels are present on the treated area especially on the upper eyelids.

8.12 The Carbon Residues

As we will see in mole removal or brown spot removal the carbon residues need to be purposely removed in order to accomplish the desired result. This is done by using a cotton pad impregnated with non flammable antiseptic.

In the case of skin tightening and especially eyelid tightening, the carbon residues should not be purposely removed. This is because throughout our extensive experience we have seen that the best and fastest recovery is achieved when the carbon residues are not intentionally removed. This is probably due to the micro traumas caused by rubbing the cotton pad while trying to remove the carbon residues. Therefore while performing skin tightening and especially eyelid tightening, do not intentionally rub the area you treated with the cotton pad as you would do in other aesthetic applications.

If you are applying an appropriate sterile topical product soon after the treatment, including antiseptic, make sure you do not rub it on the area you treated. Just apply the product very gently including any sterile cream.

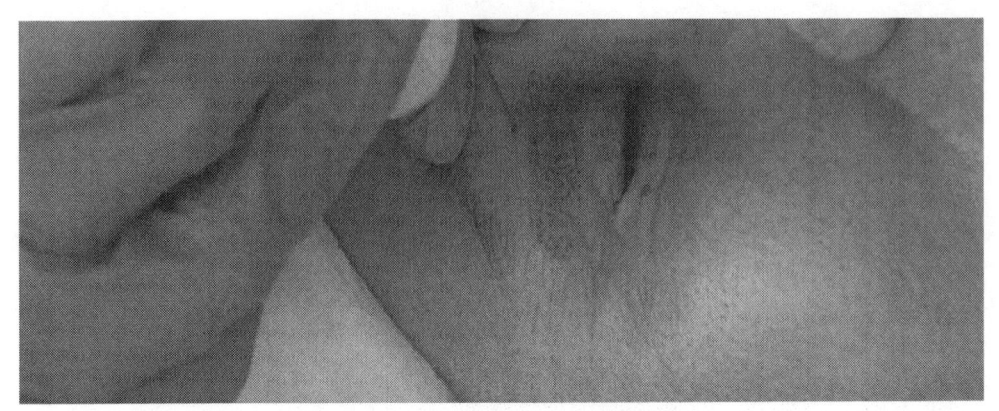

Illustration 33: Click here to watch video

As you can see (if you are using our website voltaicplasma.com) in the video, no effort is made to remove the carbon residues. This is deliberate.

In case you have applied a sterile cream (most commonly a sterile soothing topical product), you will find that the carbon residues will mix with the cream making the cream brownish, this is normal. The carbon residues are sterile anyway as you have cleaned and disinfected the area before applying the numbing product.

8.13 Immediate apparent skin contraction during eyelid tightening

The immediate noticeable effect of eyelid tightening is an apparent skin contraction. Please note that this is not permanent and not representative of the end results of the particular session you are carrying out. The results will become apparent only once the area has fully recovered after the swelling has subsided and the scabs have fallen off or the peeling process is over. This apparent immediate skin contraction can result in the fine lines to apparently disappear completely, however this is not a permanent effect because this is simply due to the superficial dehydration effects of the electrical arcing.

(If you are using our website voltaicplasma.com you can watch a video). In the video above, we can see how the skin contraction due to dehydration effects lead to the fine line to apparently disappear. Once again please note that this apparently dramatic effect is temporary and it is not strictly representative of the end results after the area has recovered.

Sometimes (in 40% of the cases) as the arc is applied the area around the skin reddens noticeably. This means that the skin reaction to the treatment can be quite significant and the swelling following the treatment can be quite intense. Swelling usually starts the day following the treatment.

8.14 Swelling and downtime

Swelling is characteristic to eyelid tightening using electrical plasma (or lasers) and it should be always expected after this type of aesthetic procedure. Swelling can be minimised using <u>certain techniques</u> but never completely avoided, because in order to produce the desired <u>localised skin tightening</u> a deliberate controlled burn has to be caused to the eyelids. Also swelling is associated to the perceived downtime because the client prefers to withdraw from social activities until the area looks normal again and make-up can be used as usual.

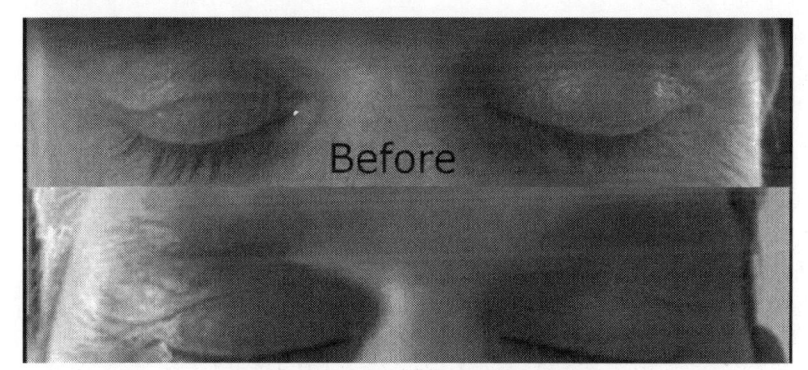

Illustration 34: Swelling and downtime

Please note that the swelling should not be cured because it is not a disease and it is a direct transient consequence of the controlled burn caused by the aesthetic treatment. A common mistake made as after care treatment is the use of antihistamines to try and alleviate the swelling. However this type of swelling does not respond to antihistamines.

During the downtime some clients can experience a certain degree of discomfort. The degree of discomfort depends on the sensitivity of the skin to the treatment as well as the overall treatment intensity. The higher the treatment intensity the more the swelling and the discomfort which can be experienced by the client during the period of time in which the swelling is most pronounced. As the swelling start to subside so will the discomfort levels.

Swelling starts on the following day and usually peaks on the second day. The third or fourth day after the treatment the swelling usually starts to subside slightly and in most cases the swelling will have subsided completely on the fifth day. While the swelling starts to subside the scabs starts to form. Please note the scabs do not always forms however they do in most cases. The scabs will normally have fallen off by themselves on the sixth or seventh day after the treatment. The swelling intensity and discomfort levels are not only dependant on the intensity of the treatment but also the individual skin reaction.

In case of high intensity treatments blistering can also develop. The fluid inside blister can also be transferred to the under eyelids (eye-bags). Sometimes the blistered eyelid can give up some fluid during the recovery period. This is when the after-care is very important and it has to focus on avoiding possible causes of infections. This is simply done by keeping the area clean, avoid possible causes of infections, and applying the appropriate antiseptic twice a day. One again, swelling is a normal reaction to be expected after high intensity treatment and it normally starts to subside three to four days after the treatment, by itself.

8.15 How to reduce swelling and downtime

We have investigated all possible ways to reduce the swelling period, consequently reducing the perceived down time and discomfort to a minimum. It is important to emphasise that due to the very nature of this type of aesthetic treatment including those using lasers, swelling can be attenuated but never eliminated. In order to minimise the downtime after any type of laser treatment for skin tightening, a soothing product is used in order to alleviate the burning feeling soon after the treatment. Any treatment focused to reduce the burning sensation and later attenuate the swelling has to be carried out immediately after the treatment to be most effective. Typically within 5 minutes from the time you have completed the treatment.

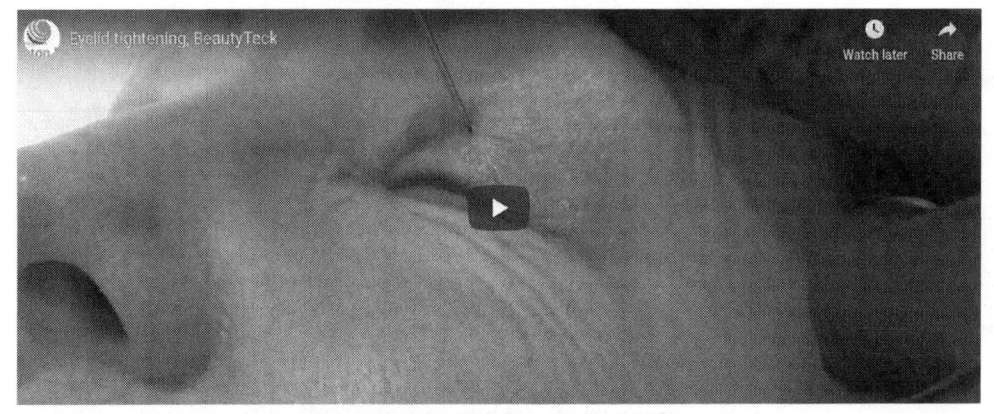

Illustration 35: Click here to watch video

We have found that if the treatment is carried out at minimum/medium intensity and an appropriate numbing product is applied both soon after the treatment and at intervals a few hours after the treatment and the following day, the swelling is reduced to a minimum. If the treatment is carried out at the right intensity, the skin is not particularly sensitive and the right product is applied then the swelling is reduced to such a minimum that it is hardly visible and most clients do not feel any discomfort during the skin recovery period.

- ➢ **How to perform the treatment with our device:**
  - ➢ Set the device at minimum power level (three battery configuration if you are using the earlier version of the **BeautyTeck**)
  - ➢ Apply the arc in instantaneous bursts (approximate arc duration, one quarter of a second).

- only increase the intensity of the treatment by reducing the distance between spots to a minimum. You can apply the spots one beside the other as shown in the video above.
- Do not use a higher power setting than the one recommended here otherwise the swelling will be substantial despite the soothing product or soothing technique used.
- Do not treat an area larger than the one shown in the video above.
- **Apply the suitable soothing product immediately after the treatment.** Please bear in mind that this is the most important application of the soothing product. This is when the skin will be most receptive to the soothing treatment. Make sure you do not deliberately remove the carbon residues and you do not rub the area too hard (as this could cause micro traumas which could delay the recovery process). Keep spreading the soothing product very gently until the gel or the cream has been completely absorbed.
- Instruct the client to reapply the product before going to sleep in the same fashion as you have done at your premises. The product then has to be reapplied the next day, first thing in the morning, in the afternoon and before going to sleep. This soothing product has to be used also the the second day after the the treatment three times a day. The soothing treatment can be discontinued the third day after the treatment once (if they form) the scabs start to become apparent.

Please bear in mind that certain skin types are particularly sensitive and reactive to the treatment, therefore, in these cases the clients may show the normal signs of swelling despite the method used in order to soothe the area after the treatment. This particular type of skin reaction is predictable especially if the surrounding area you have treated reddens visibly a few minutes after the treatment.

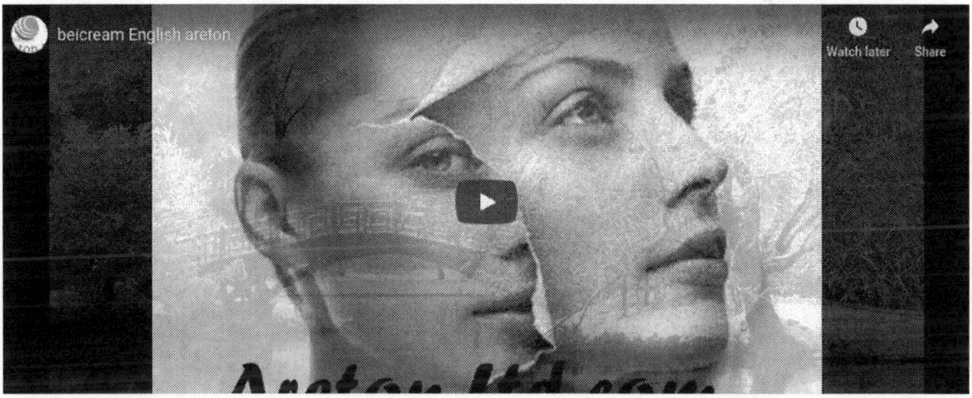

Illustration 36: Beicream Soothing Cream, Click here to watch video

About the soothing product to be used. There are several soothing products on the market and this is not a heavily regulated product type, therefore you have a wide selection. Please make sure that the products you use are sterile and are suited for purpose. Some products although advertised as soothing skin products are not suited for this particular purpose, therefore check with the manufacturers before selecting each specific soothing product. Please be aware that using products that are not manufactured using appropriate methods and hence not suitable or packaged appropriately can increase the likelihood of infection. Therefore make sure the soothing product you are using is fit for purpose. We have made a specific product for this particular application, for more information **please click here.** Please bear in mind that the most effective application of these soothing products (or solutions) is right after the aesthetic treatments are carried out. The subsequent applications are effective but not not as effective as those applied immediately after the aesthetic treatment has ended.

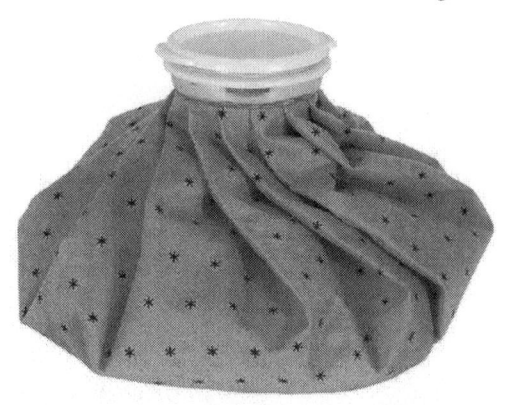

Use of intense cold as a soothing solution. Some beauty practitioners use ice packing as a soothing solution. This is an effective option used soon after burns of any type to soothe the part and decrease the adverse reactions to the burn, and this is also most effective immediately after the burn has occurred. Hence, intense cold, is most effective if applied immediately after the aesthetic session has ended (within 5 to 10 minutes).

8.16 Scabbing process

As swelling subsides, normally scabbing develops. It usually develops in place of the voltaic spots which you have previously applied during the aesthetic treatment. In certain circumstances, especially when particularly low intensity treatments are carried out, scabbing may not develop. As the scabbing develops also the feeling of discomfort will be replaced by minor itchy feeling which will slowly fade away as the scabs start to fall off by themselves.

If scabs develop, it is important they are not picked by the client. Picking the scabs may not only delay the recovery period but also may lead to long term marks on the skin.

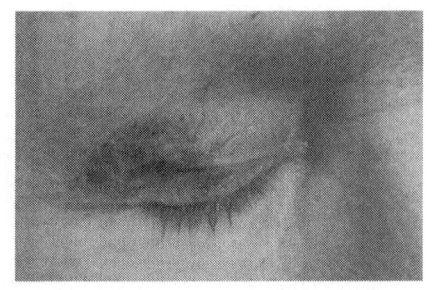

Illustration 37: Scabbing

8.17 Pink skin

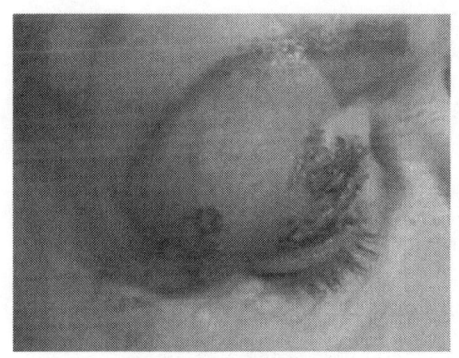

Illustration 38: Pink Skin

Once the scabs will have fallen off by themselves the area which has been treated will be slight pinker, this is a normal reaction to most skin resurfacing treatments including voltaic arcing skin tightening. This is because the new skin formed after the treatment has not enough melanin to match the rest of the skin. Amongst all professional skin resurfacing devices or products, this also occurs with most professional skin peel products. After a while the pinker skin will gradually develop the normal skin colour of the surrounding skin. This is happens gradually over the following weeks.

8.18 When can the client use make-up?

The use of any type of make up (including mineral make-up or make-up products advertised as suitable after laser treatment) is strictly forbidden after until all the scabs have fallen off by themselves.

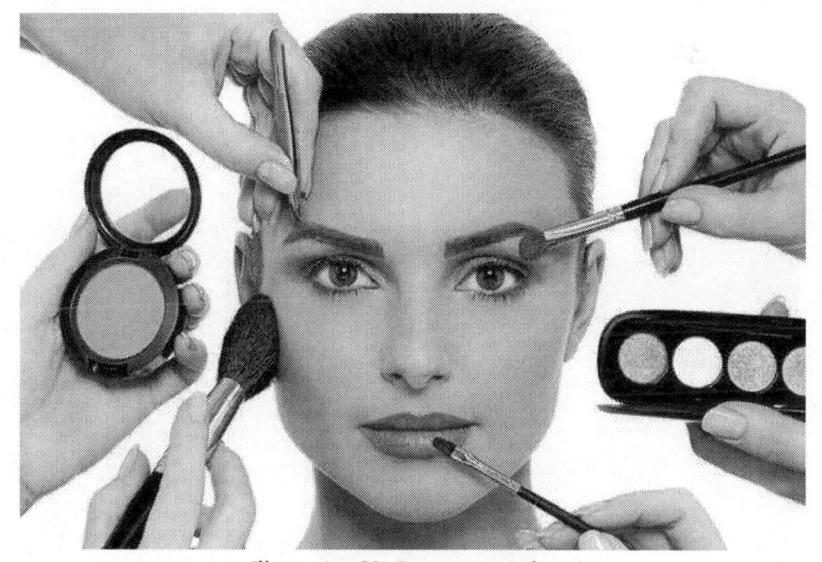

Illustration 39: Permanent makeup

www.voltaicplasma.com   Author: Andreas Russo

This is for two reasons:

1. most make-up products are not sterile and it has been shown that their use clearly jeopardise the healing processes or also referred to skin recovery. This leads to adverse reactions including infections, which can lead to scarring. Often the use of make-up before the right time lead to term hypo-pigmentation or cause the formation of red dots.
2. even if appropriate sterile products are used, the area becomes occluded for an extensive period of time, and this can increase the likelihood of bacteria proliferation inside the area that is supposed to be recovering in the fastest possible way. This delays the normal skin recovery process and increases the chances of developing undesired long terms effects including hypo pigmentation.

8.19 Broad spectrum sun screen

The use of sun screen (preferably physical protection) is mandatory for at least three months

UV protection must be worn, on the treated area, in the morning before going out and in the early afternoon.

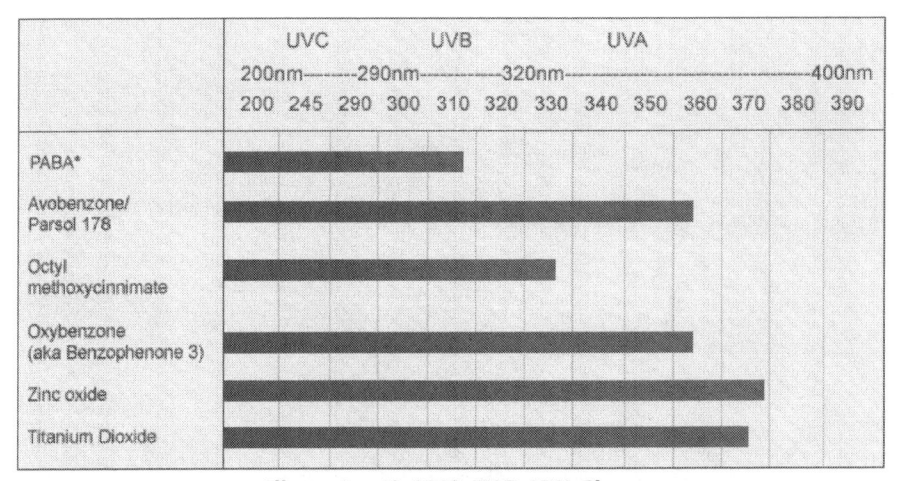

Illustration 40: UVC, UAB, UVA Chart

Exposure to UV sources have been shown to increases the likelihood of developing long term hyper pigmentation not only after the use of skin tightening by using voltaic arcing but also after the use of glycolic acid peels, lasers and other skin tightening procedures including skin resurfacing in general.

www.voltaicplasma.com   Author: Andreas Russo

8.20 When to repeat the treatment

The long-term effects of eyelid tightening by using electrical arcing is a long-term targeted tightening of the eyelids. This improves the appearance of saggy eyelids. The skin tightening effects are cumulative therefore repeating the treatment leads to very good long term results.

The treatment can often be repeated after 8 weeks provided that no adverse reactions have been reported and only low/medium intensity treatments were carried out. Although high intensity treatments should be avoided, in case they have been carried out, the wait time between treatments should be 6 months.

Ask the client if the treated area feels tender to the touch or over sensitive. If this is the case do not repeat the treatment until the area feels normal again. Different people have different skin reactions to the treatment and the beauty therapist has to ensure the area has recovered fully. If the area is somewhat tender to the touch or particularly sensitive then this means that the treated area is still undergoing some recovery or regeneration process. Once the recovery is completely over, the skin will feel normal again.

By "skin recovery" we refer to the downtime (the period while swelling or scabs are still developing, while the area looks unsightly and make-up cannot be worn). The skin will still be recovering and forming new collagen a few days and sometimes weeks after the scabs have fallen off.

8.21 Long term adverse reactions to the plasma eyelid tightening treatments

Despite the heavy advertising as completely safe and carefree treatments, plasma eyelid lift treatments are never completely risk-free despite the device used or the way the treatment has been carried out. This is not currently a topic covered in the main marketing literature as this puts the interest of manufacturers at stake. **The potential adverse reactions are:**

1. Hyperpigmentation. This is only due to the exposure of the area to UV radiation while the long-term healing process is taking place. This is never due to the type of device used or the way the treatment has been carried out.
2. Pink Aptrophic spots (where the spots were applied) which last up to 6 months after the treatment. It is not completely clear what causes this long-term adverse reaction however so far this has ultimately subsided on its own over the log term. It is thought this is likely due to the use of makeup or inappropriate products during the short-term healing process.
3. Protracted long-term healing process coupled with inflammation of the area. This adverse effect has been reported only after high-intensity treatments. Also, for this reason, it is highly advisable to only carry out low or medium intensity treatments.
4. Protracted periods of skin laxity on the upper eyelids where high intensity treatments were carried out. The laxity is also associated with a mild feeling of discomfort on the area treated.

This adverse effect has been reported after treatments with all devices especially after high-intensity treatments.

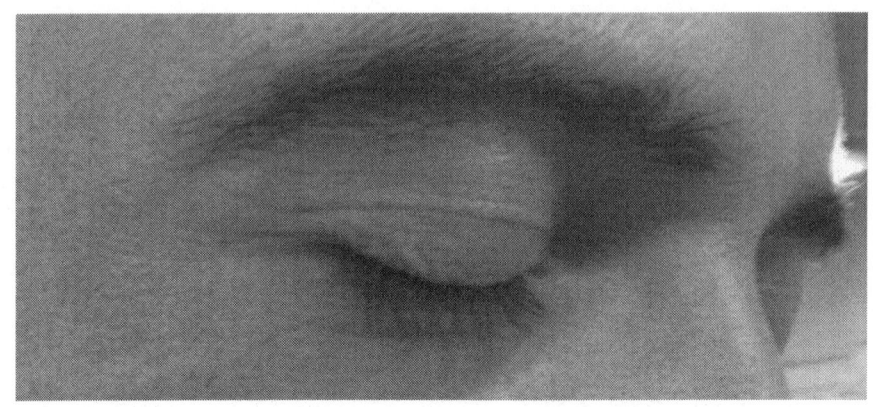

Illustration 41: Laxity a few weeks after a high intensity eyelid tightening procedure.

Points 3 and 4 are due to the overall intensity of the treatment, therefore it is highly recommendable to avoid high-intensity treatments in all cases. As mentioned earlier the slight advantages of performing high-intensity plasma treatments on the upper eyelids are seldom worth the protracted swellings, pain discomfort and the increased likelihood of protracted long-term healing and skin laxity. This can easily discourage clients from undergoing further treatments.

Eyelid Tightening and a Rare case of Hyperpigmentation due to UV Exposure

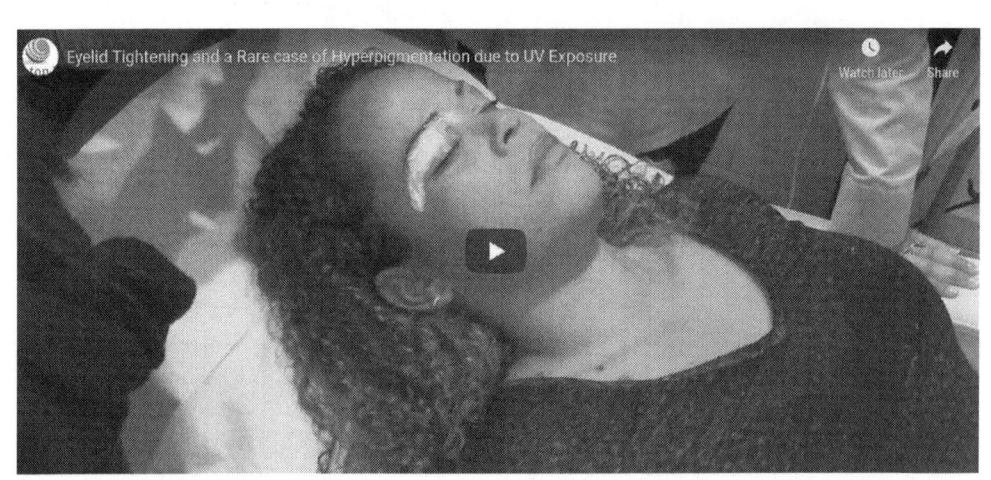

Illustration 42: click here to watch video

8.22 Claims of non surgical blepharoplasty

Some manufacturers are advertising plasma eyelid tightening as non surgical blepharoplasty. We have had the opportunity to use those devices and we have noticed the common trait with all other plasma devices for similar intended used on the market. The real results of plasma eyelid lift is a minor improvement of the appearance of the saggy skin and after several trials with those devices it is believed it is not practical to achieve the same results as surgical procedures using electrical plasma. Although the long-term results after a number of eyelid tightening treatments may be good this is seldom comparable with the result of any surgical blepahroplasty intervention.

The temptation of making these claims is easily understood given the large demand to achieve surgery-like results without surgery, however seldom plasma treatments can match the results of surgical procedures despite the techniques and device used.

The claim which seems more appropriate and has been more widely accepted is: "Plasma Eyelid lifts leads to a minor improvement in the appearance of saggy eyelids."

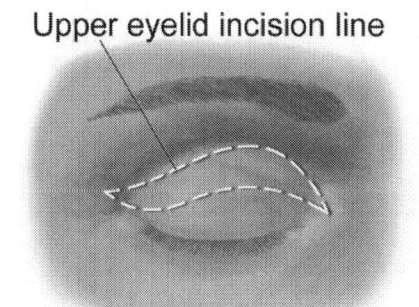

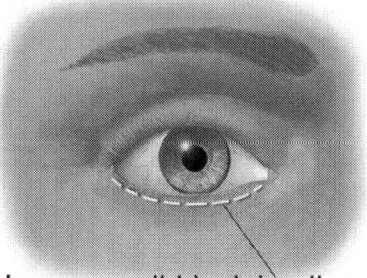

Illustration 43: blepharoplasty

It is recommended to all aesthetic practitioners to make realistic claims in their advertising of plasma procedures despite promises made by others. It has now been accepted that people are willing to undergo these treatments even if the claims made about these treatments are realistic. Reviews of these types of Voltaic plasma procedures made by professionals without vested financial interests in selling these types of devices or the treatments all have felt that it would not be realistic to expect results which are equivalent to surgery in cases of a great amount of loose skin to be removed. Every time one undergoes a plasma treatment he/she will go through the healing process and the long terms healing. During the healing process (both long-term and short term) a number of adverse reactions could take place, therefore if the improvement sought by the individual is dramatic, surgical procedures should be the recommended instead.

www.voltaicplasma.com   Author: Andreas Russo

Not all cases are suitable for these types of procedures. Although several people would like to have the same results as surgery with the use of Plasma eyelid tightening, in case of considerable skin laxity this procedure should not be recommended. This is because several number of sessions may be required in order to achieve the results desired by the client.

Every time the client undergoes a plasma eyelid tightening treatment he/she undergoes a number of potential adverse reactions, therefore repeating the treatment a number of times exposes the individual a number of times to the same potential adverse effects. Therefore the higher the number of treatments to higher the likelihood of an adverse reaction to occur. For this reason plasma treatment should not be replacing surgical dramatic improvements.

On the other hand if the improvement sought is only minor then medium mild intensity treatments can be far more advisable to surgical interventions in the first place. One to two treatments can achieve the desired results like in this case presented below where the tightening was satisfactory after only two treatments

People with minor laxity are the perfect candidates for these types of aesthetic procedures. This is because one or two low/medium intensity treatments are usually sufficient to achieve their desired results and they will not be exposed to the inherent risks of the procedure several-times.

8.23 Further advice

Do not use any type of injectable anesthetic as a numbing solution for upper eyelid tightening.

The main after-care principle after eyelid tightening are:

1. Avoid infections. The skin will recover on its own accord without any product, provided that no infections develop. The use of inappropriate products including make-up or unsuitable creams before the scabs have formed can be detrimental and lead to undesirable effects.
2. Appropriate broad-spectrum protection must be worn every day. While the use of broad-spectrum total sunscreen increases protection against the possible adverse effects of rays exposure, these adverse effects are still possible even using broad-spectrum protection. Hence, direct or indirect exposure to ray sources must be purposely avoided whenever possible. Any form of tanning including artificial must be avoided for at least three months after the last treatment.

Do not use any medicinal products. Only use those sterile products suggested in the after-care product list of the manufacturer. If you would like to use different after-care products, consult with the specific manufacturer whether their products are suitable to be used after this type of aesthetic treatments. If in doubt do not use any products other than mild antiseptics.

No antihistamines, swelling is not an allergic reaction. Swelling is a normal and "to be expected" reaction to the superficial burn caused by the electrical arcing treatment. Do not use topical antibiotics as a precautionary measure. Remember that antibiotics are used to cure infections and they are not supposed to be used to prevent them. It has been shown that indiscriminate use of antibiotics will eventually lead to bacterial resistance to the specific antibiotic used due to bacteria's natural selection process.

Avoid the treatment on those clients with herpes simplex even if there are no flare-ups at the time. If the Herpes Simplex is dormant the client should undergo an antiviral therapy before any eyelid tightening using either lasers or electrical arcing.

Do not use plasters of any type. No other forms of occlusion like bandaging shall be used during the downtime.

9.0 How to perform plasma upper eyelid tightening for the first time

Here you will find all the important instruction which will help you carry out your first plasma eyelid tightening in complete safety and avoid the most common treatment mistakes.

We will take you through the best way to use our plasma devices for aesthetic uses correctly step by step, providing you with clear video examples that you can take as reference when you carry out these types of aesthetic treatments. We will make clear the distinction between low, medium and high intensity treatments. We will provide you with the necessary visual reference experience for you to carry out your first plasma upper eyelid tightening procedure with confidence. Before going ahead and study this section please study the Plasma Eyelid Tightening Module.

9.1 Preface

One of the most common aesthetic practitioners' initial challenges is that they are not confident carrying out their first plasma eyelid tightening procedures on their own. Here we will clarify this issue and as we will see, it is relatively easy to carry out your first eyelid tightening in complete safety. As we have already learned, the preferred technique for upper eyelid tightening is the spot mode or the spot operation. This has been used extensively around the world and it is very easy to learn.

There are other ways to use plasma for eyelid tightening like the spray operation but this is not always straightforward to learn. When you start using plasma for eyelid tightening for the first time you should use low-intensity treatment. There is no clear-cut distinction between low/medium/ high-intensity treatments. A low-intensity treatment can fall into a medium intensity treatment only by changing a few parameters of the treatment like duration of the arc and/or distance between the spots. Similarly, a medium intensity treatment can fall into a high-intensity treatment and vice versa a high intensity treatment can become a medium intensity treatment too by changing some parameters.

Even if there is no clear-cut definition of low, medium and high-intensity treatments it is easy to recognize the intensity of the specific treatment by looking at them as they are being performed. At live training sessions, you are shown how these types of treatments are performed on one person only, this webpage will show you several examples so that you will have more reference experience in order to perform these types of treatments in complete confidence and safety. Given the number of examples you will be able to watch in this webpage and our YouTube Channel, you will be equipped with the tools you require to recognise the difference between the different types of intensity treatments and learn how to carry them out for the first time.

9.2 How to carry out your first plasma upper eyelid tightening procedure

Please note that this page has been made for the use of the BeautyTeck and or the devices marketed by Areton Ltd. For instructions of other devices please refer to the original manufacturer's instructions and training.

1. The first step for you is to familiarise with the way the plasma devices are used on "familiarise with the use of electrical arcing devices web page on Voltaicplasma.com" there is extensive information on how become accostuimed to the use of these devices for the very first time. Once you have completed the exercises on the "test meat" and you are comfortably able to use the device at the minimum power level, then you can start the use of the device for eyelid tightening for the first time.
2. If you have the BeautyTeck, set the device at minimum power level with three battery configuration. In any case, do not be tempted to use a higher power setting than the lowest one. If you are using devices sold by other companies use their instructions for this procedures.
3. Use only short bursts duration of less than a 1/4 of a second (as seen in the video below)
4. Distance the spots between 3 to 2 mm apart. You can also distance them 4 mm apart if you wish.
5. Cover a relatively small area of the upper eyelid.

It is easier to understand what we mean by watching a video example. The following video is your reference for low-intensity treatment when you carry it out for the first time. Watch youtube video

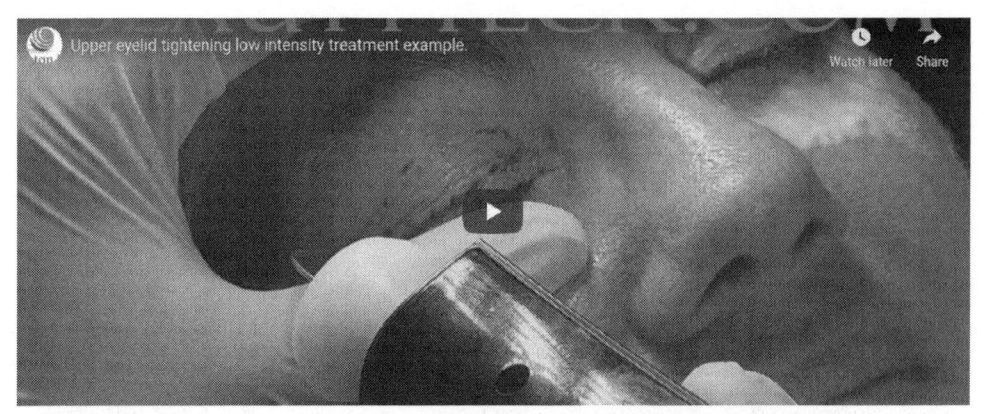

Illustration 44: Click here to watch video

9.3 Medium intensity

Once you have performed your first low-intensity upper eyelid tightening treatment and you have seen the results, then you can move to performing medium intensity treatments. Normally medium intensity treatments are performed by only changing the duration of the arc slightly and reducing the distance between the spots. Also, the area treated will increases slightly.

1. If you are using the BeautyTeck the device setting is level 1 with three battery configuration.
2. The distance between the spots is decreased slightly and ranges between 1 to 2 mm.
3. The duration of each spot is in the region of 1/4 to 1/2 of a second.

The video below will provide you with some reference treatments to emulate in order to reproduce these types of treatment intensity. Watch youtube video.

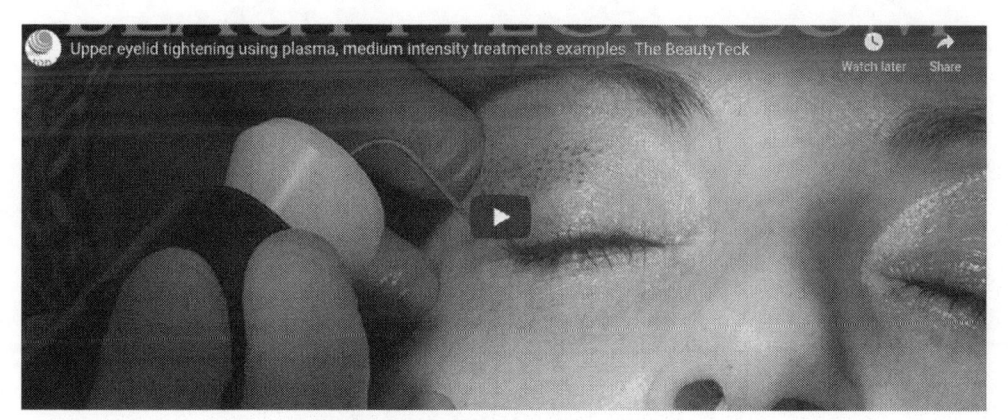

Illustration 45: Click here to watch video

9.4 High intensity treatments

After witnessing the results of low and medium intensity treatments you may be tempted to perform high-intensity treatments in order to achieve far better results. Please remember that the results of plasma eyelid tightening cannot be rushed and the improvements achieved due to the treatment cannot produce the miracles that many short lived markets advertise. There are limits to what it is realistically possible due to the physics of this type of treatment.

The problem with high-intensity treatments is that while the results may be marginally better than low and medium intensity treatments the immediate reactions and increased likelihood of potential longer-term adverse reactions can discourage people from undergoing further plasma tightening treatments.

Additionally, it has become clear that high-intensity treatments do not bring significant improvements compared to medium intensity treatments. In other words, high-intensity treatments do not bring about proportional improvements to the tightening sought by the clients. In terms of results, high-intensity treatments only bring about a minor long-term improvement compared with the long-term results of medium intensity treatments.

The immediate transient adverse effects of high-intensity treatments are:

1. Major swelling which is inevitable after high-intensity treatments even using appropriate soothing products. Soothing products can sometimes alleviate the severe swelling.
2. Pain following the first 24 hours after the treatment.

This does not mean that low medium intensity treatments do not lead to the same short-term swelling and pain, however, they are far more moderate than what occurs in high-intensity treatments.

Watch our video on High Intensity Plasma Treatment

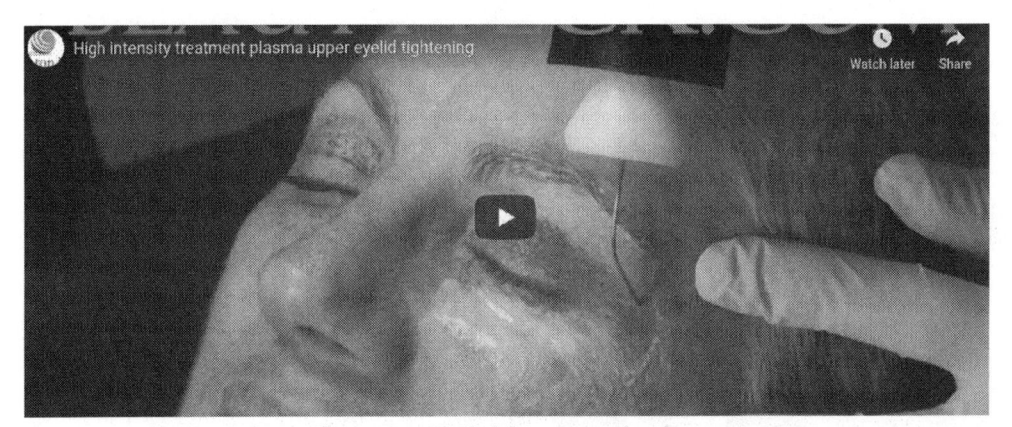

Illustration 46 Click here to watch video

Unfortunately, it is not true that adverse effects cannot occur after these procedures. The treatment itself consists in inducing a controlled burn of the upper and lower eyelids, therefore, depending on the way the burn has been carried out and the particular type of skin, the likelihood of adverse effects differ. As a general rule of thumb the higher the overall intensity of the treatment the higher the likelihood of adverse effects occurring after the upper eyelid tightening procedure. We have carried out thousands of high-intensity treatments over the years without major adverse reactions. However, although rare, the few adverse reactions reported over time have only followed high-intensity treatments. One of the main problems with high-intensity treatments is that the swelling and pain are the most intense after these types of treatments and this alone may dissuade people from undergoing further treatments despite the results.

9.5 Rarely high-intensity treatments can lead to some of the medium-term adverse effects:

1. Prolonged period of redness (also referred to long-term healing), this can last up to 6 to 8 weeks after the treatment.

2. Long term laxity lasting up to 3 months after the high-intensity treatment. This has been reported to occur after high-intensity treatments and it takes place during the long-term healing but it is transient. However in some rare cases it can last for several months. It is as if the area gets worse in the long term instead of getting better. In most cases, this is coupled with long periods of inflammations.These adverse reactions have not been reported after medium/ low-intensity treatments. Therefore high-intensity treatments should always be avoided in a commercial environment. Please note that the main cause for people to be discouraged from undergoing further treatments has been the severe swelling and pain following the treatment, the long-term healing and laxity are very rare occurrences.

Please remember that despite the amazing expectations and promises made by different manufacturers these types of treatments have their inherent limitations due to the skin physiology and the inherent physics of the treatment itself. Plasma treatments cannot shorten the skin because electrical plasma simply does not cut the skin. Some manufacturers bring forward the immediate carbonisation (therefore deep dehydration) to show that the "there is immediate shortening of the skin", however, please note that the immediate skin contraction of the area after the carbonisation (also referred to as sublimation for marketing purposes) is only transient because the dehydration will be over as soon as the swelling takes place.

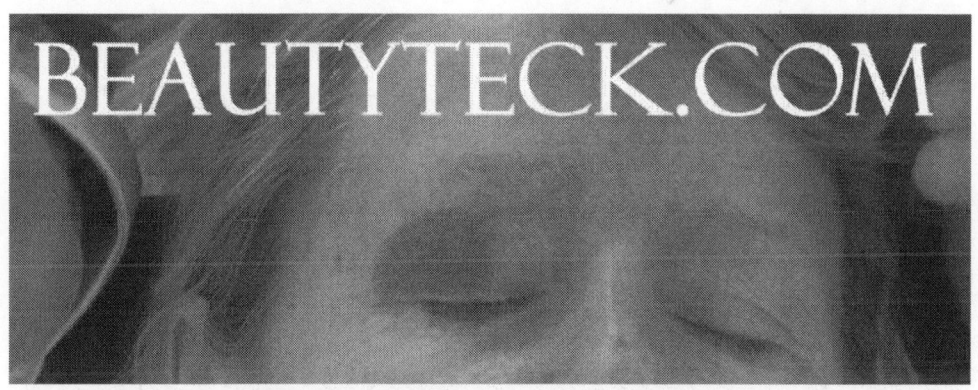

Illustration 47: As you see the fold of the right upper eyelid has disappeared. Example of immediate skin shrinkage advertised as "permanent skin shortening" by some manufacturers. Please note that these types of results are neither permanent nor representative of the actual results. The area is dehydrated immediately after the treatment and it will be subject to change over the coming days and sometimes months.

www.voltaicplasma.com   Author: Andreas Russo

9.6 Conclusions

After examining the effects of most high-intensity treatments using voltaic plasma with different devices we have come to the conclusion that performing high-intensity treatments are more disadvantageous than advantageous. This is because the minor added tightening are overshadowed by the increased pain and swelling, also the likelihood of potential adverse reactions is higher. The intense swelling and pain after high-intensity treatments are sufficient to discourage people from undergoing further necessary eyelid tightening treatments to achieve the desired effects. High-intensity treatment, on rare occasions, has led to long-term inflammation of the area lasting up to 3 months and laxity.

Laxity is the opposite of tightening and its likelihood of occurring can be minimized by only performing low/medium intensity treatments. Laxity can be corrected by further eyelid tightening treatments. The most common adverse reaction is hyper-pigmentation, however, this is never due to the way the treatment is carried out. It is only to do with the early exposure to UV radiations. To learn more about the effects of high intensity treatments versus medium or low intensity treatment please study the section "Long Term Healing".

10.0 Long-term healing after plasma upper eyelid lift high-intensity treatments

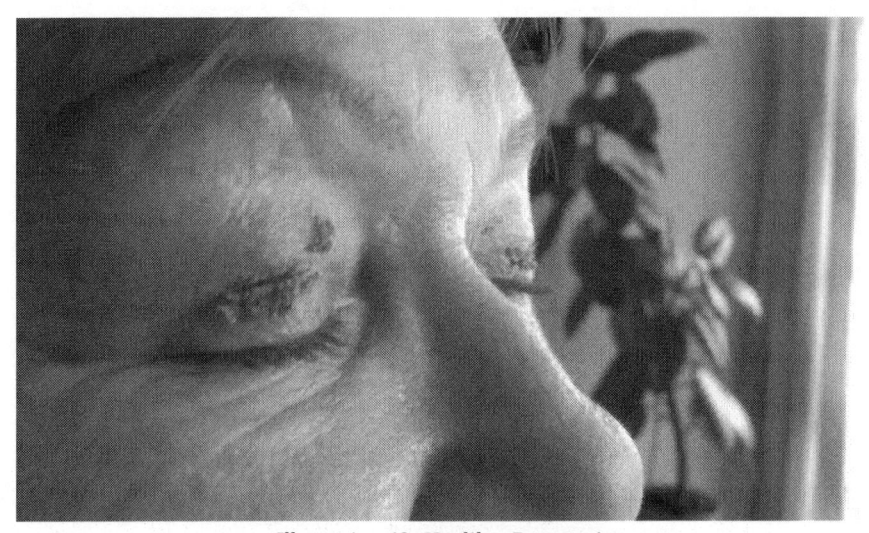

Illustration 48: Healilng Progression

10.1 Overview

There are two healing phases in localised skin tightening using electrical Plasma:

1. Short-term healing
2. Long-term healing

While the short-term healing results in swelling and the scabbing, the long-term healing deals with the long-term regeneration and remodeling of the skin. While the former takes place immediately after the treatment and it is over within a few days, the latter usually takes place over the course of weeks, and sometimes even months.

During the long-term healing, the skin is still subject to redness, tenderness and it is still being remodeled. The remodeling lasts as long as the feeling of tenderness is still occurring.

The long-term skin recovery period depends on several factors, in particular:

- The intensity of the treatment (remember that the treatment intensity is dependant on a number of factors, and not only the power setting of the device). In particular the longer the duration of the arc the deeper the heat will be propagated inside the skin. The closer together the spots the more intense the heat. Generally, the higher the intensity of the treatment the more intense is the redness after the procedure and the longer it takes for the long-term healing to be over.
- The duration of the long-term healing is also dependent on the individual skin recovery ability.

Certain appropriate soothing or healing products can reduce the time required for the long-term healing process.

10.2 What is the long-term healing process anyway?

While the short-term healing process can be easily explained by comparing it to the effects of skin burns and small injuries, the long-term healing process has to refer to something slightly different. We relate the long-term healing process to the all familiar topic of skin regeneration after mole removal or minor skin wounds recovery process soon after the scabs have fallen off. After the scabs have fallen off following plasma aesthetic treatments or minor skin injuries, the new skin is usually red and has a different texture to the rest of the skin. The area can also be itchy and tender for a while.

Also, the long-term skin recovery process is similar to that which occurs after deep skin cosmetic peels. Like in skin peels the deeper the peel penetration the longer the redness after the treatment, however generally the long-term skin recovery period after plasma treatments take longer. While a peel long-term recovery can last up to three weeks (with a feeling of tenderness and dryness of the skin) the redness and tenderness and dryness can last up to 3 months, this is normal and to be expected after plasma high-intensity treatments.

While the skin is still red and tender it is still being regenerated and remodelled. In order to understand what it is happening during the long-term healing, we will take the mole removal example. When the new skin regenerates it is of a different red/pink colour and it lacks pigmentation. Also, the texture is different.

Illustration 49: Area a few days after plasma mole removal. The area is red soon after the scab has fallen off. The new skin will eventually return to its normal colour and texture, consequently blending with the surrounding skin.

Over time the skin texture and colour will return to normal and it will be difficult to tell any treatment was carried out at all. After mole removal, the scabbing takes place. Once the scab has fallen off the area will be red and have a noticeably different skin texture to the surrounding skin. This is because the new skin has formed instead of the old skin lesion. When the new skin forms it is usually of a vivid colour and it also has a noticeably different skin texture.

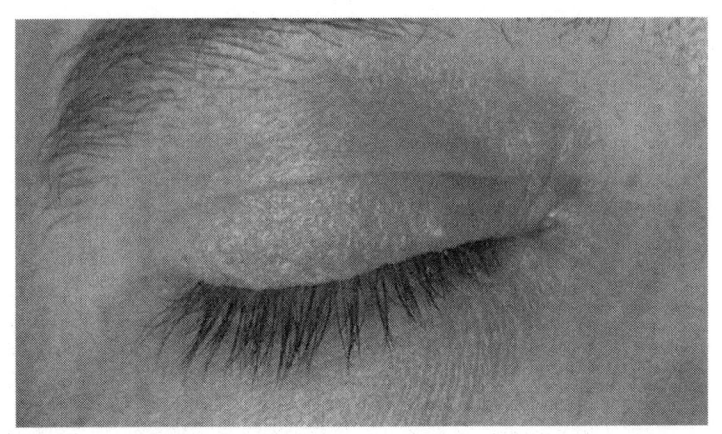

Illustration 50: Detail of the right eyelid a few days after a benign skin lesion removal procedure using electrical plasma. The area is red/pink after the scab has fallen off.

The difference in colour between the treated area and the surrounding skin will slowly fade away over the following weeks. Similarly, the new skin texture will blend with the surrounding skin over the course of the following weeks.

10.3 Redness after localised plasma skin tightening

In a similar fashion to mole removal, after localised tightening treatments (including plasma upper eyelid lift), the new skin will be red after the scabs have fallen off. The same applies to localised skin tightening using electrical plasma. Once the scabs have fallen off the area has an intense red colour like the one seen in mole removal. Additionally, in case of localised skin tightening, the skin will tend to regenerate due to the thermal stimulation caused by the burn inflicted by the electrical arc.

Therefore the redness (inflammation) is caused by two factors:

1. the new skin being regenerated after the minor injury caused by the electrical arc and
2. the heat stimulation caused by the treatment.

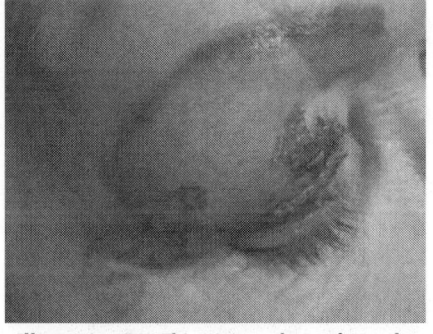

Illustration 51: This picture shows the scabs falling off after an intense plasma upper eyelid lift procedure. Some of the scabs are still present and this picture shows clearly how as the scabs fall off, the area is noticeably red from the plasma eyelid lift procedure.

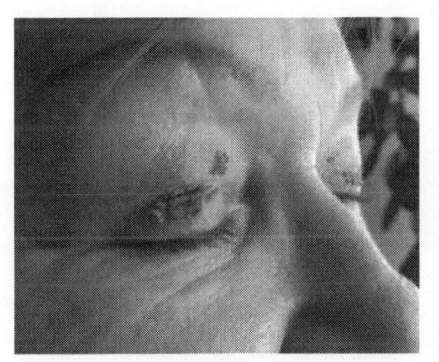

Illustration 52: "Red Meat" type pf colour after the scabs have just fallen off. This is a normal occurrence after plasma localised skin tightening.

After the short-term healing, the new skin is naturally red, furthermore, the skin undergoes a further continuous slow process of regeneration and remodeling during the time it takes for the area to recover from the thermal stimulation (burn) caused by the plasma superficial skin burn. In other words, inflammation, redness and skin remodeling are an "all in one" effect of the long-term skin healing process.

www.voltaicplasma.com   Author: Andreas Russo

Since the redness is due to the skin regeneration process, exposure to intense UV light, during the long-term healing can lead to hyper-pigmentation. As a rule of thumb, when the redness has completely subsided, then direct sun exposure is less likely to lead to hyperpigmentation. Furthermore, if the treatment is repeated before the long-term healing is completely over (while the area is still tender), the treatment becomes unbearably painful even using most common "over the counter" topical numbing products. Therefore as a rule of thumb, if the area is still red or tender, the treatment should not be repeated until the area has returned to normal and the tenderness faded completely.

Please note that the end of the redness does not mark the end of the long-term healing. The area may still be still subject to the long-term healing even while not appearing red at all. What marks the end of the long-term healing is the end of the tenderness instead. In any case, the redness is not permanent and it subsides over time.

10.4 What does the long-term healing feel like

Tenderness and redness should not be cause for concern, because it is a normal part of the long-term recovery process. It will eventually subside on its own accord without leaving a trace as long as no exposure to intense UV light has taken place.

The following applies to high-intensity treatments without the use of any soothing or healing products:

1. **Itchiness.** The initial feeling is of itchiness, this starts during the scabbing process and continues soon after the scabs have fallen off. It usually lasts approximately 7 to 10 days after the scabs have fallen off.
2. **Tenderness.** While the itchy feeling subsides slowly, it is replaced by a feeling of tenderness. The degree of tenderness and its duration is dependent on the treatment intensity. The end of the long-term healing process is marked by the end of the feeling of tenderness.
3. **Dryness.** This feeling can occur as soon as the scabs have fallen off and it can last all throughout the long-term healing period.
4. **A stinging** feeling is also common all throughout the long-term healing when applying creams, sunscreen and cosmetics.

Even low-intensity treatments do cause similar reactions, however, the symptoms last less and their intensity is far milder. Please note that the redness can still have subsided while the healing process is still ongoing what really marks the end of the long-term healing process is the end of the tenderness.

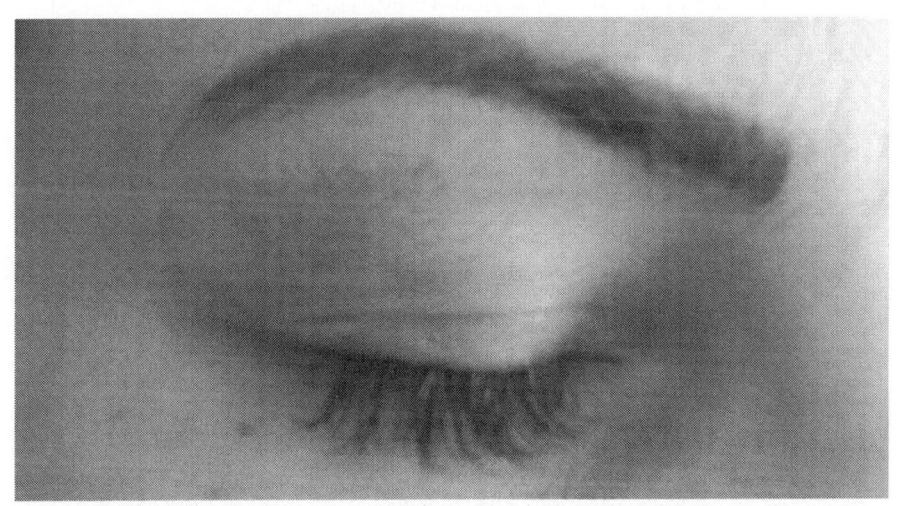

Illustration 53: This picture was taken one month after the plasma high-intensity treatment. Redness and tenderness of the area and slight laxity after a plasma high-intensity treatment.

10.5 Plasma upper eyelid lift tightening remodeling during the long-term healing period

An important aspect of the long-term healing process is the skin re-modelling. There is usually a clear change in the skin structure immediately after the scabs have fallen off. However the change at that point is evident but not permanent, the skin structure will change over the course of the long-term healing while the skin feels still tender. The following pictures are a demonstration of the re-modelling happening over the course of a few hours after the scabs have fallen off.

After the scabs have fallen off (during the long-term healing) the change becomes significant and relatively rapid. In the picture below you can see the difference (in terms of tightening) a few hours later. However, the area is still red.

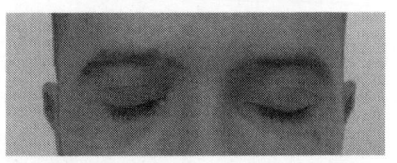

Illustration 54: The day after the scabs have fallen off completely the area is significantly red. Some results may be apparent already in most cases, however, the area is still subject to change over the following hours and days.

www.voltaicplasma.com   Author: Andreas Russo

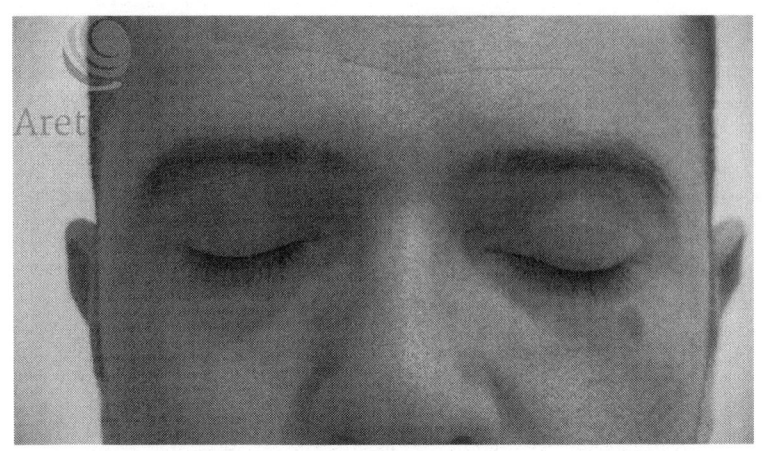

Illustration 55: A few days after the scabs fell off after plasma eyelid lift treatment using the spray operation. The area is still red and still subject to remodelling. The area has tightened further compared to the picture taken immediately after the scabs had fallen off.

The area will be still subject to change over the course of the long-term healing. Once the tenderness is over the results can be regarded as virtually permanent.

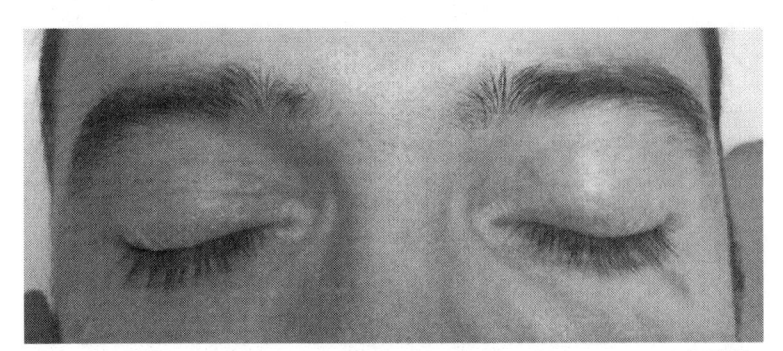

Illustration 56: Eyelids over one year after the last plasma upper eyelid lift procedure November 2016. This is the long-term result of the plasma procedure.

Please bear in mind that the skin is a live organ and subject to change over the long-term, therefore, however, slow the skin will change over the long period even after the long-term healing process is over. Once the desired results are achieved, the treatment can be repeated when required, usually several years later.

Skin laxity is a temporary adverse reaction to plasma eyelid tightening treatment. Please note that in all cases examined so far, skin laxity has been a transient effect only observed during the long-term healing process while the area was still very tender. This transient effect has been observed only after high-intensity treatments.

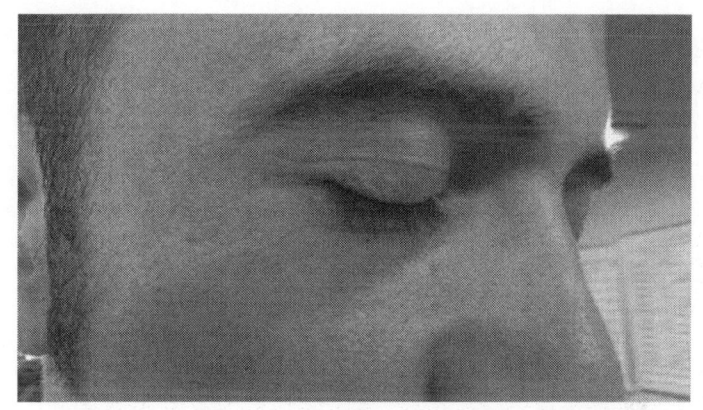

Illustration 57: Upper eyelid laxity 3 weeks after a plasma high-intensity upper eyelid tightening treatment. This was a transient effect and it was part of the skin remodeling during the long-term healing. This effect has only been observed. after high-intensity treatments and in all cases observed this was transient. The picture was taken at the end of November 2016. The treatment was performed at the beginning of November 2016. Treatment date 7/11/2016

If skin laxity occurs, it starts to take place a few days after the scabs have fallen off on their own accord. In any case, even if the laxity is taking place the skin tightening will still occur in the long-term. Skin laxity has subsided in all cases observed.

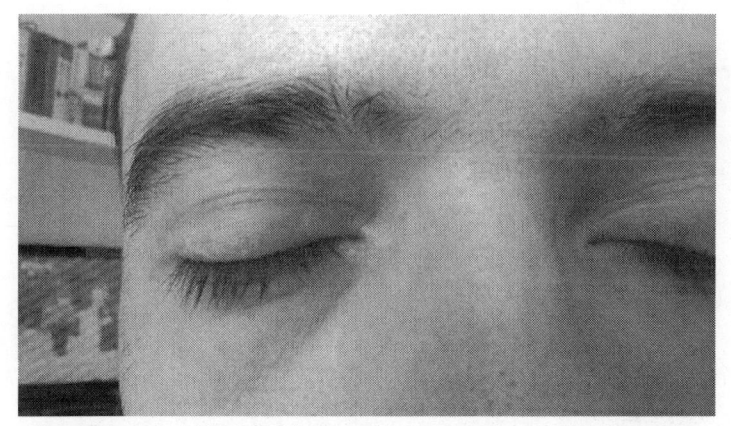

Illustration 58: 14/01/2017 laxity reducing over time. Tightening taking place during the long-term healing.

Therefore, because high-intensity plasma treatments lead to:

- Extended periods of redness
- Extended periods of tenderness
- Skin laxity

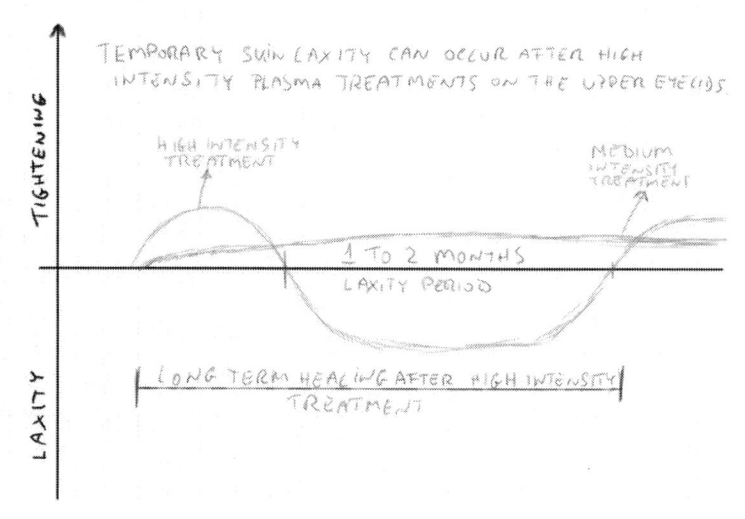

Illustration 59: Long term healing After High Intensity

carry out low/medium intensity treatments instead. If the plasma eyelid rejuvenation treatment is carried out at low medium intensity, the minor improvements may be achieved without the need of going through extended periods of inflammation which can discourage people from undergoing further treatments. Therefore even if you are an experienced practitioner in these types of procedures this is a further reason for always opting for a medium intensity treatment.

In all cases observed the redness and tenderness always subsided, hence these symptoms are all transient. To date, no case of chronic tenderness or redness has been reported despite the several thousands of high-intensity treatments performed the world over. Additionally, in case of high-intensity treatments, the temporary laxity is not a cause for concern as it is also transient.

The skin remodelling lasts as long as the area is still tender (long-term healing). Once the tenderness subsides the skin remodelling is over. This is when the results become representative.

Also, another problem reported is the presence of small atrophic red spots (sometimes lasting a number of months) where the voltaic plasma spots were applied. They are most likely caused by the use of makeup during the short-term healing process.

All the effects discussed here are transient, however, hyperpigmentation is the only undesired effect which may become permanent, despite that, it can be easily removed by using certain other aesthetic products.

www.voltaicplasma.com   Author: Andreas Russo

11.0 Upper Eyelid Tightening AferCare

The main principle of after-care after eyelid tightening using Plasma is very simple:"Any possible source of bacterial infection has to be deliberately minimized". Anyone who is about to undergo Plasma Eyelid Tightening should read this topic. There is more about aftercare in the section <u>Aftercare</u>

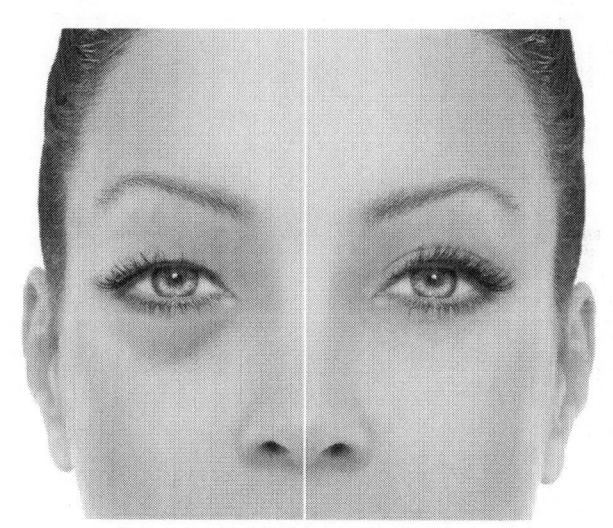

Illustration 60: After Care

11.1 Swelling

Swelling is characteristic of this type of aesthetic procedure and it should always be expected after using voltaic plasma on the upper eyelid area. This is because the area will be recovering from an intentional burn, therefore, the natural side effect is swelling. Swelling can be minimized using <u>certain techniques</u> but never completely avoided, because a deliberately controlled burn has to be caused to the eyelids in order to induce the desired <u>localized skin tightening</u>.

Although swelling is to be expected there is no reason to try and cure it because in all circumstances it will subside on its own accord. Therefore the use of any ointments or medicine is only detrimental. Several people without the appropriate training have suggested even the use of antihistamines which its only used to treat allergic reactions and other uses which have nothing to do with this type of aesthetic treatment.

The few adverse effects have been caused by the use of incorrect creams and products in order to minimize or "cure" the swelling. Please note that the swelling should not be cured because it is not a disease and it is a direct transient consequence of the controlled burn caused by this type of aesthetic treatment.

11.2 Healing Progression

This is a general account of the healing progression after plasma upper eyelid tightening. More detailed information can be found on Plasma Upper Eyelid tightening healing process case study where we examine in detail three different healing progressions after upper eyelid tightening.

Howeve the following will provide an overview of the healing progression.

Day 1. The Swelling peaks the day following the treatment. Some clients might find it harder to open their eyes as soon as they get up in the morning the first day following the treatment. Gradually, throughout the day the swelling will subside slightly. Discomfort, pain and slight discharge can occur but this is normal.

Day 2. The swelling is the same or slightly less than the previous day (Day 1). The swelling peaks soon after waking up and subsides slightly throughout the day. Sometimes swelling also spreads to the eye-bags even if no plasma aesthetic treatment was carried out on the lower eyelids, this is normal because the upper eyelid communicates with the lower eyelid and some fluid inside the upper eyelid can spread to the eye bags. This is normal and this undesired swelling of the lower eyelid will subside over the following days.

Day 3. The swelling should start to subside noticeably and the spots where the electrical plasma was applied will start turning into scabs. The scabs must not me picked and should fall off on their own accord. The discomfort experienced during day 1 and day 2 should have subsided dramatically. No further pain should be experienced on the third day following the treatment. For those people who experience eye-bag swelling, this should still be present during the third day.

Day 4. No discomfort or pain should be felt the fourth day following the treatment. Some residual minor swelling can still be on the upper eyelids. No more pain or discomfort should be felt.

Day 5. All swelling should have subsided and some scabs may still be present. The minor swelling on the eye bags should have almost subsided.

Dy 6. The scabs should have started to fall off. In most cases during Day 6 people will struggle to tell whether any aesthetic treatment has ever been performed.

Day 7. Almost all scabs should have fallen off. At this point, it is ok to start using total physical sunscreen and apply makeup as usual.

Week 2. The area although has healed it may feel more tender to the touch than usual and people may experience a stinging sensation while applying creams or washing normally. The area may look pinker than usual.

Week 3 and 4. The treated area maybe still slightly tender and pinker than the non treated area.

Month 2. Tenderness should have subsided and the area should have fully blended with the surrounding skin.

11.3 AfterCare at Home

The main principle to follow in the after-care is just minimizing the likelihood of contracting any bacterial infection or scratching the area while the scabs have formed.

The Eyelid Tightening after-care during the three days while the swelling is present consists of:

Do's

- Washing the area with **neutral soap** (there are several on the market) twice a day at night before going to sleep and in the morning immediately after getting up. Wash the area as gently as possible. Rinse profusely with cold water (do not use warm or hot water to rinse). Dry the area using a CLEAN towel, patting the area gently but never rubbing. Wash the eyelid area during the day only if the area had been exposed to dirt or dust.
- Make sure all linen in your bed are very clean and try to minimize contact with bacteria while sleeping.

Don'ts

- Do not use makeup of any type.
- Do not touch your eyelids (or the area treated in general) with your hands. In case of accidental rubbing or touching wash the area immediately as directed above.
- Do not use any creams of any type. The use of creams can lead to bacteria proliferation, delayed healing and some minor adverse effect. The use of inappropriate creams can lead to infections especially if used before the scabbing takes place.
- Do not use ice packing at home as this is could cause the area to get in contact with bacteria. The use or ice packing can be soothing but the added risk of making the area in contact with bacteria can be more detrimental than advantageous.

After-care while the area has scabbed.

- Avoid picking the scabs
- Avoid sun exposure
- Avoid the use of any creams and makeup.

After-care after the scabs have fallen off.

The area will be slightly pink and sensitive. When applying creams you can have a stinging sensation.

- Apply total physical sunscreen every day before going out in the sun.
- If using make-up, apply physical sunscreen on the area treated before applying the make-up
- Avoid deliberate direct sun exposure for at lead 3 months after the last treatment. Early sun exposure, even while you are wearing sunscreen can increase the likelihood of hyper-pigmentation.

12.0 Plasma Upper Eyelid Healing Process Case Study

Plasma eyelid tightening is an effective treatment which produces results and like most effective aesthetic treatments, the area will "get worse before it gets better". In this section we are going to study

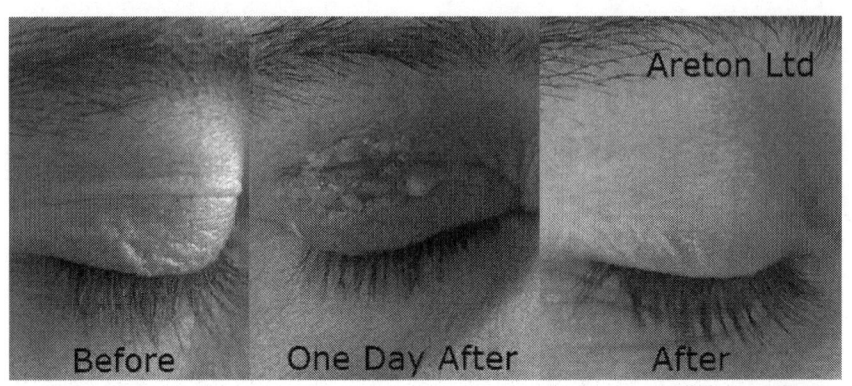

Illustration 61: The leftmost picture depicts the upper eyelid before any plasma upper eyelid tightening treatment was carried out. The middle picture is a detail of the right eyelid the day after one of the plasma upper eyelid tightening treatments. The rightmost picture is an after picture several months after the last plasma eyelid tightening treatment. As seen here, despite the dramatic immediate after effects of the voltaic plasma eyelid tightening no signs of the procedure are left.

The headling progression of plasma upper eyelid tightening. This section is very important because both practitioners and clients undergoing the upper eyelid treatment are scared when they get confronted with the immediate swelling and other natural reactions to the treatment.

Surprisingly, this is not a talked about subject anywhere, therefore we decided to focus on this issue because this has been the cause for concern to several clients who underwent this type of aesthetic procedure and were not correctly informed about these reactions to Plasma Upper Eyelid tightening.

As seen above the immediate effect one or two days after the upper eyelid tightening maybe scary but eventually the area heals and the tightening effect will take place. This section hs been written in order to shed a spotlight on the natural healing progression after plasma upper eyelid tightening. This is because the swelling is a normal transient side effects of "fibroblast" and this has been cause for unnecessary concern.

12.1 Introduction

Plasma eyelid tightening is an effective treatment which produces results and like most effective aesthetic treatments, the area will "get worse before it gets better"

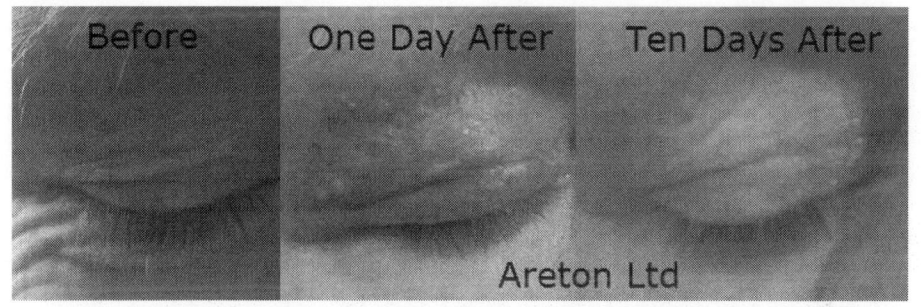

Illustration 62: In the middle of this picture there is yet is another example of dramatic swelling which occurs the day after plasma upper eyelid tightening. Inevitably the swelling subsides on its own accord without the use of any medicine or medical attention.

The swelling following upper eyelid tightening had been the major cause for concern and it has also been the source of speculation about Plasma Upper Eyelid Tightening treatments in general. As we will see this is a completely normal reaction to this type of aesthetic treatment which has to be expected in all cases.

We have grouped this information and made it openly available, so that-any one who performs these types of treatments or undergoes plasma eyelid lift can have a point of reference. In this way not only those who perform the treatment for the first time and also those who undergo the treatment are made aware in detail of what to expect.

As we will see, the symptoms during the healing process can be dramatic, however they are all transient and they do not require medical attention. They will all subside on their own accord within a few days after the treatment.

Please note that we will only focus here on the short-term healing process, the long-term healing progression is not covered here.

12.2 Difference between the healing after upper eyelid tightening and other plasma localised skin tightening treatments elsewhere on the body

The healing process after plasma upper eyelid tightening is rather similar to that of localised plasma skin tightening on other areas of the face and body. Some degree of minor swelling and discomfort are experienced after plasma localised skin tightening treatments in general, however these are not generally a cause for concern or alarm. The healing after localised plasma skin tightening on most parts of the body involves:

- Minor Swelling
- Minor Burning sensation,
- Slight Discomfort
- Scabbing.

After plasma upper eyelid tightening the symptoms are similar but magnified and dramatic. This is due to the intrinsic sensitivity of the upper eyelid, which is notoriously more delicate than the other parts of the skin. The upper eyelids are more delicate and sensitive than the order parts of the body.

After plasma upper eyelid tightening using voltaic plasma, swelling is much more dramatic that the one experienced after localised plasma skin tightening. Everything is magnified, rhe burning sensation is more accentuated, more intense and sometimes more difficult to cope with. etc. In particular not only the swelling is more dramatic but, while in localised plasma skin tightening, where the swelling is only minor and confined to the treated area, in upper eyelid tightening the swelling can also spreads to the lower eyelids. In other words everything that happens during the healing process after plasma localised skin tightening on most parts of the face and body also occurs after upper eyelid tightening but most symptoms are more dramatic when the procedure is applied on the upper eyelids.

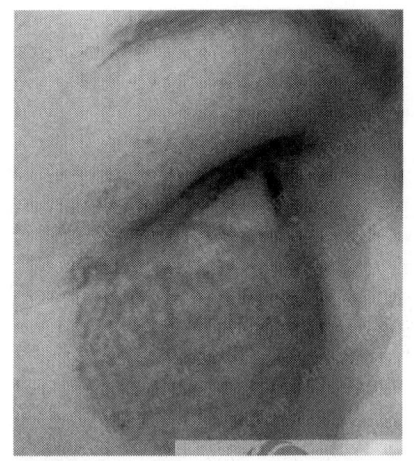

Illustration 63: Minor swelling experienced the day following lower eyelid tightening. This is only minor compared to the swelling experienced after upper eyelid tightening.

12.3 Upper plasma eyelid tightening healing process overview

In Plasma Upper Eyelid Tightening the area "gets worse before it gets better". Because of this, one of the main issues is the dramatic reactions which occur following the treatment, especially the swelling of the upper eyelids. However swelling is a natural reaction to the burn induced by the voltaic arc and it is not only to be expected but it is exactly what is needed in order to achieve the upper eyelid tightening sought by the clients.

Also, some of the aesthetic practitioners new to this type of procedures, can sometimes be caught by surprise by these reactions during the healing period.

The confusion about the healing process after plasma upper eyelid tightening is primarily due to the fact that there has not been sufficient structured information exploring in detail the healing process, this has caused unnecessary anxiety to some people undergoing the treatment.

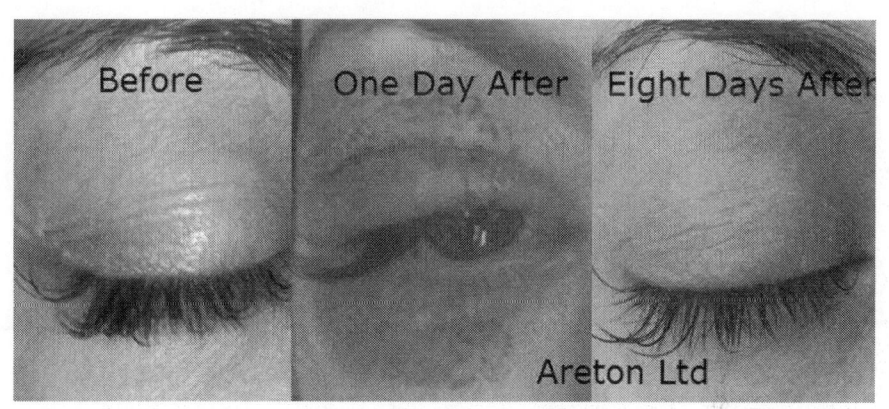

Illustration 64: In the middle we can see how the severe swelling can make it difficult to open the eyes fully. This occurs only the morning following the plasma treatment. This is a normal reaction to be expected after this type of aesthetic treatment.

The normal healing process of Plasma Upper Eyelid tightening involves:

1. Major swelling of the upper eyelid the day following the treatment (lasting 24 to 48 hours). The swelling of the lower eyelids (eye-bags) can occur even if the lower eyelids have not undergone any treatment (lasting up to 72 hours).
2. Intense burning sensation (lasting 12 to 24 hours).
3. Discomfort (lasting 24 to 48 hours).
4. Pain (lasting 12 to 24 hours).

The sometimes dramatic upper eyelid swelling and discomfort experienced after plasma eyelid lift had been cause of worry (and even distress at times) to those people undergoing plasma upper eyelid lift but were not well informed about the immediate effects of procedure. Although they may appear dramatic, such as pain, discomfort and swelling these symptoms should not be cause for concern.

www.voltaicplasma.com   Author: Andreas Russo

As we will see these symptoms are all normal effects which are transient and to be expected in all cases. None of the above effects can be completely avoided because they are caused by the very nature of the plasma aesthetic treatment itself (i.e. an intentional controlled skin burn). However they can be somewhat attenuated by using certain products and lowering the overall intensity of the treatment.

12.4 Pain

The information reported about the pain experienced is based on the feedback received by the people who underwent these types of aesthetic treatments over the years (several hundreds).

As we know the pain is caused by the burn inflicted during the treatment, therefore this is a normal reaction to this type of aesthetic procedure. Pain lasts up to 24 hours in most cases. The second day following the treatment is mostly pain-free and the pain is replaced by a feeling of slight discomfort first and itchy sensation after.

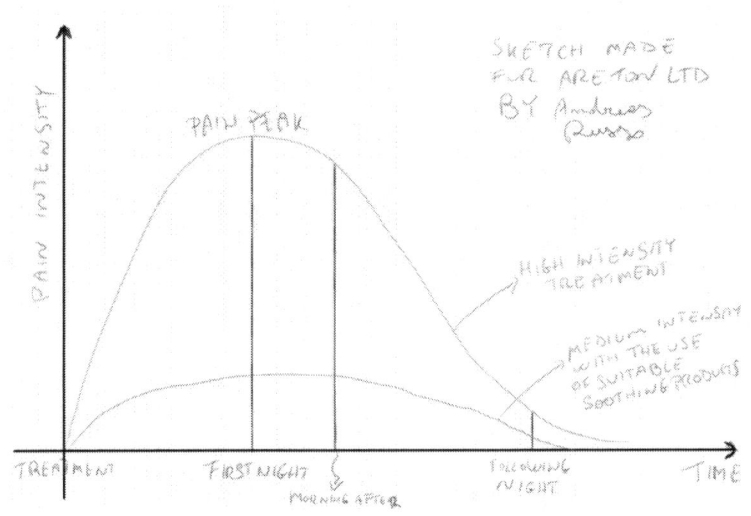

Illustration 65: The pain after plasma upper eyelid lift is very subjective, however this representative sketch provides an idea of the way pain is experienced

While discomfort is experienced by everyone undergoing plasma upper eyelid lift in different ways, on the other hand the pain experienced after the treatment is dependent on the particular individual sensitivity to pain. Sometimes pain is not reported at all. In fact there had been several cases where the individuals never reported pain as such, just discomfort.

The level of pain experienced (by people who are particularly sensitive to pain) also goes hand in hand with the level of swelling. Generally, the more the swelling the more the pain experienced.

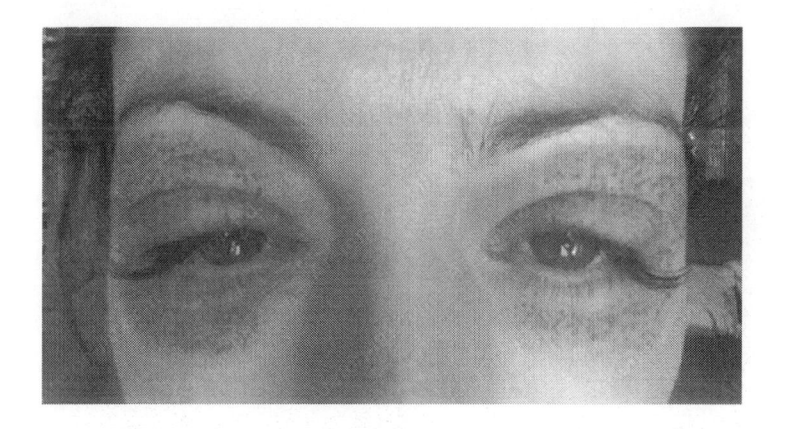

Illustration 66: The upper eyelid swelling can make it difficult to fully open the eyes the morning following the treatment. The pain experienced and swelling go hand in hand. When the swelling is at its peak this is also when the pain experienced is at its highest. As the swelling subsides the pain and discomfort subside too. The pain and discomfort are replaced by an itchy sensation when the scabs start to develop.

In general the level of pain experienced is dependent on:

- the sensitivity of the particular individual to pain,
- the intensity of the voltaic plasma treatment. The lower the intensity of the treatment the less pain experienced during the day following the treatment. The higher the overall intensity of the treatment the more the pain felt after,
- the use of soothing products immediately after the treatment and during the healing process, including the use of ice packing.

Please note that the use of drugs for pain relief is possible, however seldom necessary and not as effective as the use of the appropriate topical soothing products.

12.5 Comparison of three swelling cases

Three cases will be presented here and as we will notice the pattern in the skin recovery is similar, the upper eyelids swell in very similar ways. The degree of predictability of the swelling is relatively high.

Also the swelling subsides in similar ways making its development a very predictable phenomenon. Furthermore, it can also be reliably predicted when the swelling is supposed to subside completely.

In the cases presented:

- No ice packing or any soothing products were used.
- The treatment intensity applied was also particularly high.
- The healing occurred without the help of any medication or drugs.

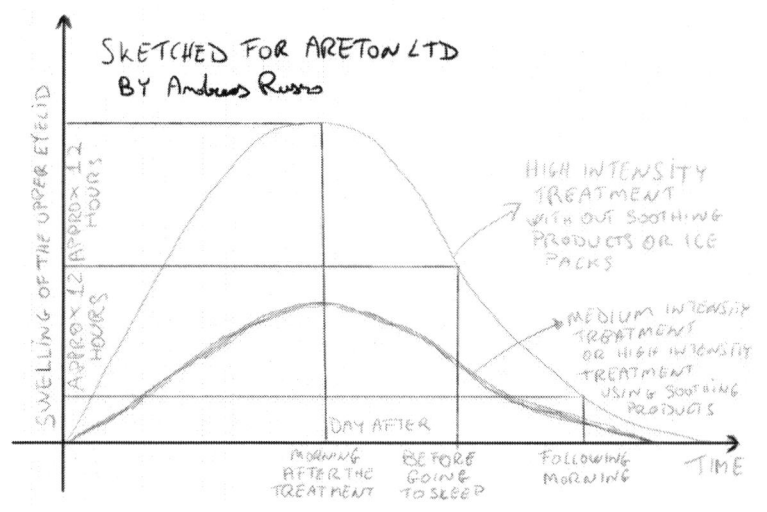

Illustration 67: representative cases are presented here with photographic evidence, over 300 cases were also examined and they reported the same or very similar healing patterns. Given the high number of cases examined these are deemed sufficient to bring forward reliable conclusions about the issue of swelling after plasma upper eyelid tightening. There could be some minor statistical deviations, however these are not considered to be very significant given the large number of cases observed and feedback reported to date.

12.6 Day one after the procedure

This is the swelling which occurs the day following the treatment. As seen in the pictures below the degree of swelling is very similar in all three cases.

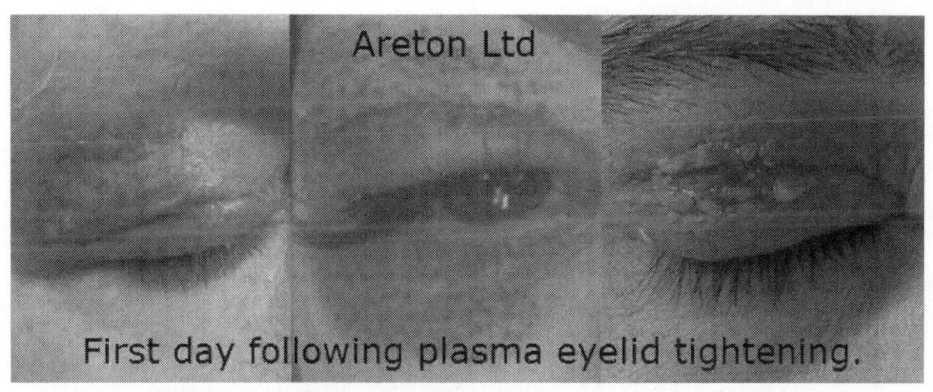

Illustration 68: The day following the treatment is when the swelling is at its highest. The peak occurs first thing in the morning and it subsides throughout the day.

12.7 Day two after the procedure

The day following the treatment is when the swelling is at its highest. The peak occurs first thing in the morning and it subsides throughout the day.

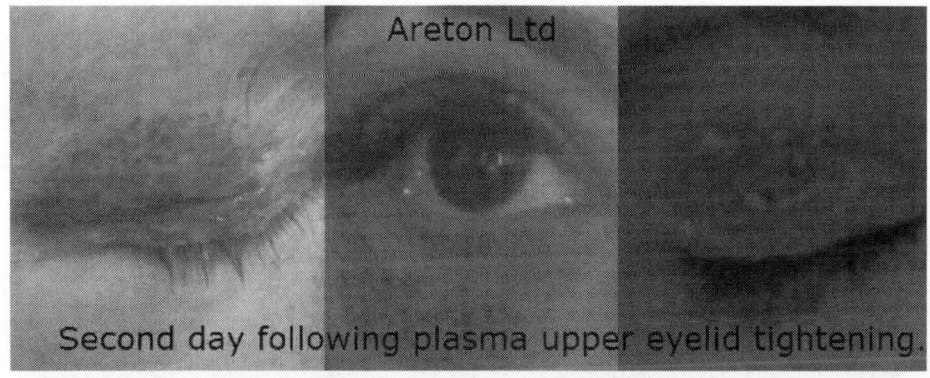

Illustration 69: The second day following the treatment, the swelling on the upper eyelid has either subsided completely or almost completely. Every body who underwent the treatment could open their eyes fully or almost fully.

12.8 Day three after the procedure

On the third day all swelling subsided completely. The residual swelling of the lower eyelid has either subsided or almost subsided. In all cases the eyes can be fully opened. No more discomfort is reported and it is replaced by an itchy sensation instead. The scabs have fully formed.

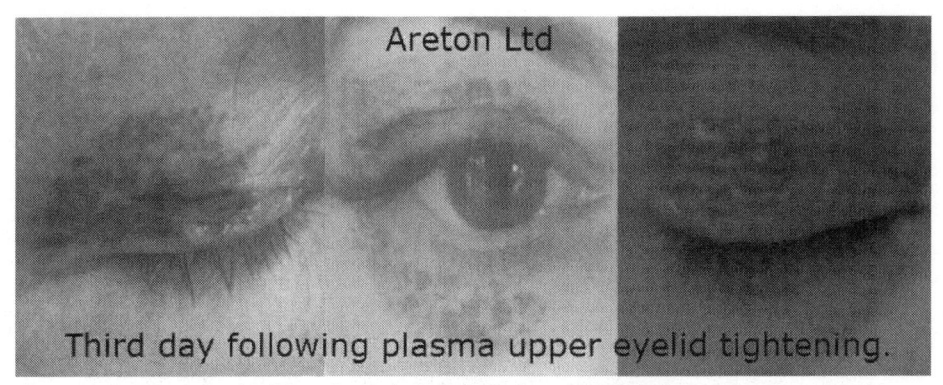

Illustration 70: On the third day, the scabs have fully formed and the discomfort is replaced by an itchy sensation.

12.9 Day four after the procedure

The scabs have fully formed and they start to fall off on their own accord. No more discomfort is felt and the itchy sensation has intensified.

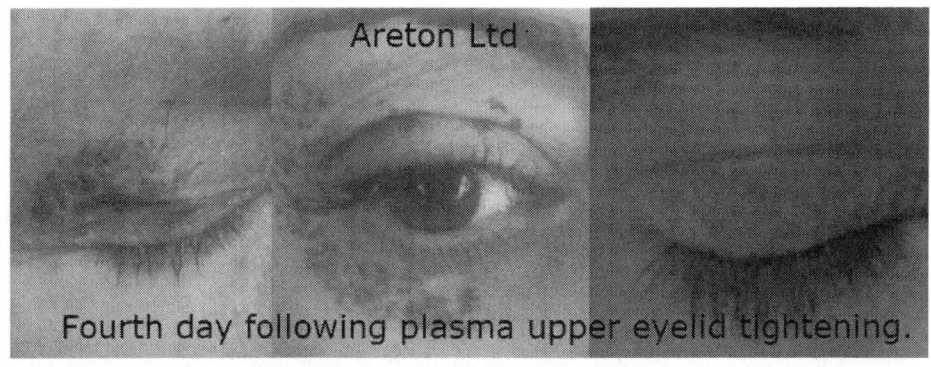

Illustration 71: The fourth day the scabs start to fall off the itchy sensation intensified. In some cases like the one on the right, the scabs fall off immediately depending on the skin type and how the treatment is performed.

12.10 Day Five after the procedure

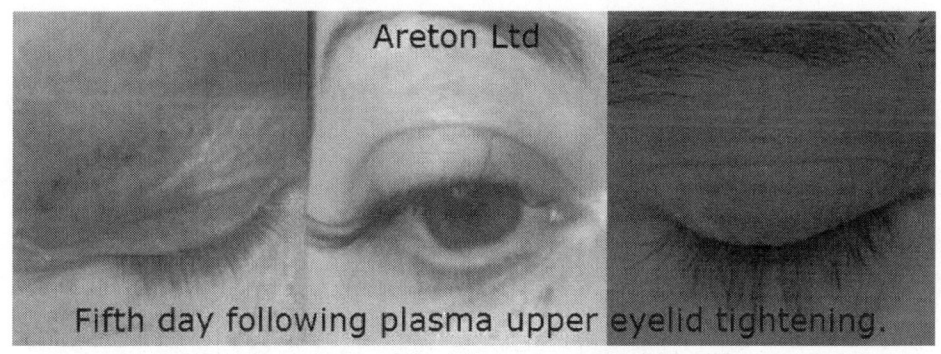

Illustration 72: The fifth day the scabs should have almost fallen off on their own accord. No discomfort only an itchy sensation

Almost all scabs have fallen off. This is when it is possible to start applying make up and sun screen. In most cases this marks the end of what it is commonly referred to as "Downtime".

12.11 Day six after the procedure

The area looks slightly irritated but returned to almost normal and the long-term recovery takes place. At this point most people will be unable to tell the area had undergone any aesthetic treatment at all.

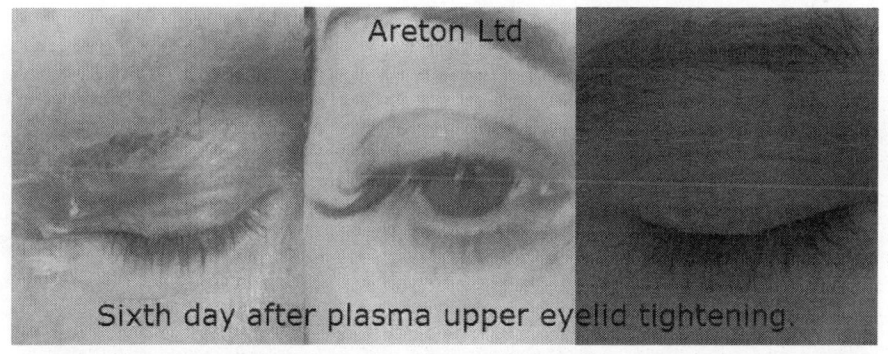

Illustration 73: The sixth day all scabs are normally fallen off. No signs of the treatment are normally noticeable. Only on some rare cases some residual scabs are still to fall off as shown on the leftmost picture.

At the time of the treatment, the individual on the left was 66, 44 in the middle and 34 years of age on the right respectively. The pictures show how the healing appears to occur faster on the youngest subject and slower on the older ones. No sufficient cases have been examined in order to bring forward a conclusive opinion on the matter of speed of healing relative to the age of the individual.

12.12 Swelling of the lower eyelid (or eyebag swelling) following upper eyelid lift

Eyebag swelling is another reaction to be expected after the plasma upper eyelid lift. This has also been a cause for concern to those who had undergone these types of treatments but were not aware of this type of short-term reaction.

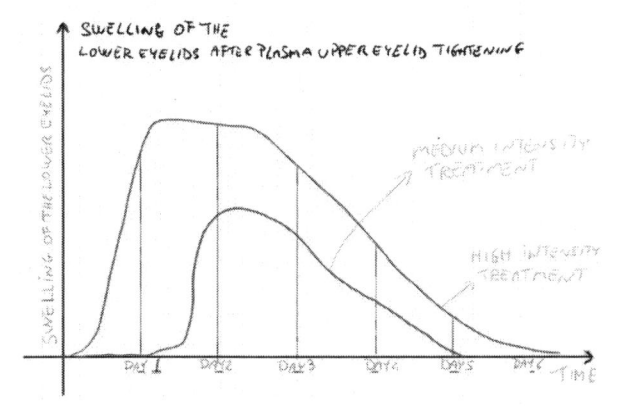

Illustration 74: Swelling Graph After eyelid tightening using high intensity and low intensity

During the healing process, although the lower eyelids had not undergone any treatment at all, they often swell too. It is interesting that the lower eyelids (or eyebags) swell even if no treatment has been performed to the area. This is because the upper and lower eyelids are interconnected, therefore the fluid produced, after the controlled burn on the upper eyelids tends to travel to the eyebags. The way the lower eyelid swelling can occur varies from person to person and sometimes it may even not occur at all, especially in case of low/medium intensity

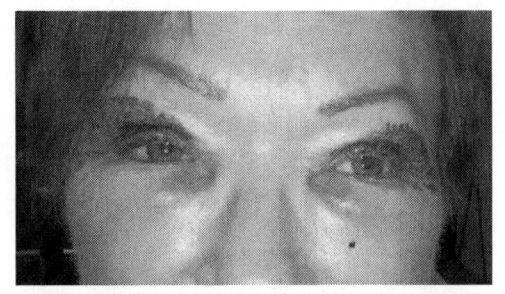

Illustration 75: Second day following plasma upper eyelid tightening high intensity treatment. The upper eyelid swelling has almost completely subsided but the swelling appeared on the lower eyelids (eyebags instead). The fluid is transferred to the eyebags.

www.voltaicplasma.com

Author: Andreas Russo

treatments coupled with the use of the appropriate soothing products.

However, this reaction has to be expected in any case. The swelling of the lower eyelid can occur either the day after the treatment coupled with the swelling of the upper eyelid but it often occurs the second day after the treatment. The lower eyelid swelling is caused by the fluid on the upper eyelids transferred to the eyebags during the second night after the treatment. As we know in any case the fluid will be naturally absorbed by the body and will leave no trace. In conclusion, the swelling of the lower eyelids is transient and will subside completely on its own accord without the use of any treatment of any type or medication.

12.13 Plasma upper eyelid lift healing process table

The following table goes through the healing progression after plasma upper eyelid lift in detail. The table has been built based on our experience and feedback received after treating hundreds of people using plasma devices for aesthetic purposes.

Please note that any individual reaction could differ to a certain extent from what described therein based on:

- technique used
- overall treatment intensity
- individual reaction to the treatment
- and device used

However as a rule of thumb, if the swelling has not subsided completely by the fourth day after the treatment and the scabs have not formed yet, contact your aesthetic practitioner.

Swelling will subside further throughout the night	You will be able to have a good night sleep and the pain or discomfort will be usually gone by the morning	Rinse and wash with mild soap before going to sleep	apply the soothing product before going to sleep for the last time; no more need for ice packing	During the second night following the treatment	
Swelling should have almost completely subsided. You may find that your eyebags have swollen instead. The scabs should start to form where the treatment was carried out; there maybe minor traces of swelling on the upper eyelids; you will be able to open your eyes as normal.	The discomfort should have gone completely and being replaced by an itchy sensation instead	Keep the area clean and avoid the use of any make-up	Not Applicable	Second day following the treatment.	
Swelling has subsided completely on the upper eyelids. You will be able to open your eyes fully as normal. Some minor swelling may still present on the lower eyelids (Eyebags). The scabs should have fully formed and they should start falling off on their own accord	No more discomfort should be felt; this is replaced by an itchy sensation	avoid sun exposure and do not wear any make up	Not Applicable	Third day following the treatment.	
Scabs have started falling on their own accord. If previously swollen the eyebags should be returned to normal	Itching sensation at its peak.	Do not pick the scabs and avoid the use of all make-up	Not applicable	Fourth Day following the treatment.	
Scabs should have fallen all off on their own accord. It is hard for most people to tell people you have undergone any treatment. However the area is still red and subject to further change over the coming weeks.	Itching sensation should start to subside. You usually find the area tender for a few weeks after the treatment. This is normal. You should not repeat the treatment before all tenderness is has subsided. When you apply creams you may feel the area still stinging. This is also normal.	You can start using make up and you must use total sun screen before being exposed in the sun. Avoid exposing yourself to the sun as much as possible.	You can apply Petroleum Jelly (e.g. Vaseline) if you feel the are being too dry	Fifth day onwards.	

Illustration 76: Click here to see the table

12.14 Conclusions

Pain, discomfort, swelling of both upper and lower eyelids are all normal reactions to plasma upper eyelid tightening. Generally, they are all to be expected, however they all subside on their own accord without the help of any medical treatment or medication of any type.

In all cases examined, swelling pain and discomfort peaked throughout the night after the treatment and the following morning. The day following the treatment is also the most challenging as this is when the pain, discomfort and swelling peak.

Swelling of the lower eyelid was observed in some occasions the day following the treatment, especially when the treatment was carried out at high intensity and/or no soothing product or ice packing were applied to the area to soothe it. When the swelling of the eye-bags occurred, it was most often observed two days after the treatment. Mostly, the swelling of the lower eyelid started to subside the third day after the treatment. In all cases the lower eyelid swelling subsided by the fourth day.

In most cases the scabs were fully formed on the third day after the treatment. However it has to be noted that scabs do not always form during the healing process.

In most cases the area returns to normal within 5 days (when all scabs have also fallen off by then). This usually marks the end of what most people perceive as "downtime". In all cases examined pain, discomfort and swelling subsided without the help of any particular remedy or medication and the area eventually returned to normal.

No medical treatment was carried out in all cases (i.e. no medical consultation or use of any drugs or ointments of any type) and the area healed on its own.

Please bear in mind that most of the undesired reactions are due to poor after-care during the healing period.

13.0 Crow's feet attenuation

Previous knowledge on Skin tightening using electrical arcing is required. One of the several applications of skin tightening using electrical arcing or fibroblast is crow's feet attenuation.

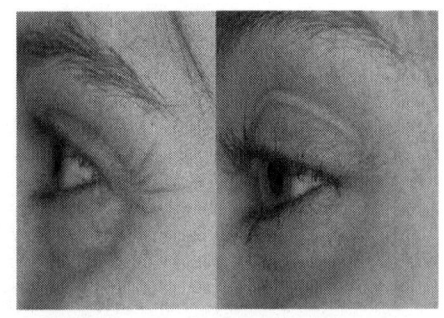

Illustration 77: Crown's Feet attenuation example

13.1 Botox and periorbital lines attenuation using plasma

It is important to differentiate this type of treatment from the effects of botox. Botox is the preferred way to attenuate the crows feet by simply relaxing the periorbital muscles, therefore, preventing the formation of these wrinkles while smiling or making other facial expressions.

In case of crow's feet attenuation using electrical arcing the effect is a minor improvement in the appearance of wrinkles while the muscles are relaxed. Therefore the effects will be visible while the muscles are relaxed. This treatment can be also combined with Botox, however, any Botox treatment must be carried out at least 40 days away from the last crow's feet attenuation using electrical arcing.

13.2 How to perform crow's feet attenuation using plasma

Apply the normal pretreatment routine before carrying out the aesthetic treatment.

Use skin tightening between the lines and do not apply the voltaic arc on the lines themselves.

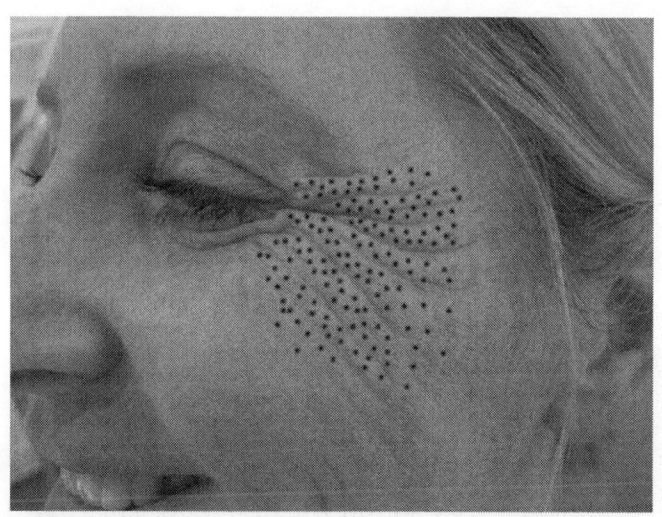

Illustration 78: The black spots represent where we would place the voltaic spots in order to accomplish the skin tightening on the crows' feet.

When you first start this type of aesthetic treatment if you use one of our devices, set it at minimum power and apply very short bursts lasting approximately one-quarter of a second (if you are using the spot mode). The distance between the spots must be approximately 2 to 3 mm.

www.voltaicplasma.com   Author: Andreas Russo

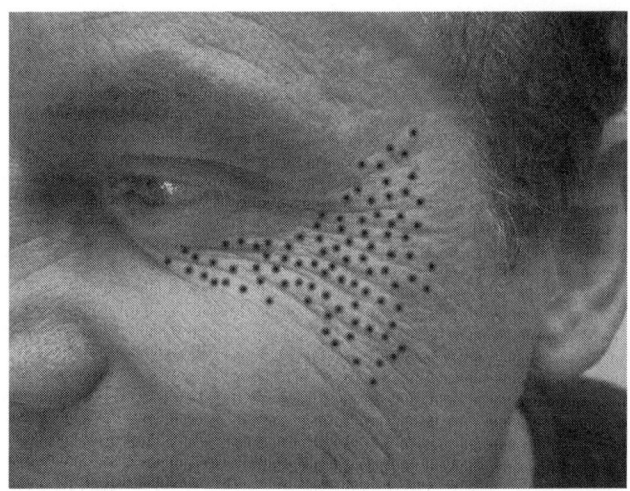

Illustration 79: Another example of where the voltaic spots would be placed in a low-intensity treatment. The spots are always applied randomly. In this example, you can see how lower eyelid tightening can be naturally integrated as part of the aesthetic treatment.

Unlike upper eyelid tightening this particular application of skin tightening does not cause the pronounced swelling characteristic of eyelid tightening. Therefore the use of a soothing product is not recommenced. Remember **not to** remove the carbon residues intentionally by wiping them off during the procedure.

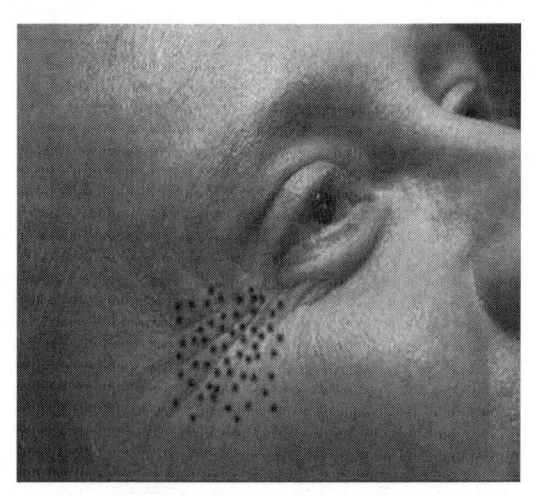

Illustration 80: The voltaic spots are applied randomly between the lines and never inside the wrinkles themselves.

www.voltaicplasma.com   Author: Andreas Russo

Sometimes scabs form two to three days after the treatment. Let the scabs fall off by themselves. You can repeat the treatment at 4 to 6 weeks intervals. Remind the importance of the aftercare to your clients.

14.0 MiniFacelift

Previous knowledge required, Skin tightening using electrical arcing.

The main principle applied to mini face lift using electrical arcing or Plasma is localised skin tightening. Use skin tightening between the lines and do not apply the voltaic arc on the lines themselves. Mini-facelift by using electrical arcing (or plasma) is usually carried out by applying the skin tightening where the skin would be pulled during a normal face lift procedure, which is close to the ear as shown in the video above. Also if you prefer you can apply the voltaic arc spots on to the entire face and this has lead to very good results. However for the sake of this section we will focus the treatment on the classic areas of a normal face lift.

It is important to manage the client expectations for this type of procedure because the improvements will only be minor and cannot be compared to the dramatic results achieved with surgery. However since, the localised skin tightening effects of electrical arcing are cumulative, repeating the treatments a number of times will lead to good results.

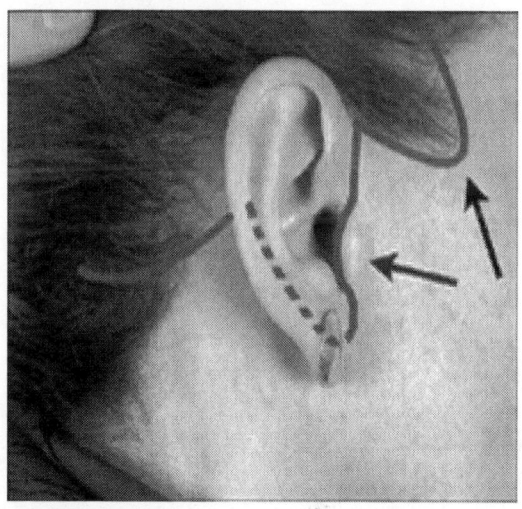

Illustration 81: The incision during a standard facelift surgical procedure is carried out along the hair line and around the ear to achieve the desired pulling effect. While using electrical arcing the voltaic spots are applied close to the ear to reproduce a similar "pulling" effect.

Although in the examples in the videos you can see how high-intensity treatments are usually carried out to perform mini-facelift using electrical arcing, when you first use electrical arcing devices for this type of treatment it is highly recommended you use low intensity treatments.

The first time you use electrical arcing for mini-facelift, if you are using one of our electrical arcing devices, set it at the minimum power level. Apply the spots distancing them 2 to 3 mm apart and use an instantaneous spot duration (approximately one-quarter of a second). As you gain experience you can then progressively increase the intensity treatment by decreasing the distance between the spots.

www.voltaicplasma.com　　　　　　　　　　　　　　　　　　　　Author: Andreas Russo

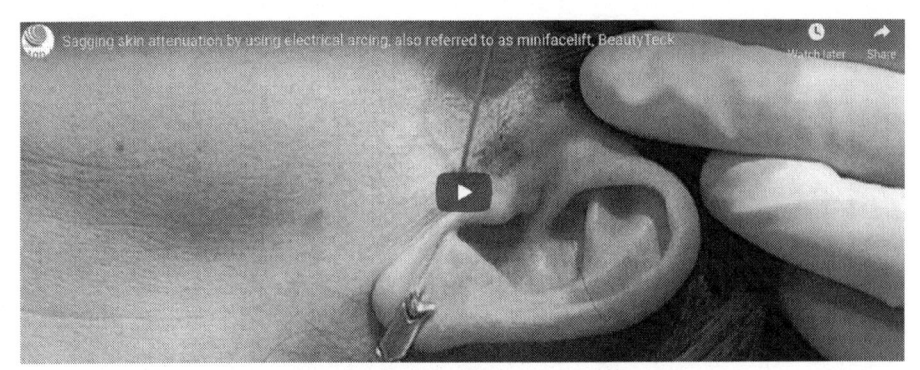

Illustration 82: Click here to watch video

Sometimes scabs form two to three days after the treatment. Let the scabs fall off by themselves. You can repeat the treatment at 4 to 6 weeks intervals. Remind the importance of the aftercare to your clients.

15.0 Jowl Line

Plasma Skin tightening can also be used to improve the appearance of the wrinkles around the jowl line. The main technique used is the spot operation. Like in normal skin tightening the intensity of the overall treatment is determined by:

1. The power level of the respective device you are using.
2. The distance between the spots
3. The duration of each voltaic burst
4. and the overall area you treat.

To revise the section in connection with the localised skin tightening please cick here.

If you want to watch a couple of examples of jowl tightening please watch the following videos.

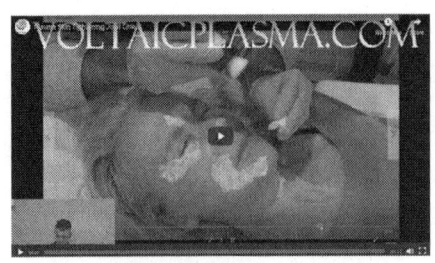

Illustration 83: Click here to watch video

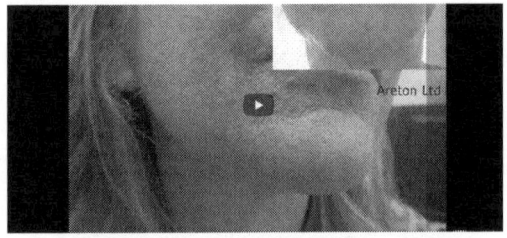

Illustration 84: Click here to watch video

www.voltaicplasma.com   Author: Andreas Russo

16.0 Atrophic Scar Attenuation

Improving the appearance of depressed or atrophic scars, like acne and chickenpox scars is easy using AC electrical arcing. The previous knowledge required is skin tightening using Plasma.

In this section you will be able to learn how to assess the type of atrophic scar you are dealing with and have the knowledge base at your disposal to best choose the method to remove or attenuate them.

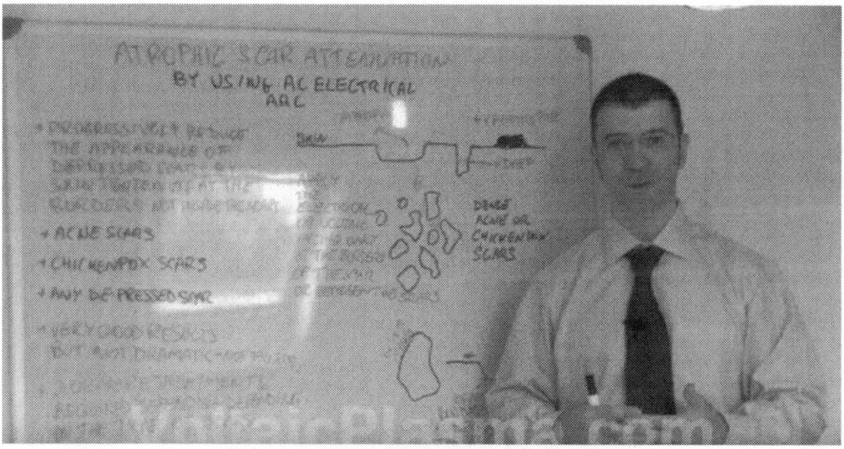

Illustration 85: Click here to watch video

16.1 Scars can come in different shapes and forms , in this section we will discuss the most common type of scars

The main distinction made between scars is the differentiation between Hypertrophic and Atrophic Scars. A Hypertrophic scar is raised (protruding), whereas an Atrophic scar is a visibly depressed part of the skin. A Hypertrophic scar is left after a deep skin injury (i.e. deep wounds inflicted during surgery, superficial wound followed by an protracted infection) and in case of Atrophic Scars, these are usually left after Acne, Chickenpox or other types of skin inflammation. Burn scars are not discussed here and they are referred to as contractures to learn more about this type of scars please **read this section**.

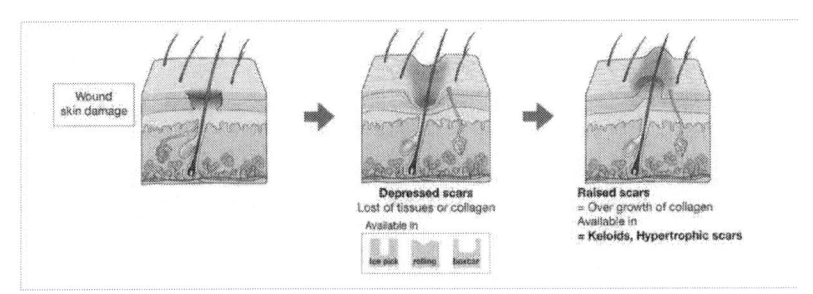

Illustration 86: The two main types of scars "Atrophic" or "Depressed scars" and "Hypertrophic" or "Protruding scars".

In illustration 86 we can see the main two types of scars which can develop after an injury or traumatic event has occurred to the skin, Atrophic (depressed scars) or Hypertrophic (raised scars).

It is important to emphasise the difference between Keloids and Hypertrophic scars, because they are often mistaken for one another.

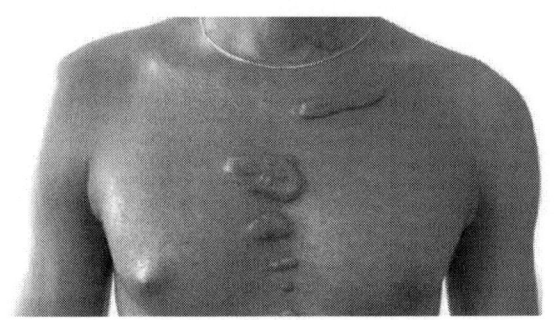

Illustration 87: Example of Keloidal formations not to be confused with normal Hypertrophic scars.

Keloids and Hypertrophic scars are fundamentally different. To learn more about the difference between Hypetrophic scars and Keloids, please **Read this section on keloids**.

16.2 Types of atrophic scars, "ice pick", "box scars" and "rolling scars"

Atrophic scars are those depressed areas (or missing part) of the skin left after a certain skin traumatic event, typically dermal inflammations. The likelihood of developing an Atrophic scar depends on how deeply the inflammation has developed and the healing process. In some cases an Atrophic Scar can also develop after a skin injury.

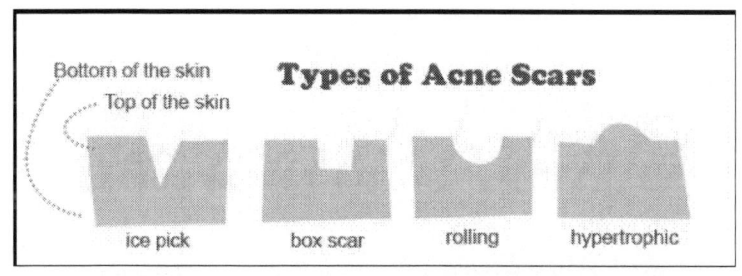

Illustration 88: Depending on the type of skin inflammation the scar which can develop can have different characteristics. In case of atrophic scars this can be classed into: "Ice pick", "Box Scars", "Roll/ing Scars". In certain other cases, especially when an infection persists for a long time or a deep wound has been inflicted a Hypertrophic scar can develop.

Atrophic scars are usually classed into three categories: "Ice Pick Scar", "Box Scar" and "Roll/ing Scar". There are several types of skin inflammation which can lead to Atrophic Scar formation. The most common cause of Atrophic Scars are severe acne and chickenpox. However, other types of injuries can cause atrophic scars as well. More generally atrophic scars are produced by skin conditions that cause an endured inflammation of the dermis. The most common atrophic scar formation process typically begins as a mild form of acne, called comedone. This comedone is formed when oil secreted from the sebaceous glands combines with the dirt or skin cells in the hair follicles. This combination creates a plug that blocks the hair follicle. After the comedone forms, bacteria begin to multiply inside the blocked hair follicle. The white cells of the body rush to the site of the infection in order to destroy the bacteria. With the build-up of white blood cells, pus is formed.

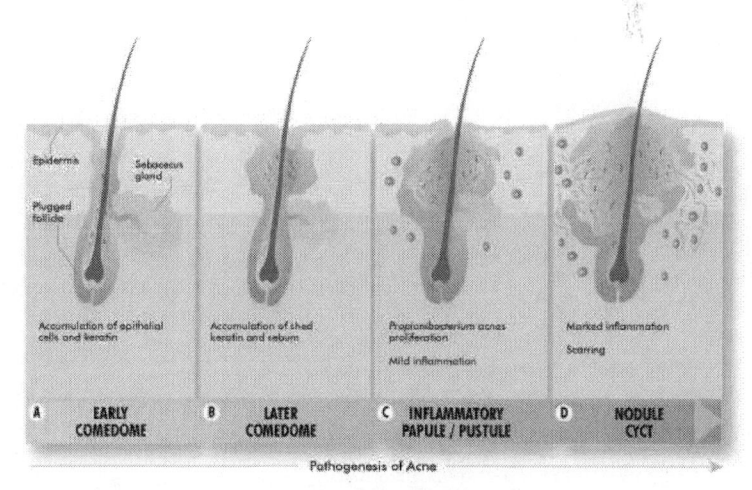

Illustration 89: Pathogenesis of Acne

In a few cases, the bacteria, white blood cells and sebum can burst into the surrounding skin and cause further skin inflammation. With the aggravation of inflammation, pressure is created and this pushes the inflammation deeper into the skin. This in turn causes severe damage and can lead to the formation of nodules or cysts. The inflammation on the skin damages the skin tissues and disrupts the structure of the collagen.

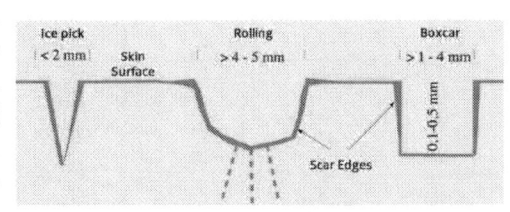

Illustration 90: The main difference between the three types of scars is not merely in the depth of the missing skin. It is mostly the with of the scar itself and the shape of the scar edges.

When the resultant scar tissue is formed after the severe inflammation, it sinks into the skin and appears as an atrophic scar. Depending on the extent and depth of damage to the dermis the type of atrophic scar can develop into, Ice pick, Box or Rolling Scar.

The deeper the damage caused to the dermis the higher the likelihood of the formation of "Ice Pick Scars". In case the damage is not involving the hypo-dermis then "Box Scars" can develop. If the damage to the dermis is superficial then the atrophic scar can evolve into a "Rolling Scar".

Small depressed atrophic scars of a diameter less than 2mm are usually referred to as "Ice Pick Scars". If the edges of the scar are sharp, then they are classed as a "Box Scar" (usually the diameter of Box Scars are between 2 to 4 mm). When the edges are not very well defined then the atrophic scar is usually referred to as "Rolling Scar". Rolling scars are normally over 5 mm in diameter. The difference in classification of atrophic scars is not always very well marked, whereas the difference between Atrophic and Hypertrophic Scars are very well defined and recognisable. In case of Atrophic Scars the difference between "Ice Pick Scars" and "Rox/Rolling Scars" is quite marked. On the other hand the difference between "Box Scars" and "Rolling Scars" can blur sometimes. This is because the edges of "Box Scars" tend to have a different degree of sharpness.

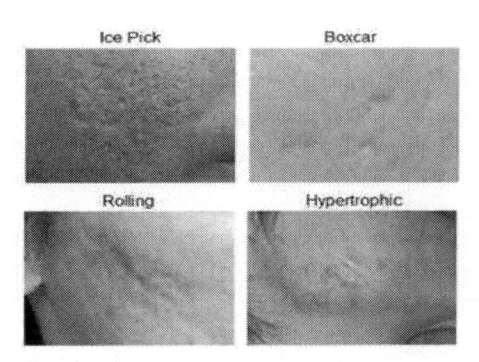

Illustration 91: The difference in classification of atrophic scars is not always very well marked, whereas the difference between Atrophic and Hypertrophic Scars are very well defined and recognisable. In case of Atrophic Scars the difference between "Ice Pick Scars" and "Box/Rolling Scars" is quite marked. On the other hand the difference between "Box Scars" and "Rolling Scars" can blur sometimes. This is because the edges of "Box Scars" tend to have a different degree of sharpness.

In **illustration 92**, you can see an example of "Ice Pick Scars" on the face caused by severe Acne. These type of scars are clearly indented, typical of "Ice Pick Scars". The missing part of the skin can be reconstructed using minor skin grafting.

"Ice Pick Scars" appear on the face and other parts of the body, after a severe episode of skin inflammation and are sometimes difficult to cover up. As the name itself suggests, this type of scar looks as if your skin has been pierced by an ice-pick or a sharp instrument because they are deep and very narrow. Not all acne, chickenpox or skin inflammation develop into "Ice Pick Scars". This type of atrophic scars appear only if the inflammation has affected the deeper parts of the dermis (Hypo-dermis). Usually the deeper the inflammation the more the likelihood of forming an "Ice Pick Scar". Very often, "Ice Pick Scars" appear after the formation of an infected cyst, which destroys the innermost parts of the dermis.

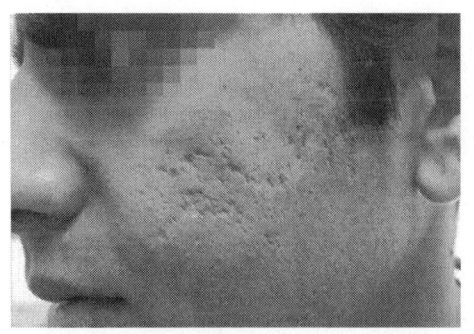

Illustration 92. "Ice Pick Scars" or indented scars are generally caused by severe acne, where the inflammation has affected the hypo-dermis. "Ice Pick Scars" are deep, small and narrow. The scar appear as if the skin has been injured by a sharp instrument such as an ice pick. Some people may have deep holes or large open pores. Often, "Ice Pick Scar" treatments can involve minor skin grafting to reconstruct the missing part of the skin.

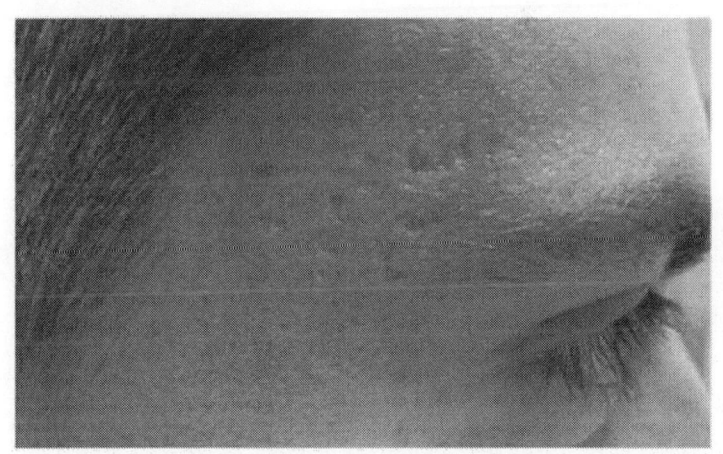

Illustration 93. Typical example of "Box Scars". Their edges are very sharp and well defined. Normally they are 3 to 4 mm in diameter.

www.voltaicplasma.com						Author: Andreas Russo

"Box Scars" occur when an inflamed acne lesion destroys the skin tissue, leaving a sunken area on the skin. They have an oval shape and look like depressions in the skin. Unlike Ice Pick Scars, "Box Scars" do not taper to a point. Depending on how severe acne was, the depth of the "Box Scars" varies. This kind of scar is most frequently seen on temples and cheeks. Normally on young skin when the scar have recently formed the edges of the Box Scar are very sharp and very well defined. This is what characterises "Box Scars" when they are recently formed.

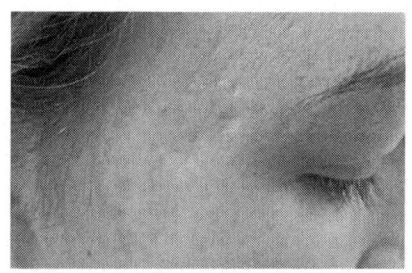

Illustration 94: Over time or after collagen regeneration treatments (i.e. cosmetic peels, laser resurfacing, plasma resurfacing etc) the edges of the box scars become less defined. Therefore over time, the line between box scars and rolling scars becomes less and less defined as shown in the atrophic scars displayed in this picture

The difference between "Box Scars" and "Rolling Scars" can be blurred at times as seen in the figure below when the edges become less defined over time.

Almost all Box Scars over time will transition to "Rolling Scars". This is due to the natural collagen regeneration process which occurs over time. This process can be speeded up by using collagen regeneration treatments like cosmetic peels, plasma skin resurfacing, laser resurfacing, micro-needling etc.

Normally all aesthetic treatments for atrophic scar attenuation which does not involve minor skin grafting or subcision, focus on accomplishing this first transition, from "Box Scars" to "Rolling Scars" by using collagen regeneration techniques.

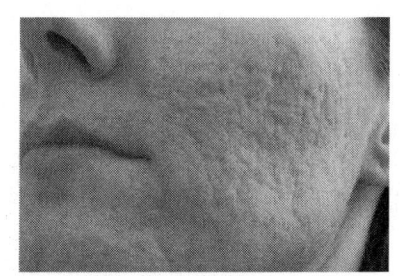

Illustration 95: Rolling Scars grouped close together. Over time or after a few skin resurfacing treatments the edge of the scars start to smooth progressively.

"Rolling Scars" are much larger in diameter than Box Scars, and because their edges are not as sharp and defined as those of the Ice Pick or Box Scars they are much easier to fade using most skin resurfacing techniques. See illustration 96 Typical example of "Rolling Scars".

So to recap Atrophic Scars are usually distinguished into three categories:

1. Ice Pick Scars
2. Box Scars
3. Rolling Scars

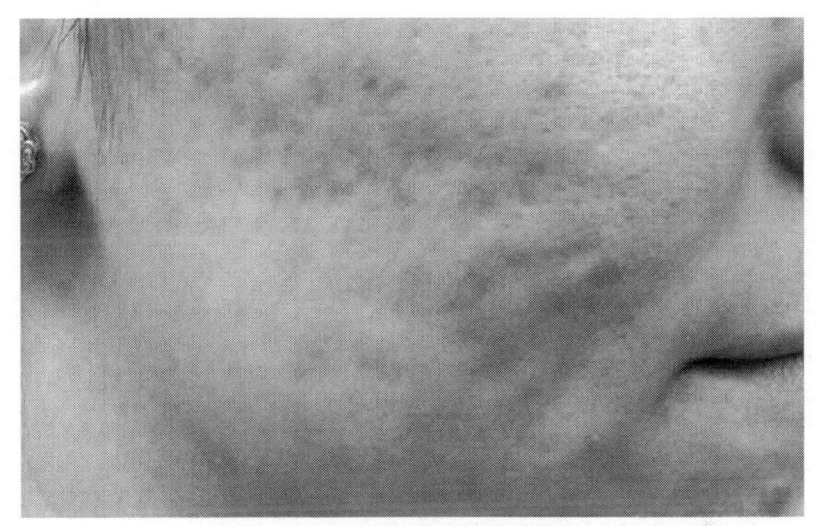

Illustration 96. Typical example of "Rolling Scars". Where the depressed areas have become blurred over time.

The differentiation between Box Scars and Rolling Scars fades over time due to the slow smoothing of the scars edges.

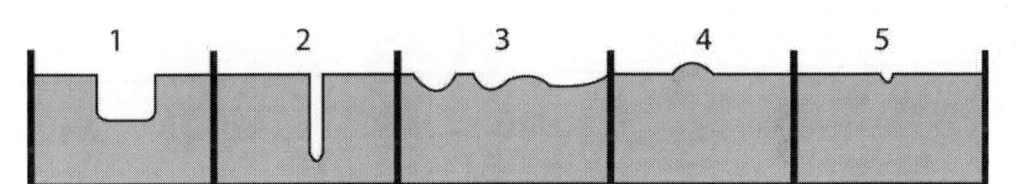

Illustration 97. Box Scar 1, Ice Pick Scar 2, Various types of rolling scars 3, Small Hypertrophic scar 4, Small Atrophic scar 5.

In the next sections we will explore the most effective aesthetic treatments used to remove the scar types 1, 2 and 3. Scars Types 4 and 5 are usually attenuated by using skin resurfacing treatments. Electrical arcing can be very easily used to remove small scar types 4 and other minor Hypertrophic skin imperfections.

16.3 Atrophic scar removal and attenuation treatments

Atrophic scars are not as easily removed as Hypertrophic scars are, however there are a number of effective treatments available for atrophic scar removal and atrophic scar attenuation. Atrophic scar removal generally is more complex than normal Hypertrophic scar removal. In the case of Hypertrophic scar removal, the ablative process focuses on removing the raised part of the scars using various methods, Laser, Electrical arcing (Plasma), Excision etc. Also **occlusion is another effective method for Hypertrophic scar attenuation** over time, this is used as a home treatment solution which is scientifically proven to lead to good results.

First of all, it is important to make a clear distinction between atrophic scar removal and atrophic scar attenuation. The two main techniques are fundamentally different. Atrophic Scar removal focuses on finding ways to "fill" or removing the skin depression which causes the atrophic scar, as we will see this can be done effectively in various ways. The best and most cost effective method depends on the type of each atrophic scars and where it is positioned. Some atrophic scar removal techniques are surgical while some others are straight forward non surgical procedures. Atrophic scar attenuation are generally aesthetic non surgical treatments and focus on finding ways to gradually improve the appearance of atrophic scars.

Atrophic scars, sometimes, can be challenging to remove completely because the aesthetic procedure has to focus on finding the best way to reinstate the the missing part of the skin. Depending on a number of factors, this cannot be always straight forward. Sometimes, atrophic scar removal can involve some degree of minor skin re-constructive technique in order to achieve the best possible results in the least number of treatments.

The strict requirement for reconstructing the depressed part of the skin is not always necessary because in certain cases a satisfactory result can be accomplished by using simple skin resurfacing methods or other very simple aesthetic treatments. As we will see, this is specifically the case for superficial rolling scars treatment.

Generally in case of box scars the natural skin regeneration process (which occurs over time or induced by using skin resurfacing techniques) leads to a progressive smoothing of the sharp edges of the atrophic scar and

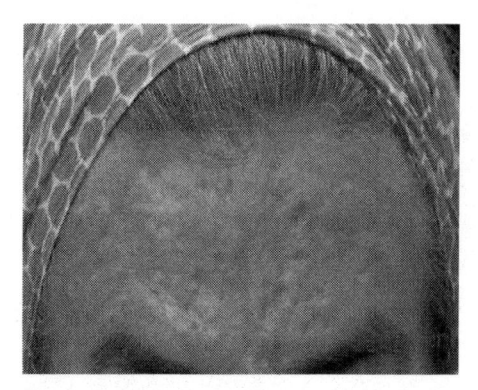

Illustration 98: Typical atrophic scars left after severe acne

therefore Box Scars normally progress into Rolling Scars over time. In case of superficial rolling scars, a number of skin resurfacing treatments generally lead to further smoothing of the "Rolling Scars" until satisfactory results.

The Above picture (ilustration 98) shows the typical atrophic scars left after severe acne. In illustration 68 the depressed areas of the skin typical of atrophic scars are evident. The best first line of treatment for these type of atrophic scar removal procedures maybe surgical. The type of removal treatment for each scar maybe different depending on each type of atrophic formation. The choice of the best type of treatment for each type of scar is left to the practitioner. The second line of treatment is the use of skin resurfacing techniques, localised skin tightening or collagen regeneration treatments in general. These are used to fine tune the results of the main scar removal treatments.

1. **Atrophic scar removal treatments.** The use of minor surgical procedures and atrophic scar removal procedures are usually the first line of treatment. These procedures focus on reconstructing the missing part of the skin caused by the acne or injury that produced the atrophic scars in the first place. As we will see, not one type of removal treatment suits all types of atrophic scars. For example in case of very deep relatively large box scars, the best technique can be minor skin grafting where the a small section of the skin is "implanted" into the depressed part of the scar. In case of deep Ice Pick Scars instead, the use of targeted potent cosmetic peels is usually effective in the removal of this type of atrophic scar.

2. **Atrophic scar attenuation treatments.** These are all aesthetic non surgical treatments. These aesthetic procedures focus on the use of collagen stimulation techniques or skin regeneration principles (skin resurfacing) and sometimes localised skin tightening. This is done using laser and voltaic plasma skin resurfacing, micro-needling, cosmetic peels etc. These are usually the second line of treatment after the main atrophic scar removal treatment. They are used as to perfect the results accomplished by the removal treatments. Also scar attenuation treatments are used as first line of treatment in cases of superficial rolling scars. In this case simple skin resurfacing procedures can lead to satisfactory results without the need for using minor surgical procedures.

16.4 Ice pick scars removal

In case of very deep indented Scars (Ice Pick Scars), the smoothing effects of skin resurfacing procedures will be effective in improving the appearance of this type of Atrophic Scars, however the missing part of the skin cannot be reconstructed by using traditional skin resurfacing methods. Traditional skin resurfacing treatments using lasers, micro-needling, repeated cosmetic peels or skin tightening using electrical arcing at the borders of the ice pick scar usually lead to a degree of improvement in the appearance of this type of atrophic scar, however the this type of aesthetic treatments on their own seldom lead to satisfactory results in the treatment of very deep "Ice Pick Scars". Additionally these methods on their own are classed as "Ice Pick Scar Attenuation", instead of "Ice Pick Scar Removal". This is because on their own, traditional skin resurfacing techniques cannot remove deep "Ice Pick Scars". In fact traditional skin resurfacing treatments, on their own, do not lead to the reconstruction of the deep missing part of the skin in deep "Ice Pick Scars".

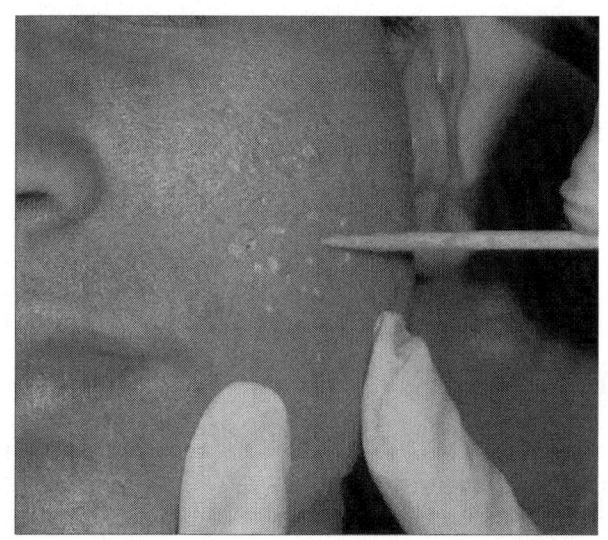

Illustration 99: Use of TCA for "Ice Pick Scar" Removal. The use of suitable potent cosmetic peels inside the scars is the preferred option for Ice Pick Scars removal. This method is referred to as "Bridging" the ice pick scars. Although this is considered the best practice for Ice pick Scar removal, this is an easy non surgical technique

A very effective method used to reconstruct the missing part of the skin in deep and narrow "Ice Pick Scars" is a technique called "Bridging". Throughout the years this method has been used the world over with great success for "Ice Pick Scars" removal. It is referred to as "Bridging" because this technique takes advantage of the fact that the internal walls of "Ice Pick Scars" are very close together.

Because of this, when a superficial ex-foliation is carried out inside the "Ice Pick Scar" during the healing period the internal walls of the scar tend to join together as extra collagen is produced to "Bridge" the small "gap" of this type of atrophic scar. In other words, the highly concentrated cosmetic peel delivered inside the narrow scar, causes a very superficial small "wound" inside the narrow walls of the "Ice Pick Scar". As the internal walls of the atrophic scar heal, the effect is as if the scar starts to "fill up" with new skin tissue which is formed between the walls of the scar (Bridging Effect). Therefore the depth of the scar decreases visibly due to the new collagen formed inside the scar.

The preferred product used for this application, in many aesthetic clinics with very good and repeatable result is TCA. Highly concentrated Trichloroacetic Acid solutions (over 80% in concentration) are delivered in small droplets inside the ice pick scar. Immediately after the TCA solution has been delivered the atrophic scar turns white. This "whitening" will last in the region of 3 hours. It will then be followed by redness around the "Ice Pick Scar".

A couple of days after the treatment the scars treated will start turning black, a sign that the scabbing process (and bridging) is taking place. The scars usually recover completely within one week. Please note that other specialised cosmetic peels other than TCA can be used instead, leading to similar results in "Ice Pick Scar" removal.

Over several years, tooth picks impregnated with the potent cosmetic peel have been used to deliver the cosmetic substance inside the "Ice Pick Scar". Some aesthetic practitioners prefer the use of small conventional mesotherapy-type of syringes to deliver the small droplets of potent peel inside the "Ice Pick Scars".

Please note that the Cosmetic peel is NOT injected but simply purred in droplets inside the "Ice Pick Scar". The use of the Syringe allows a faster and more effective delivery of the the cosmetic peel.

In the video below you can appreciate how this easy method is applied on a real case.

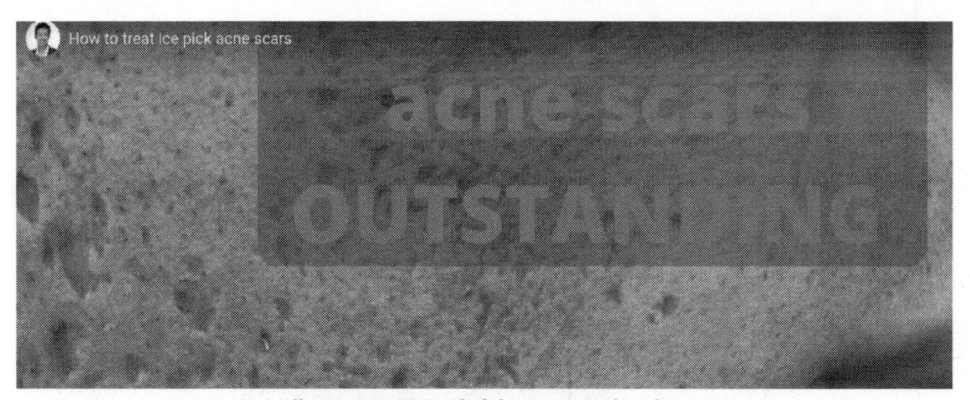

Illustration 100: Click here to watch video

During the healing process, the part has to be kept free of infections and disinfected twice a day. Sun screen must be worn for at least 3 months after the last treatment and exposure to sun light or UV sources deliberately avoided for at least that period.

This type treatment has to be repeated a number of times in order to achieve good results. On average two sessions are normally sufficient. This treatment is usually followed by the skin resurfacing treatments, using Lasers, Electrical arcing, or cosmetic peels. These techniques are used to fine tune the results and correct minor skin imperfections.

If using one of our AC Electrical arcing devices to fine tune the results after the "Bridging" treatment for Ice Pick Scar removal, set the device at minimum power level and apply the spot mode on the edge of each scar and between the scars. Do not apply the spots inside the depressed part of the scars themselves.

In the following video you can see a voltaic arcing treatment for acne scar attenuation. As you can see the arc is applied between each scar and never inside the scar itself. Please note that in this case no Bridging treatment was used before this voltaic arcing treatment.

www.voltaicplasma.com   Author: Andreas Russo

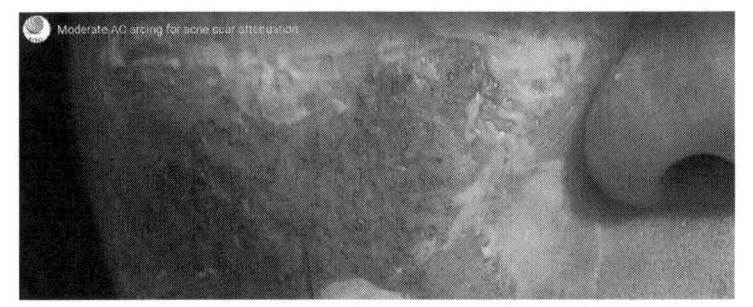

Illustration 101: Click here to watch video

16.5 Box scars removal

Before you perform any "Box Scar" removal treatment, make sure the area is vascularised (properly reached by blood vessels). This is especially important in recently formed scars, as some of them may not be ready for scar removal treatments (scar tissue hard to the touch). Appreciating whether the scar tissue is properly vascularised is done simply by touching the scar tissue itself, if it is soft to the touch and not stiff then this is a sign that the scar is adequately vascularised. If the area is stiff then a number of skin resurfacing treatments are recommended before performing any of the following procedures. The preferred option to vascularise stiff scars is the use of micro-needling. Other options involve laser resurfacing, voltaic arcing resurfacing, cosmetic peels.

Illustration 102: Different size and shapes of "Box Scars". Some can resemble Ice Pick scars while others can resemble Rolling scars

If the skin is soft to the touch and you can pinch it with your fingers without encountering any stiffness, then you can go ahead and perform any of the box scar removal procedures described here.

We have seen how the preferred method for Ice Pick Scar removal is the use of suitable highly concentrated peels to accomplish the "Bridging" effects between the internal walls of the Ice Pick scars. This is possible due to the proximity of the internal walls of the Ice Pick Scars.

In case of "Box Scars", because the walls of the scar are further apart, than Ice Pick Scars, the technique of "Bridging" may not be the most suitable to accomplish the best results because the internal walls of Box Scars are too far apart to join after the use of highly concentrated TCA or other suitable cosmetic peels.

Currently, the most popular treatments available for box scar removal are:

- **Minor Skin Grafting or Punch grafting (floating),** when the Box Scar is particularly deep and placed on an area of the skin not particularly subject to stretching, like the forehead, temples or chin area.
- **Punch excision, discard and close**. It is done by making a little punch excision of the scar. This is the same technique used when performing skin excision to send the sample for histological examination to verify a lesion is benign. After the excision is performed, the area is stitched up and heals by **primary intention**.
- **Subcision. Subcision** is used when the "Box Scar" is quite swallow, or it is placed on an area of the face particularly subject to stretching or wrinkling. This technique focuses on making a wound inside the scar itself in order to trigger a Hypertrophic scarring formation which would elevate the depresses part of the scar.

Fillers. Also some aesthetic practitioners use fillers to try and elevate the depressed part of the "Box Scar". Although effective, this technique is not explored here as it is not a permanent solution and it requires ongoing treatments due to the fact that fillers will naturally be reabsorbed over time (within 12 to 24 months after the treatment). Therefore every time the filler is absorbed, the treatment has to be repeated. Because the use of fillers is not a permanent solution and there are effective permanent Box Scar removal solutions available, we prefer to explain and explore those instead.

Generally, there is no right or wrong removal treatment choice for Box Scars. This is because Box Scars come in different part of the face, in different shapes and depths. Sometimes they resemble Rolling Scars if they are large, sometimes they can resemble more Ice Pick Scars. Therefore it is the choice of the aesthetic practitioner to use the technique that it is deemed best suited for the particular Box Scar, based on its shape, position on the face and depth of the depressed area.

16.6 Minor skin grafting or punch grafting (floating)

Skin grafting is used in many areas of skin reconstruction and it is particularly useful and effective in reconstructing the missing skin in a "Box" type of scar. Punch Grafting is a simple minor surgical technique used to "fill" the missing part of the skin inside the atrophic scar. Another part of the skin is implanted into the missing part of the atrophic scar.

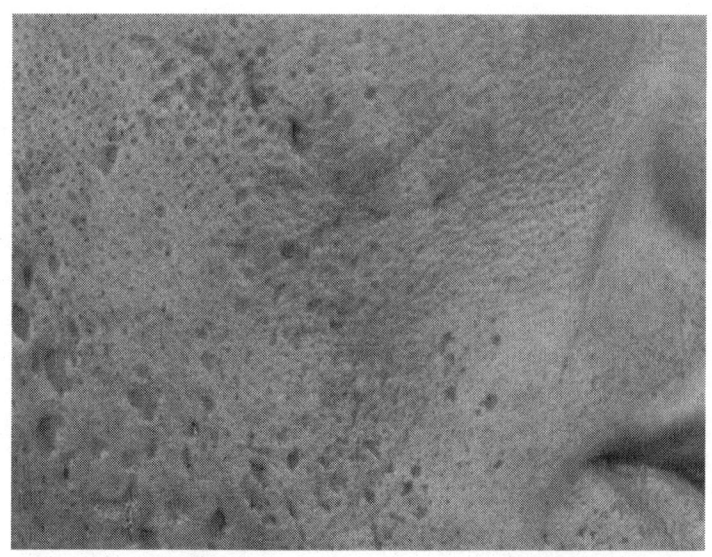

Illustration 1023: Typical Box and Ice Pick Scars on the face. Based on the individual type of scar the treatment can be different. This is a classical example of the various types of scars that a single individual can present. In this case we have many Box Types of scars and some other Box Scars can resemble Ice pick scars. So the practitioner has to choose the type of scar removal treatment for each individual scar based on their experience and specific type of scar. There is never a right or wrong type of scar removal treatment for each scar.

This "Punch Grafting" technique is generally used when subsicion would be quite difficult to carry out especially in case of particularly deep Box Scars. However, if the Box Scar is deep and located on an area of the face prone to stretching or wrinkling (i.e. periorbital area, cheeks etc) then this technique should be avoided as the new skin may not implant properly in place of the missing part of the skin. In this case the **"punch excision, discard and close"** technique should be used instead.

Minor Skin Grafting or Punch grafting (floating) provides the most optimal results in less mobile areas of the face such as the forehead and temples. Punch floating is the treatment of choice for most deep "Box Scars" and usually heals in 3 to 4 weeks without a trace of the circular incision used to make the punch.

In the video below we can see how skin grafting is used to regenerate the missing skin of the depressed area of an atrophic scar.

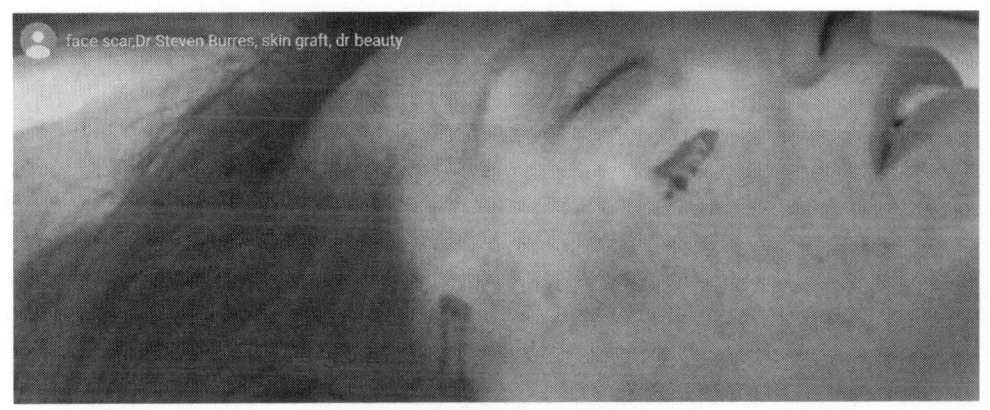

Illustration 104: Click here to watch video

The surgeon deliberately inflicts a wound into the "Box Scar". Once the wound is made, the small skin graft (punch graft) is implanted on to the fresh wound and stitched up. Stitches are used in case of large "Box Scars". The stitches are removed within 15 days. In case of small Box Scars, given that the use of sutures would be impractical, **skin glue** is the preferred option used instead of stitching.

Once the part has healed, usually further skin resurfacing treatments are used in order to correct minor imperfections left after this minor surgery. The main treatments used are laser resurfacing to smooth out the skin in general. In case of protruding imperfections voltaic arcing and laser ablations can be used to level off these imperfections. Also a course of home peeling treatments can be performed by the client at home.

16.7 Punch, discard and close

This is another easy and effective technique used with great success in the removal of Box Scars. It is carried out by excising the scar itself and closing it with stitches. The part is then left to heal by primary intention. The stitches are removed 7 days after the procedure. This technique is used when

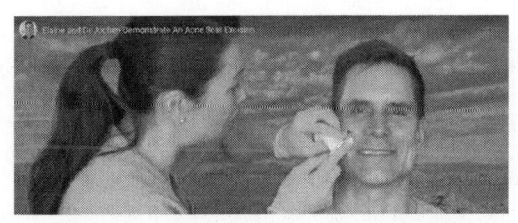

Illustration 105: Click here to watch video

Minor Skin Grafting or Punch grafting (floating) is not the most suitable option for Box Scar removal (i.e. the scar is too large, or the practitioner would deem the grafting to probably be unsuccessful). One downside with this procedure is that this technique will usually lead some other form of scar-tissue due to the stitching. Fortunately, if the procedure is carried out correctly, the new scar tissue is normally slightly Hypertrophic and hence very easily removed like any minor skin imperfection. This then allows simple skin resurfacing treatments (scar attenuation) to blend in the new small scar with the surrounding skin area.

In case Voltaic Arcing (Plasma), is used after this procedure to smooth the area, then the arc is used on top of the new hypertrophic scar in order to level it off with the surrounding skin area. Please note that not all scars left by the sutures maybe hypertrophic and the beauty practitioner has to choose the best technique for the specific skin imperfection left after the area has healed.

Other skin resurfacing method can be used too, including micro-needling, localised and overall laser resurfacing, cosmetic peels etc. As usual, these are secondary treatments aimed at fine tuning the results and help the new scar to blend in and achieve a smoother skin after the "Box Scar" removal treatment. If some minor protruding or hypertrophic imperfections are left after healing these can be easily removed by using voltaic arcing (Plasma) or Lasers.

16.8 Subcision

The main challenge in improving the appearance of atrophic scars in general, is fnding the best way to regenerate the missing part of the skin which creates the "hole' in the skin. As we have seen, there are sometimes very simple and effective techniques (Bridging) used for removing deep "Ice Pick" scars. However if the Box Scar is particularly superficial then the Punch, Discard and close or Minor Skin Grafting or Punch grafting (floating) techniques would be unnecessary (because too invasive) since there is a more simple, less invasive and effective permanent removal treatments for this type of shallow scars. This is done by achieving a minor elevation of the depressed part of the scar using a technique referred to as *subcision*. This is a technique where a conventional scalpel is carefully used to cause a deliberate wound inside the depressed part of the scar itself.

Subcision is a technique used in order to raise the depressed area of the individual atrophic scar in general. This is done intentionally inducing another process of scarification. Essentially, the atrophic scar is carefully cut at its bottom and a wound is purposely formed which is left to heal.

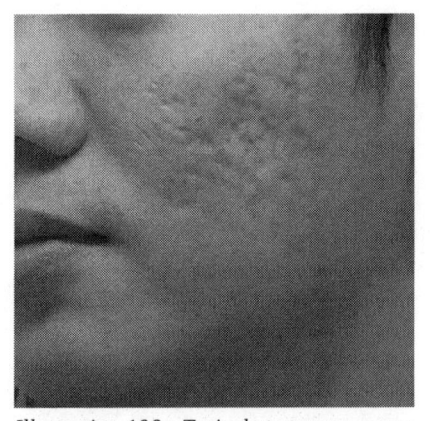

Illustration 106: Typical acne scars, some Rolling and Box Scars. The practitioner may decide to perform subsicions to raise the depressed areas of the individual atrophic scars. The procedure is quite time consuming but simple.

The natural scar generation process will produce extra collagen which in turn will raise the previously depressed area of the atrophic scar.

Scabs will form three to four days after the procedure. The scabs should fall off by themselves within 5 to 7 days and the results are typically very good and permanent. After this type of simple surgery the improvement is normally visible however further aesthetic treatments are usually recommended to correct the minor imperfections left after the surgery. In other words, surgical subsicion is used to coarsely improve the appearance of shallow atrophic scars and other aesthetic treatments (scar attenuation treatments) normally follow to fine tune the results.

Normally a number of skin resurfacing sessions are carried out once the area has recovered fully. This will allow to smooth the skin imperfections left after the subcision treatment. The skin resurfacing can be carried out by using cosmetic lasers, voltaic arcing, or a number of sessions of cosmetic peels.

Subcision **is a simple technique and it is well explained as shown in the following video.**

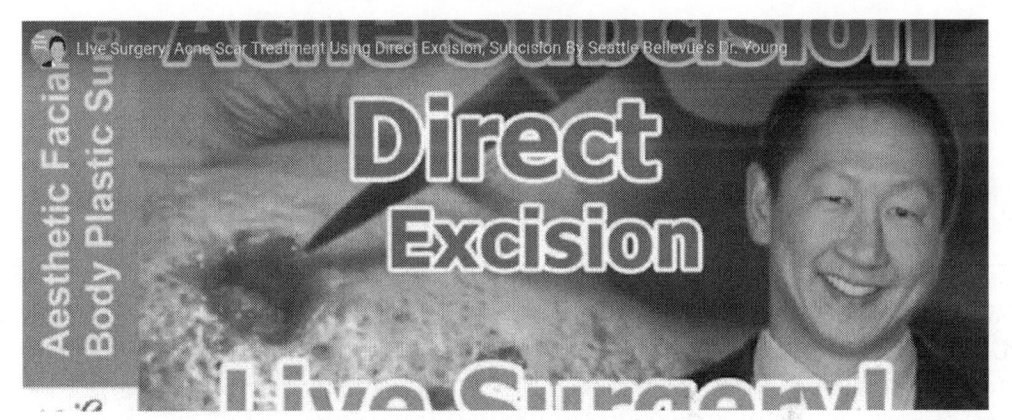

Illustration 106: Click here to watch video

This technique (subcision) is preferred when the atrophic scars (typically Box Scar and sometimes Rolling Scars) are are relatively shallow. Usually the depth of scar required to opt for subcision is between 1 and 2 mm. However, in case of particularly deep scars, this technique maybe impractical and do not lead to very good results and "punch grafting and closing" or "minor skin grafting" may be preferable instead.

The best treatments to better the results after subcision, are laser resurfacing, cosmetic peels or micro-needling.

16.9 Atrophic scar removal treatments conclusions

Bear in mind that atrophic scars are generally difficult to remove completely, therefore a certain degree of improvement in their appearance is considered to be the most appropriate expectation for this type of aesthetic treatments. No treatment both surgical or non surgical can always guarantee complete disappearance of the atrophic scars (or Acne Scars) even if carried out correctly.

Above we have discussed the types of treatments that are notoriously effective in the removal of atrophic scar of various shapes and depths. These techniques have been used around the world for several years with great success. However there is not right of wrong treatment choice for any given type of atrophic scar. The aesthetic practitioner is called every time to evaluate the type of scar individually and choose the type of treatment which he or she deems best suitable for each individual type of scar.

Often these treatments are followed by some **atrophic scar attenuation treatments** to fine tune the results and get rid of minor skin imperfections.

16.10 Atrophic scar attenuation treatments

Above, we have discussed the first line of atrophic scar removal treatments. They are effective and usually lead to very good results. These treatments aim at finding the most effective way to either "Bridge" the small gap in the narrow scar (Ice Pick Scars), reconstructing the missing part of the skin (Large and Deep Box Scars), stitching up the missing part of the skin (Small and Deep Box Scars), trying to elevate the depressed part of the skin by using Subcision (Shallow Box Scars).

However, although effective, these techniques may leave some residual imperfections, hence in order to accomplish the best possible results other follow up treatments may be required. This is because almost any scar removal treatment can leave some degree of imperfections both atrophic or hypertrophic. Sometimes the imperfections could present themselves as minor hypertrophic formations, other times as atrophic formations most commonly resembling shallow rolling scars formations. The type of imperfections left depends on the type of scar removal treatment performed, the after-care and the reaction to the removal treatment itself.

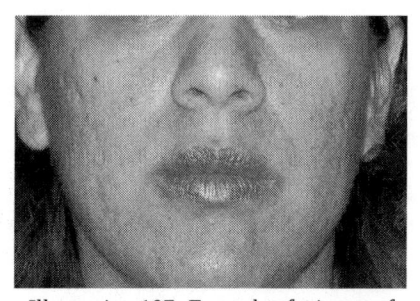

Illustration 107: Example of mixture of box and superficial rolling scars. The superficial Rolling scar can be treated using the atrophic scar attenuation techniques described here. While the deeper "Box Scars" should undergo scar removal procedures before carrying out any scar attenuation treatment. Please bear in mind that in cases like this one 4 to 6 treatments may be required in order to attenuate the deeper atrophic scars, unless a scar removal treatment is carried out for the deeper scars before hand.

These imperfections can be smoothed off using various techniques. If the imperfections are hypetrophic the best post treatments are either Voltaic Arcing or Laser Removal of the protruding imperfections. If the imperfections are atrophic or depressed there are several options for Atrophic scar attenuation treatments. Atrophic scar attenuation is performed as a second line of treatment after the main removal procedures with the techniques described above. Typically, atrophic scar attenuation treatments focus on collagen regeneration and sometimes also localised skin tightening.

This is done in various ways:

- Using laser resurfacing techniques. Suitable to remove minor hypetrophic imperfections and smooth atrophic areas.
- Voltaic Arcing also referred to as Plasma. Suitable to remove minor hypetrophic imperfections and smooth atrophic areas.
- Micro-needling. Suitable to stimulate collagen regeneration, therefore smoothing shallow rolling scars.
- Cosmetic peels. Suitable to stimulate collagen regeneration, therefore smoothing shallow rolling scars.

The aesthetic techniques presented below, although they should be used as second line of treatment, namely to attenuate the appearance of atrophic scars, they are very often used as the first and only line of treatment. This is because in several aesthetic clinics the minor skin grafting technique, punch and close or bridging are not used, very often due to to the personnel unfamiliarity with these removal treatments or lack of qualifications to carry them out. However even if these scar attenuation techniques are used as first and only line of treatment they often lead to very good results on their own after several treatments.

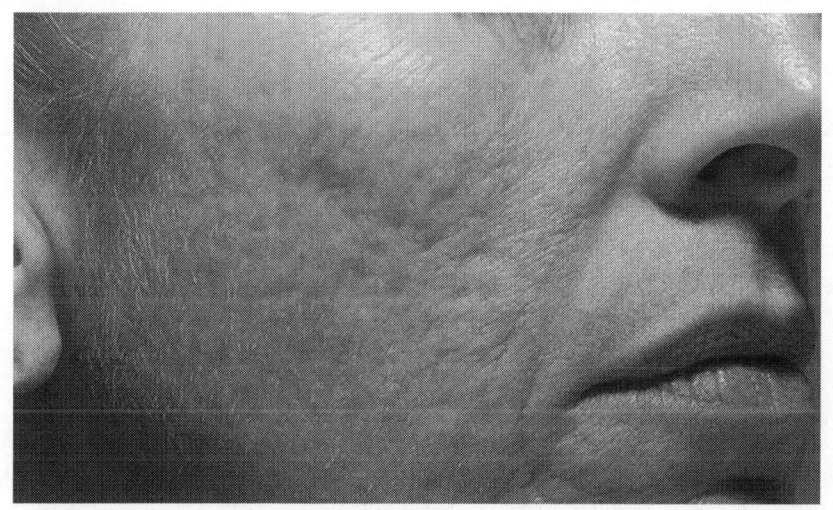

Illustration 108: Typical example of superficial rolling scars which can be treated within one to two session with a good atrophic scar professional attenuation treatment.

Even thought many times the atrophic scars attenuation techniques are presented as the first and only line of treatment, whenever possible it is recommended to use them as the second line of treatment after the major atrophic scar removal treatments. Experience shows that coupling the scar removal treatments with the atrophic scar attenuation presented below accomplish the best results using the least exposure to aesthetic treatments.

The fact that atrophic scar attenuation procedures are advertised, in several aesthetic clinics, as "*all in one*" effective scar removal treatments, shows that they are effective because their repeated use eventually satisfactorily fade the atrophic scars. However, in several cases, given that there are more effective techniques to achieve the desired results in less treatments and sometimes in a more cost effective ways it is advisable to use the techniques presented below as a second line of treatment and market them as atrophic scar attenuation procedures. If using both the scar removal techniques presented above in conjunction with the appropriate scar attenuation procedures, satisfactory results are usually achieved minimising the number of treatments and therefore minimising the costs to the client.

Below we explore the use of Voltaic Arcing (Electrical Plasma) treatments in special detail. Voltaic Plasma like Lasers present the triple benefit of being used for:

1. Removing minor hypertrophic imperfections left after the scar removal treatments.
2. Collagen regeneration stimulation.
3. Localised skin tightening.

16.11 Laser resurfacing for acne scar attenuation

Lasers (normally CO_2 and Fraxel) are often used for atrophic scar attenuation. These treatments are often advertised as scar removal treatments. Laser treatments stimulate collagen regeneration by causing a controlled burn into the skin. This burn causes a natural collagen regeneration and skin tightening effect. Depending on the laser wavelength, the burn (or heat transferred into the skin) can be more or less superficial. The higher the laser's beam wavelength, the deeper the heat penetrates into the skin. Conversely the shorter the wavelength the more superficial the heating effects. In the following video you can see a CO_2 laser treatment for superficial rolling scar attenuation.

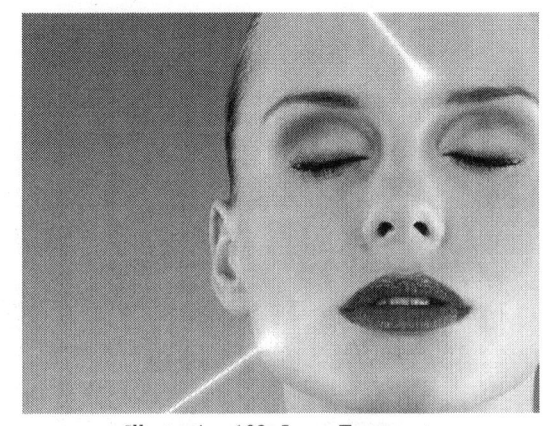

Illustration 109: Laser Treatments

Click here to watch video

A number of treatments may be required to accomplished the best possible results. Mostly 4 to 5 treatments are usually required in order to achieve the desired results in case of deep scars. Please note that although they are often promoted as surgical treatments in aesthetic clinics (to increase their perceived value) they are clearly non invasive, non surgical treatments.

16.12 Voltaic arcing atrophic scar attenuation treatment (plasma)

Voltaic Arcing (Plasma).

The use of electrical arcing for atrophic scar attenuation is for:

- Removing the small imperfections left by the minor surgical procedures (i.e. minor skin graft and/or punch/close). If used for removing minor hypertrophic imperfections (i.e. the minor hypertrophic scars naturally left after the use of minor skin grafting, or punch and close), the common spraying technique can be used to ablate the minor hypertrophic formation with the view of levelling it off with the surrounding skin. This is the same technique used for Moles Removal.
- Like Lasers, it is also used for its skin tightening and collagen regeneration properties to smooth the shallow rolling scars or the shallow atrophic imperfections left after atrophic scar removal treatment. Therefore voltaic arcing treatments are very good for atrophic scar attenuation in general.

Attenuate shallow atrophic scars.

When using Plasma (or Voltaic Arcing), use the typical spot technique on the borders of the scars and never inside the scars themselves. What we are trying to accomplish is "pulling" the surrounding skin area so that after a few treatments the scar will be less noticeable. Please note that for treatment of *very deep scars*, using AC electrical arcing, can improve the appearance of this aesthetic condition by making the deep scar look more shallow, in most cases however, the complete disappearance of the scar is unlikely.

If the atrophic scars are isolated (or far apart from each other), apply the spots around each scar. Never apply the arc on the depressed part of the scar as doing so could eventually worsen the appearance of the scars instead of improving it.

In the video below you can see how the typical spot technique is applied for a relatively large isolated atrophic rolling scar. The scar is over 15 years old and therefore it has not preserved its original Box type characteristics (the typical sharp edges of box scars) and it has evolved into a relatively large rolling scar. In this case the atrophic scar was caused by a childhood wound and not acne or a cyst.

In this short video the voltaic spots are applied very tightly together and the device is set at minimum power level.

www.voltaicplasma.com   Author: Andreas Russo

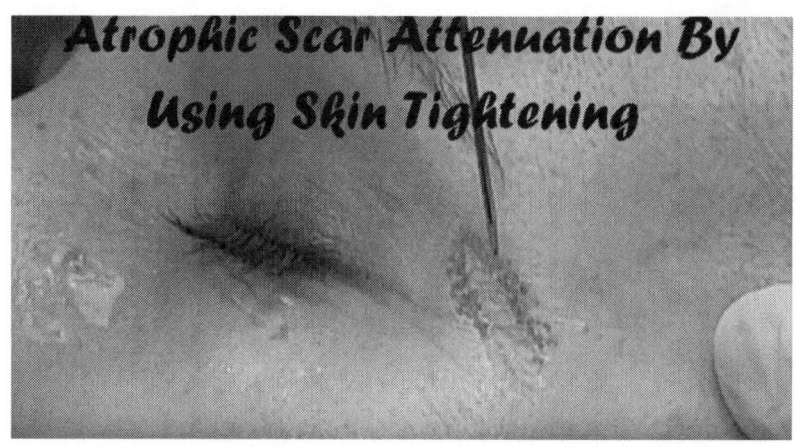

Illustration 110: Click here to watch video

In the following video we can appreciate the treatment of another isolated rolling scar using skin tightening resurfacing techniques. As seen in the video the technique used was a slight spray operation with the device set at the minimum power level. Although the preferred technique is the spot mode, some experienced users move to spray operation for skin tightening and skin resurfacing purposes.

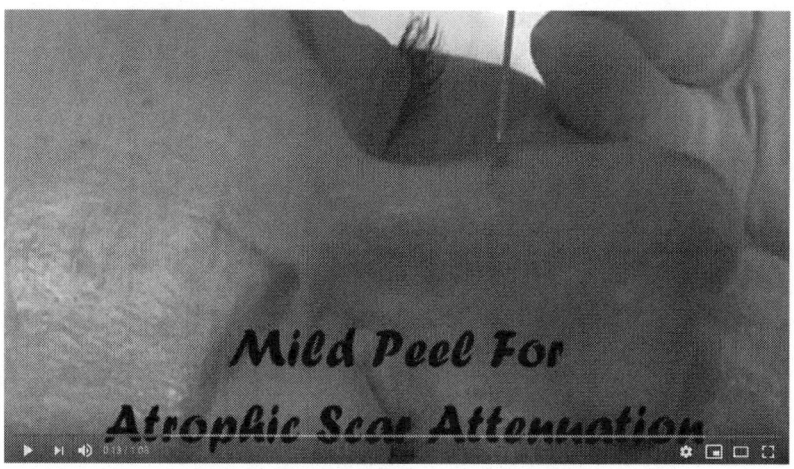

Illustration 111: Click here to watch video

The following video presents another case of minor atrophic scar attenuated using AC Electrical Arcing. As we can see in the video the arc is applied in the spot mode at the borders of the scar itself to cause the desired "pulling" effects.

www.voltaicplasma.com   Author: Andreas Russo

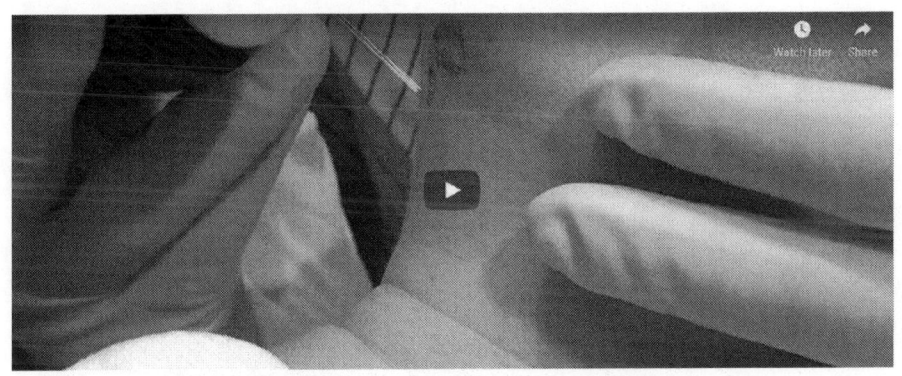

Illustration 112: Click here to watch video

As seen in the above examples the basic techniques using voltaic arcing for atrophic scar attenuation of any kind is very simple. This is a safe aesthetic treatment which does not involve surgery. Remember that for relatively deep scars it is always recommended, whenever possible, to use these attenuation techniques after the main atrophic scar removal treatments. This aesthetic procedure is also highly recommended for localised skin tightening and skin resurfacing after main scar removal procedure of deep and ice pick scars.

How to perform the treatment:

1. Apply **topical numbing cream** before starting this treatment to achieve maximum comfort to the client during this type of aesthetic procedure.
2. Use the intensity treatment you consider appropriate. Usually the the fist time you use voltaic arcing for this application it is advisable to set the power level of our device to minimum, use an instantaneous spot duration and distance between spots varying between 2 to 3 mm apart. The treatment usually lasts between 10 to 15 minutes depending on the area to be covered.
3. Downtime ranges between 5 to 6 days, however it can last longer depending on the intensity of the treatment and how the after-care is carried out. In case, Voltaic Arcing for atrophic scar attenuation, we define as "downtime" the time period during which the area looks as if is getting worse rather than better. This is the time period required for scabbing to form during which the use of cover up make-up of any type is strictly forbidden.
4. Allow a minimum 4 weeks' interval between treatments. A slight improvement after each session is generally noticeable after the scabs have fallen off.
5. In case voltaic plasma is used as a first line of treatment without prior scar removal procedure, this type of treatment has to be repeated 5 to 6 times in order to achieve reasonable good scar attenuation results. Remember that the use of plasma is recommended as a second line treatment for smoothing off imperfections of both atrophic and hypertrophic formations left after the main scar removal treatments. If Plasma is used as second line treatment, usually one or two sessions suffice in order to achieve the desired results.

6. Apply make-up only after he scabs have fallen . Apply total sun protection after any scabs have fallen off for at least two to three months after the last treatment. Avoid direct sun exposure for at least 2 months. Generally instruct your client to follow the normal **after-care instructions**.

Treatment of deep Atrophic Scars using plasma or fibroblast. In case of very deep scars, a slight improvement in their appearance will be possible by using electrical arcing, however their complete disappearance or best results would be unlikely with this technique alone. Also this applies to any other skin resurfacing technique for atrophic scar attenuation. This technique is primarily used to improve the appearance of atrophic scars in general and flatten swallow rolling scars by using the skin tightening and skin resurfacing properties of voltaic plasma. In case of medium deep or particularly deep scars, the best option to accomplish dramatic results is the combination the atrophic scar removal treatments (subsicion and/or localised skin grafting etc) followed by the plasma skin resurfacing discussed here. In this case skin resurfacing (using electrical arcing, lasers, micro-needling or cosmetic peels) is done after the area has recovered from the scar removal procedure.

16.13 Micro needling atrophic scar attenuation treatment

Micro needling

Micro-needing is extensively used to stimulate collagen regrowth. This has good applications in acne scar attenuation. This is a non surgical non invasive technique. Depending on the depth of the needles penetration into the skin and the level of vascularisation of the skin a certain degree of bleeding can occur during the treatment.

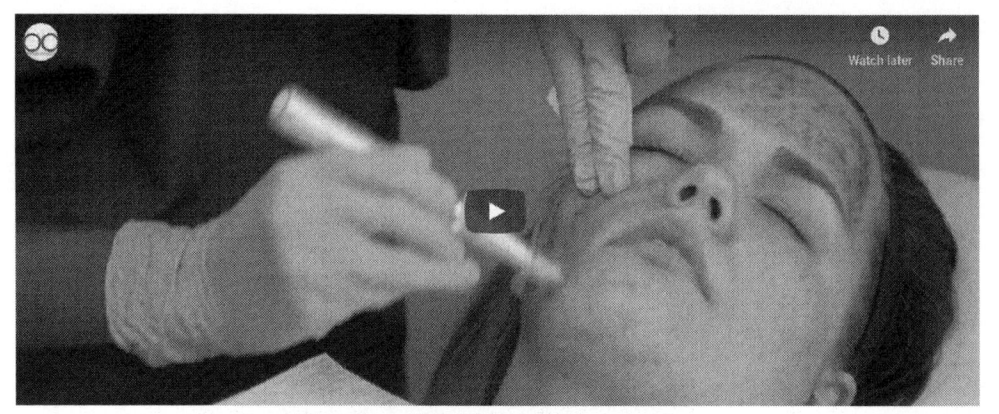

Illustration 113: Click here to watch video

In the video above we can see a micro needling device used for collagen stimulation.Click here to watch video

16.14 Cosmetic peels atrophic scar attenuation treatment

Cosmetic peels.

Collagen regeneration is at the basis of most scar attenuation treatments. As it is well known collagen regeneration can be triggered easily using simple cosmetic peels. Please note that most cosmetic peels suitable for this application are all allowed in the CosIng cosmetic European Portal and all ingrediats are normally can be freely used for this type of treatment.

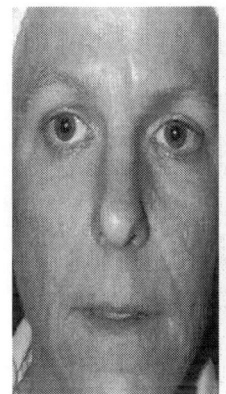

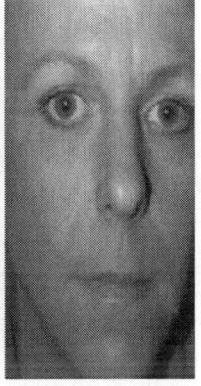

Illustration 114: Representative dramatic results of combined minor cosmetic surgery and skin resurfacing/tightening.

16.15 How to treat atrophic scars in practical cases

There are different approaches in treating atrophic scars and in general there is no right and wrong answer. Treating atrophic scars and improving their appearance can be a long process and you can combine a number of different types of treatments to improve their appearance.

The method proposed is treating the deeper scars and ice pick scars to make them shallower first and then perfect the results by using easier aesthetic treatments.

The initial treatments should be tailored to try and improve the appearance of the deeper scars. Identify the deepest and "pick scars" and apply the relevant aesthetic treatments to flatten them as much as possible. You can use subcision or punch discard and close to improve deep "Box Scars".

For "Ice Pick Scars" the most popular is the "bridging method" using TCA, This is the most popular because it is "non surgical" and TCA is widely available.

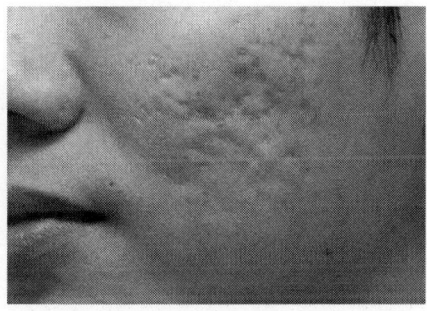

Illustration 115: Atrophic Scars

Click here to watch video

However you can also use punch discard and close to improve the appearance of Ice pick scars. If your clinic has a surgeon or medical practitioner then the "punch discard and close" method can be used. Minor skin grafting is also another option.

Once the deepest scars have been flattened and they resemble shallower box scars you can perfect the results by repeating the following aesthetic treatments:

- Voltaic Arcing Atrophic Scar Attenuation Treatment (plasma)
- Micro Needling Atrophic Scar Attenuation Treatment
- RF Micronnedling
- Cosmetic Peels Atrophic Scar Attenuation Treatment

17.0 Smoker lines attenuation

Improving the appearance of the classic smoker lines (also addressed as bar-code lines or *perioral lines*) is easy using AC electrical arcing. The previous knowledge required is skin tightening using Plasma, so please study that section before coming to this topic.

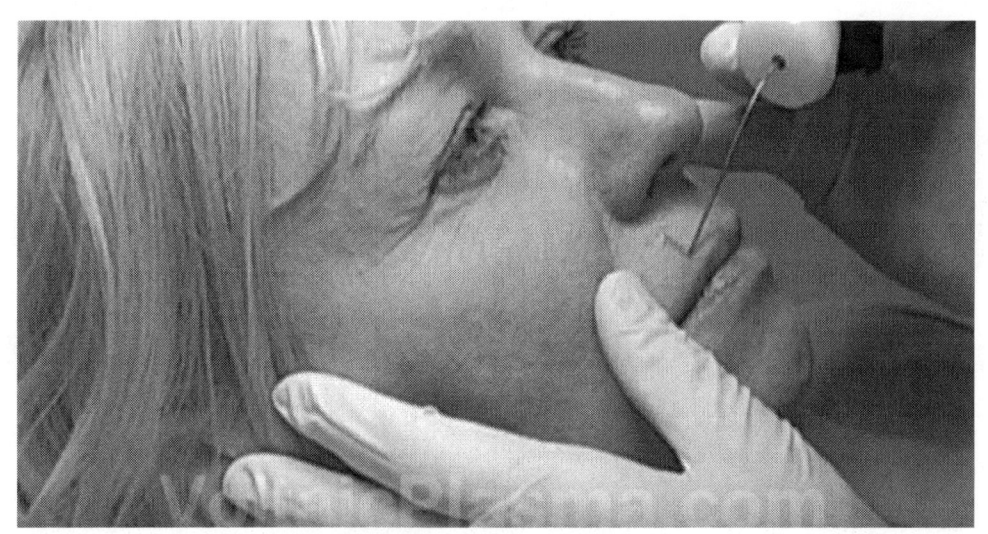

Illustration 116: Click here to watch video

17.1 Introduction to perioral lines

These types of wrinkles are generally referred to as "perioral" lines (peri means around, oral stands for mouth) because they are located around the mouth. They occur naturally due to normal facial expression of the perioral muscles. Everyone will eventually develop perioral lines over time because they are formed due to normal everyday facial expressions of the mouth. At an old age, perioral lines (or smoker lines) may not necessarily be caused by tobacco smoke; smokers just develop them much earlier, the wrinkles become much deeper and more unsightly.

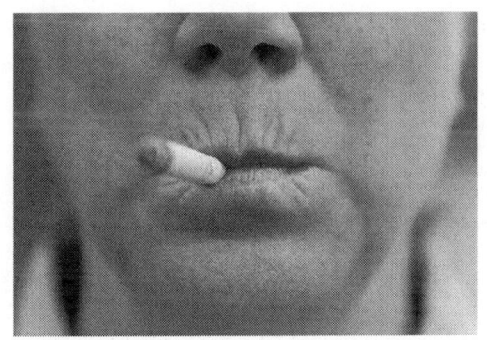

Illustration 117: Smoker lines are caused by repeated lip muscles contractions while talking, drinking from straws, smoking etc. but particularly exacerbated by the skin ageing effects of oxidation due to smoking damage.

Hence *perioral* lines are usually referred to as *smoker lines* because they are highly accentuated in heavy smokers. *Perioral* lines are just deeper and more unsightly in heavy smokers who develop them earlier and faster than non smokers (to read two interesting articles about the damage caused by cigarette smoke please click here and here).

Women are particularly are self conscious of their *perioral* lines and sometimes, women also seek aesthetic *perioral* lines attenuation treatments, even if they are non smokers. Heavy smokers over 60 years of age usually have particularly deep and sometimes unsightly *perioral* wrinkles. Smoker lines may be challenging to fix because sometimes they can be particularly deep, however there are many aesthetic treatments available to improve their appearance.

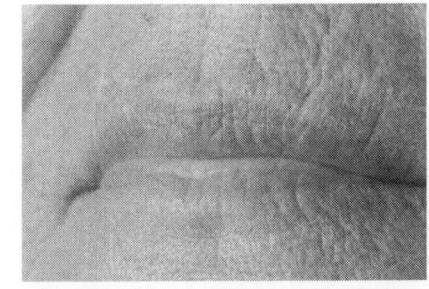

Illustration 118: Typical perioral lines exacerbated by the skin oxidation effects caused by tobacco smoke.

It is important to emphasise that no aesthetic treatment can guarantee the complete disappearance of these lines as any expression wrinkle can be attenuated (even significantly) but never removed unless the facial muscles movements are impaired both intentionally (using botox toxin) or unintentionally (due to medical conditions).

www.voltaicplasma.com   Author: Andreas Russo

17.2 The options to reduce the appearance of perioral lines

Although they can seem quite challenging to treat, there are several solutions for *perioral* lines attenuation. There are permanent and non permanent solutions. We will explore the non permanent solutions first and the permanent solutions after.

Temporary solutions

Non permanent treatments to attenuate *perioral* or *smoker lines* are accomplished through the use of Botox injections or fillers, alternatively a combined treatment of both. Botox treatments have the effect of reducing the facial muscle movement that causes the *perioral* lines in the first place. However, the effects of Botox are temporary and this treatment requires to be repeated over time. Also fillers are used in order to fill the recess of the wrinkles themselves. Like Botox, fillers are not a permanent solution and they will get reabsorbed over time. This means that the treatment has to be repeated every time the filler has been reabsorbed.

Permanent solutions

The main principle behind permanent aesthetic solutions for *perioral* lines attenuation (also referred and advertised as smoker lines removal) is skin regeneration (collagen regeneration/ stimulation) and skin tightening. Although some of these treatments may be incorrectly advertised as surgical procedures, by definition they all are aesthetic non surgical treatments. As it is well known collagen regeneration and skin tightening can be accomplished in several ways. For example using:

- Laser resurfacing.
- Electrical arcing.
- Micro needling.
- Cosmetic peels.
- Micro dermal abrasion.

Although the focus of this page is the use of Voltaic Arcing (Plasma) for *perioral* lines attenuation, we will touch briefly on each of the aesthetic treatments available for *smoker lines* attenuation.

The following video provides a good overview of the approach which can be taken in tackling *perioral* lines by the professional aesthetic practitioner.

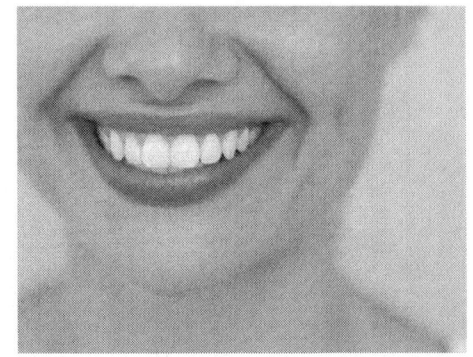

Illustration 119: *Click here to watch video*

www.voltaicplasma.com

Author: Andreas Russo

17.3 Laser resurfacing

Lasers treatments have very effective skin resurfacing and skin tightening properties. Therefore they have been used over several years for *perioral* lines attenuation . Both Fraxel and CO2 lasers are normally used for this application in aesthetic clinics.

Although they are sometimes referred to as surgical methods for marketing purposes, they are clearly non invasive non surgical procedures. Like in laser tattoo removal, a certain degree of bleeding can occur during these aesthetic treatments. Bleeding is a minor occurrence and it is temporary. This stops immediately after the treatment has ended because the minor bleeding is caused by broken superficial capillaries.

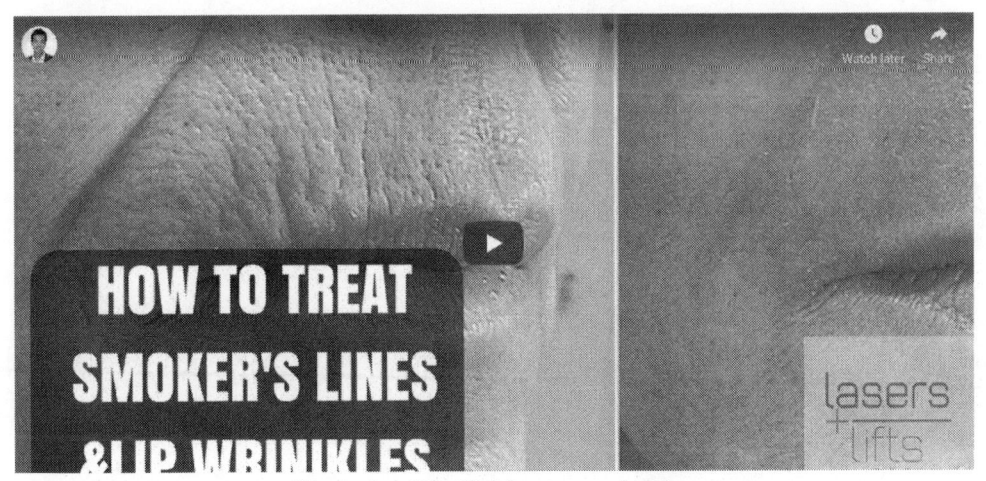

Illustration 120: Click here to watch video

Redness immediately after the treatment lasting up to 24 hours is a normal reaction to this type of aesthetic treatment using aesthetic lasers. The day following the treatment redness is followed by swelling caused by the burn induced by the laser treatment itself. The degree of swelling is proportional to the intensity of the treatment and it peaks the third to fourth day after the treatment. As the swelling subsides a scabbing/peeling process usually takes place. The scabbing can last up to 7 to 10 days after the aesthetic treatment depending on the intensity of the aesthetic treatment and the particular skin reaction. Both swelling and the peeling effects disappear on their own accord without the use of any medicines or medication. The downtime of this type of treatment varies between 6 to 10 days depending on the type of treatment and the particular skin reaction.

www.voltaicplasma.com   Author: Andreas Russo

17.4 Micro-needling

Micro needling has the notorious effect of collagen stimulation. Micro-needling reduces the appearance of fine lines including *perioral* lines as a stand alone treatment. There are also devices which combine micro needing with micro currents used to heat up the skin. This has a double collagen stimulation not only through the micro injury caused by micro needling but also due to the micro-current injected into the skin. Furthermore there are other micro needling devices which inject skin rejuvenation substances through the skin.

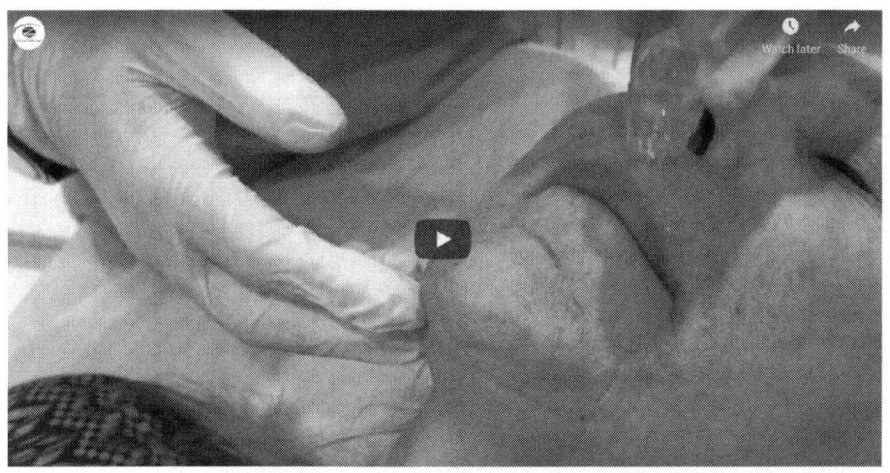

Illustration 121: Click here to watch video

17.5 Peels

AHAs (**Alpha Hydroxy Acids**) based products have well known collagen stimulation regeneration properties. These properties make AHA based cosmetic peels excellent products to reduce the appearance of fine lines and also *perioral* lines attenuation.

There are several AHAs options for cosmetic peels suitable for this type of aesthetic treatment the most popular is glycolic acid. However there are several other options for this particular application including mandelic acid, TCA based products etc.

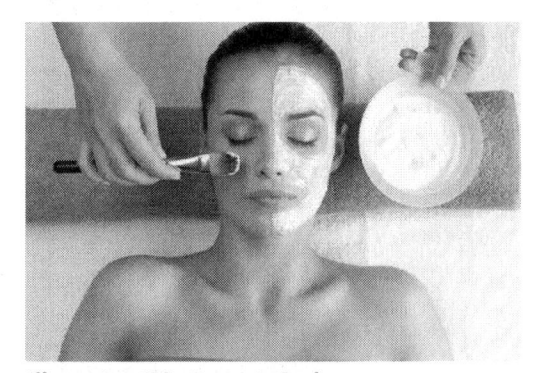

Illustration 122: Cosmetic Peels

One of the main disadvantages of this aesthetic solution is that several treatments may be required in order to achieve the best possible results. By contrast, the main advantage is that they are relatively inexpensive because they are widely available on the market and they can sometimes be used at home and not only in an aesthetic clinics, making this a very convenient home based aesthetic treatment.

17.6 Microdermabrasion

Significant improvements in the appearance of *perioral* lines can be also be achieved by using microdermabrasion treatments. By "sanding down" the skin around the *perioral* area the treatment lessen the uneven pigment and brighten the skin around the mouth, thus improving the textural appearance of the skin around the mouth. Brighter, lighter, more evenly coloured skin looks smoother and less wrinkled. Done right, these superficial treatments may also stimulate new collagen formation in the superficial dermis to help structurally reverse wrinkles too.

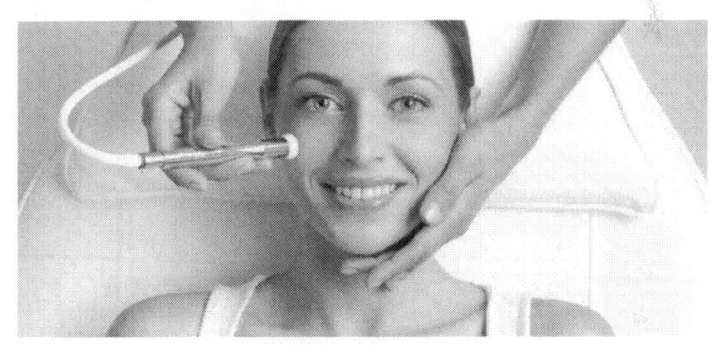

Illustration 123: Microdermabrasion

17.7 Smoker lines attenuation using electrical arcing (plasma) resurfacing and tightening

Over the years Voltaic arcing (also referred to as *Plasma* or *Micro Arcing*) has been used extensively in *perioral* lines attenuation with very good results. As you will see in this section this aesthetic procedure is safe and extremely easy to perform. It is recommended to advertise this aesthetic treatment as *perioral* lines attenuation, instead as *perioral* lines or *smoker lines* removal. Although some clinics may advertise this type of treatment with voltaic arcing devices as *perioral* lines removal or smoker lines removal this is best to be advertised as *perioral* lines attenuation as there is a mild improvement in the appearance of these lines after each treatment.

With electrical arcing the aesthetic treatment attenuates the *perioral* lines by "pulling" the area between the wrinkles taking advantage of both collagen regeneration and localised skin tightening.

Therefore, strictly speaking, Voltaic plasma cannot remove completely the vertical expression lines. With the "pulling" effect induced by the **localised skin tightening**, the the wrinkles become less and less visible after each treatment.

The best candidates for this procedure are women over 60 years of age who have been heavy smokers because, not only are they particularly motivated to have these wrinkles removed, but their vertical smoker lines are usually quite deep hence easily attenuated using electrical arcing (plasma). Therefore older women who have been smoking all their lives are usually very satisfied with the results achieved using this type of aesthetic treatment.

By using Electrical Arcing you apply the same **localised skin tightening** techniques which allow wrinkle attenuation around the *perioral* lines or at the edges. You can either use the **spot mode** or the **spray mode** for this type of **localised skin tightening**. The first time you attempt this aesthetic procedure using any or our devices, set the unit at minimum power level and apply the spots in a random fashion, with an instantaneous duration (one quarter of a second), and distancing them between 3 to 4 mm apart. As you gain experience with this type of treatment you can increase the intensity of the treatment by first decreasing the distance between the spots. Some experienced users move towards the **spray operation** as they gain experience.

In the video below we can appreciate an example of mild (low **treatment intensity)** for *perioral* line attenuation using electrical arcing. Our electrical arcing device was used at minimum power level. The aesthetic procedure in the video below is deliberately fast-forwarded. As you can see the beauty therapist in this case has removed only the part of the topical numbing product required to allow the treatment.

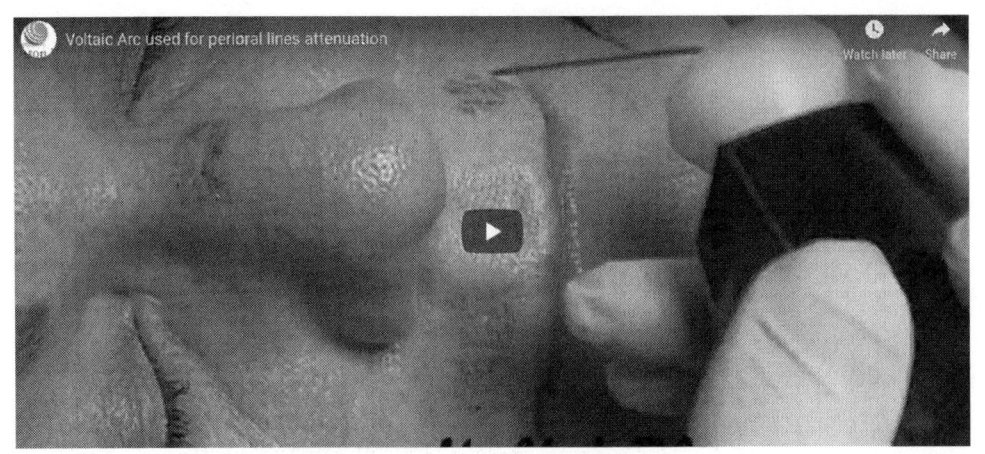

Illustration 124: Click here to watch video

Where the treatment is not being carried out the numbing product is still applied. It is highly recommended to only remove the topical numbing product in small patches to ensure the area you are going to treat is still numb at the time of the treatment. A common mistake made by beginners is to remove all numbing product all at once. Depending on the product used, the numbing effects maybe relatively short lived, therefore if the area to be treated is relatively extensive, the effects of the numbing product may have faded by the time you can treat area which previously had the numbing product applied on it. Treating an area while it is not numb can make the treatment rather uncomfortable to the client. For more information about the use of numbing products before this procedure please **click here**.

In the video below we can see the same procedure at normal speed. It is clear that the treatment is deliberately superficial (low intensity treatment). This is because the effects of the localised skin tightening do occur even when the arc has been applied very superficially (low intensity treatment). It is always advisable to apply the arc superficially when first performing localised **skin tightening using plasma**. It is far better to perform the treatment at low/medium intensity rather than using high intensity treatments. As explained in the skin tightening section the intensity of the treatment is not directly proportional to the skin tightening effects; rarely high intensity treatments are recommended for this aesthetic application. Therefore when in doubt, always apply the arc ensuring to be carrying out a very mild/medium intensity treatment. The treatment can then be repeated as required to achieve the desired results.

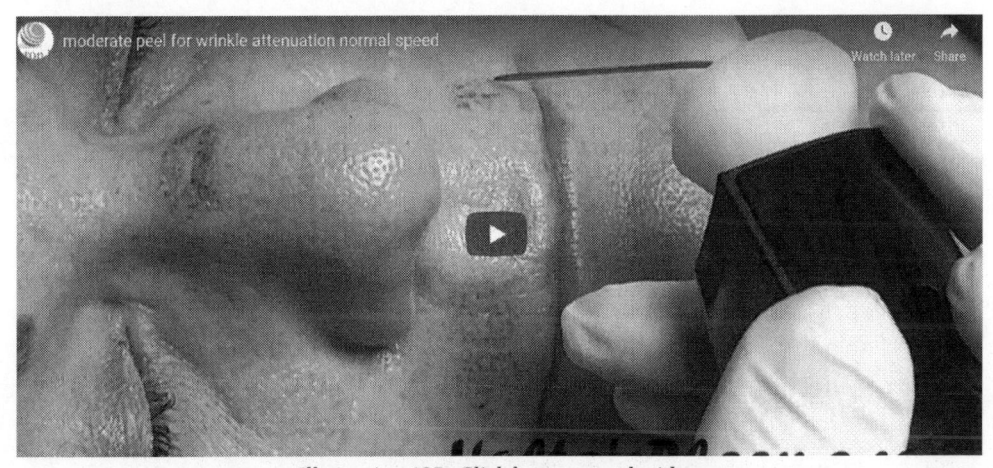

Illustration 125: Click here to watch video

Those who live a healthy lifestyle, also develop some form of *perioral* lines over time, however they are very easily attenuated due to the fact that there is no extensive skin damage caused by the oxidation effects of carbon monoxide in cigarette and tobacco smoke.

In the video below we can see an example of *perioral* lines attenuation treatment using plasma on a non smoker. In this case the client had made clear her intention to attenuate her very mild *perioral* wrinkles. Normally, the beauty practitioner would not intentionally advice this treatment to non smokers as their *perioral* lines are superficial and normally other aesthetic treatments using electrical arcing may be preferred such as Eyelid Tightening. However should the client expressedly request this treatment you can go ahead and perform it using low intensity treatments as demonstrated in the video below. The Beauty therapist in this case used a mild spraying technique. The device used was set at minimum power level. As you see in this short clip the fulguration is applied very superficially in short spraying bursts. Remember that the minimum power level of our electro fulguration devices are meant to be used for all the aesthetic treatments, it is especially recommended for beginner level.

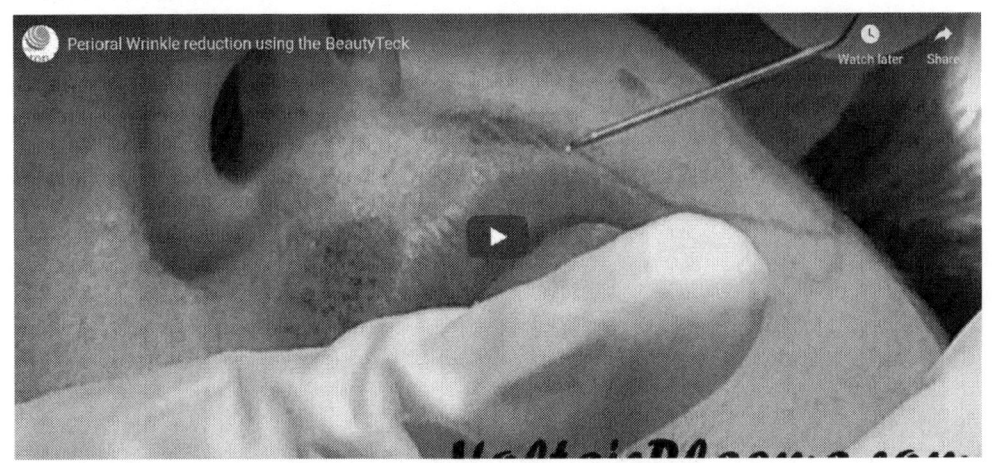

Illustration 126: Click here to watch video

In the video below we can see another example of a mild spray operation for smoker lines attenuation. The spraying motion is applied on the borders of each line. This is a mild intensity treatment.

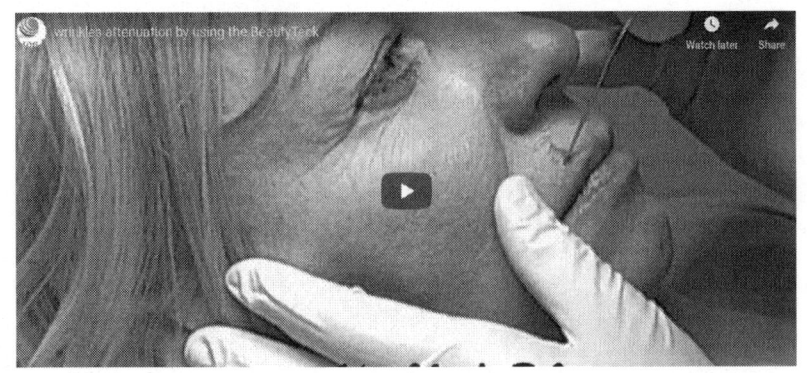

Illustration 127: Click here to watch video

17.8 Protocol for perioral lines attenuation using our electrical arcing devices

Apply the usual procedures before this type of aesthetic treatment such as screening the client, patch testing, explaining the content of the consent form and apply the appropriate numbing product before carrying out this type aesthetic treatment. The **pretreatment** procedures are the standard ones which can be found in this link **here**.

- Use the **spot mode** or **spot operation** between the *perioral* lines and not inside the lines themselves. When performing this type of aesthetic treatment for the first time apply the spots randomly distanced 3 to 4 mm apart. Apply the spots in a random fashion, with an instantaneous duration (one quarter of a second), and distancing them between 3 to 4 mm apart. As you gain experience with this type of treatment you can increase the intensity of the treatment by first decreasing the distance between the spots.
- Only use the **spray mode** or **spray operation** after you have gained confidence performing these types of treatments using the spot mode first. The user performs an epidermal superficial peel between the vertical wrinkles. Only some experienced users move towards the **spray operation** as they gain experience; most aesthetic practitioners prefer using the **spot operation** as it easy to use and leads to consistent results..
- After this procedure has been carried out, the client has to look after the area appropriately until the scabs have fallen off on their own accord. The main after care required is the use of the appropriate antiseptic to reduce the likelihood of infections during the skin recovery process. Scabs may or may not develop depending on the skin type and how the treatment has been carried out. In the spot mode the scabs tend to develop where the ablation points have been applied, in the spray mode the scabing will be replaced by a mild peeling effect instead. The scabs, if they develop they will start to form two to three days after the procedure. The client has make sure to pro-actively avoiding infections, and avoiding picking the scabs which may form and do not use any type of cover up make up until the scabs have fallen off by themselves. To review this section please read the standard **after care instructions**.
- **Treatment Downtime**. The client can resume any of their normal professional activities immediately after this aesthetic treatment, however the client should purposely avoid any activities which can increase the exposure to potential infections. Normally redness occurs immediately after this type of aesthetic treatment.There could be some degree of swelling associated to this treatment. However swelling is a rare occurrence and usually takes place after high intensity treatments and starts the day after the treatment peaking the third to fourth day subsiding on its own accord. On average the *perceived downtime* is 7 days and this varies according to the intensity treatment and the individual skin reaction.
- The treatment can be repeated every 4 to 5 weeks. Depending on the skin reaction to the treatment (ie the skin is still pinkish after 4 to 6 weeks). Wait until the skin colour is normal before repeating the treatment
- Normally for deep *perioral* lines (smoker lines) 4 to 5 medium intensity treatments may be required in order to achieve satisfactory results.

- In case of mild *perioral* lines in non smokers one to two medium intensity treatments may suffice to achieve the desired results.

17.9 Manage perioral lines after the permanent attenuation treatments

Although they maybe challenging to improve there are several aesthetic treatments available for *perioral* lines attenuation, some are temporary and others are permanent. Once the main "permanent" aesthetic treatment for *perioral* lines attenuation has been carried out successfully, you may want to delay its recurrence, this is done by tackling the two root causes of the *perioral* lines formation by

1. Reducing the muscle movements,
2. and delay the natural or induced (by smoking) Skin Oxidation (ageing).

The muscle movement cannot be impaired completely as it is necessary for normal daily activities, however **appropriate** Botox injections can help reduce the muscle action and eventually delay the recurrence of the smoker lines. Therefore the periodical use of Botox can serve as a preventative treatment to try and delay the worsening of the *perioral* lines over the long haul.

Skin oxidation can be delayed simply by quitting smoking, taking on a balanced diet, reducing alcohol consumption, avoiding exposure to UV light both from natural and artificial sources; also starting or continuing regular moderate physical exercise can be beneficial.

18.0 Brown Spots

Superficial brown spots may appear due to prolonged sun exposure without appropriate sun protection. It often appears in people over 40 years of age. Brown/Sun Spots usually disappear after superficial peeling of the epidermis by using AC electrical arcing devices or other cosmetic peels. This is because brown spots are usually quite superficial and therefore a mild skin resurfacing treatment usually suffices in order to remove them.

18.1 How to remove Superficial Brown Spots using Voltaic arc

- → Apply the appropriate numbing product for your client's maximum comfort.
- → Set the device at a minimum power level (level 1 with three batteries if you are using the BeautyTeck). Gently spray the brown spot and wipe off the carbon residues. Usually, one gentle spray motion will suffice to remove the superficial pigments of the brown spot.

- ➢ → If superficial brown spots are left untreated the pigments of the brown spots move deeper into the skin over time becoming eventually Age Spots. Age spots are usually found in clients over 60 years of age.

- ➢ → It should be noted that age spots are not going to disappear using a superficial ablation. It is highly recommended not to try and remove age spots within one session as this will require a deeper ablation that could later develop into scarring. Instead, it is recommended to perform 2 to 3 superficial treatments, spread 4 weeks apart from each other and let the part recover between treatments for at least 4 weeks.

- ➢ → Remind the importance of the **aftercare** to your clients

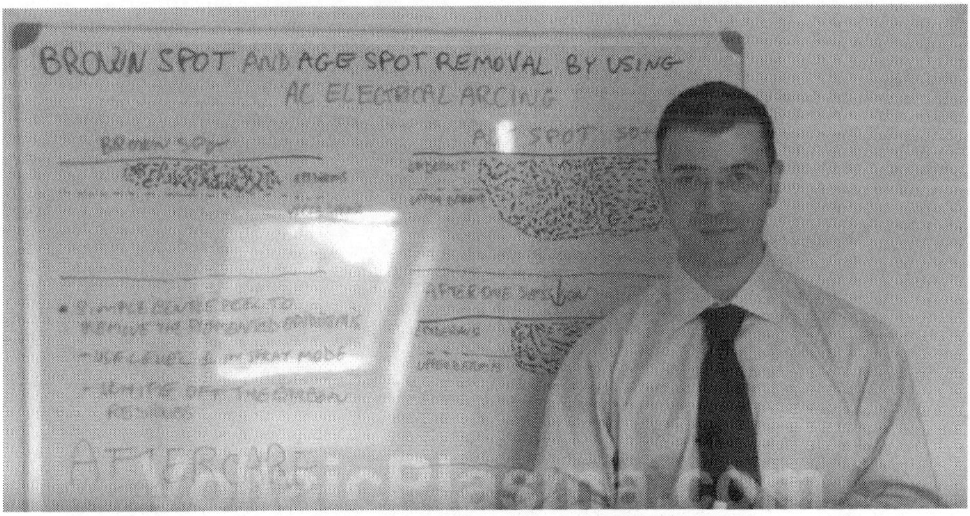

Illustration 128: Click here to watch video

19.0 Moles and skin lesions removal, make sure they are benign first

When we are working to remove moles and benign skin growths we first need to be sure that the lesion is not cancerous. This is very important, because if you removed a lesion which was pre cancerous or cancerous this could cause grave risks to the person you removed the lesions from. But why? This is because when you remove a mole for aesthetic reasons all you are interested in is achieving the best possible aesthetic results. In case the lesion you removed was cancerous, likely you may not have removed it completely and the cancer may continue to grow and spread without the person noticing it on time. Therefore, it is important to perform a correct diagnosis before removing the mole. But how is a diagnosis performed?

Page 138

Up until today, the way a skin diagnosis is made, are symptom-based. The specialist examines the colour, size, shape of a skin condition and asks you a few questions. Based on his/her experience or knowledge he/she may be able to make an educated guess of the skin condition you may have.

It is very important to understand that, up until today, it is very unlikely to have 100% guarantee that any diagnosis made in this manner is correct which is to say based on the specialist's opinion alone. Normally the easiest basic test your doctor or GP applies is the **ABCDE rule**. This is when the doctor tries to exclude that the particular lesion may be sinister.

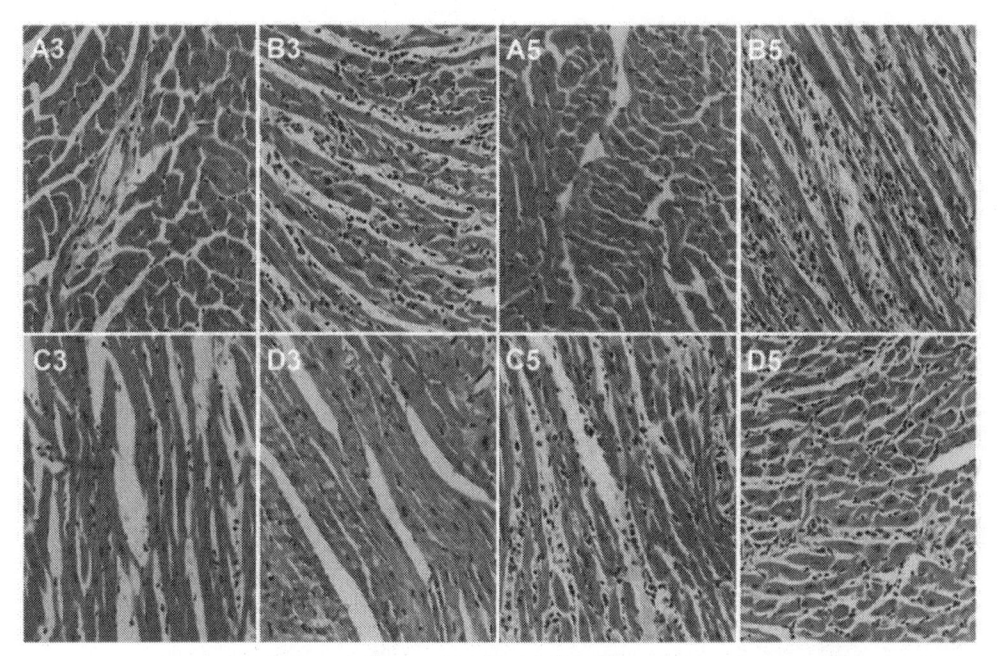

Illustration 129: Under skin

Medicine is never an exact science and currently, the only known way to have the best degree of certainty that you have a correct diagnosis of each lesion on your body is the use of histological examinations. A histological examination is a detailed observation of the tissue of a living organism's tissue under the microscope. By examining the tissue in the microscope one can have the best chances to make the most accurate diagnosis currently possible.

To this day, the problem with histological examinations is that it is still impractical to perform on all the lesions on our body for two reasons:

www.voltaicplasma.com					Author: Andreas Russo

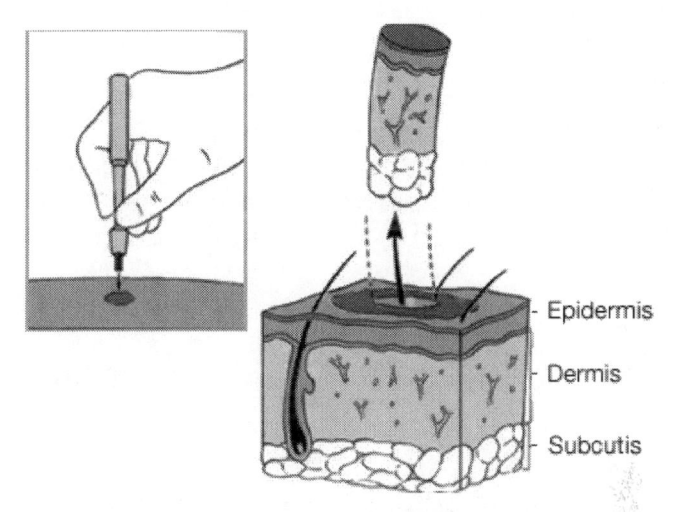

Illustration 130: A punch biopsy of the skin. The sample will be sent to the lab for histological examination. A punch biopsy is generally only performed if the doctor deems necessary to perform further investigations.

→ Generally, because in order to extract the cell of the particular lesion a biopsy is required. Biopsies are rather invasive and are very likely to leave a scar. Also, it would be impractical to perform a biopsy on each lesion on our body because there are so many of them.

→ The real resources allocated (i.e costs) to performing a histological examination itself are relatively significant.

For these two reasons (scarring and costs), the doctor or specialist, normally makes an estimation of how likely the lesions may be benign (harmless). In case the perceived likelihood of the lesion to be nonbenign is relatively high, the doctor will opt to perform a punch biopsy to send the sample taken to the lab for a histological examination.

In this way (by visual inspection), the diagnosis although not 100% accurate will provide the best compromise in terms of invasiveness and costs, while hopefully still maintaining an acceptable degree of accuracy.

To summarise, only a histological examination can guarantee the highest probability of an accurate diagnosis.

The specialist's trained eye can provide and indication but it is never guarantee of a 100% accurate diagnosis, despite his/her qualifications or experience.

So if you are not a specialist what is the practical solution? You are not capable of formulating an accurate diagnosis and even if you are, you may not be even qualified to do it!

The solution is simple:

- Learn yourself how to identify any possible cancerous mole. There is a lot of information and courses available for you to train your eye and ask the right questions. If you suspect the lesion may not benign, immediately refer your client to a dermatologist.

- Make sure you include in your consent form a clause that states that you do not make any diagnosis and you remove any skin lesions under the assumption that each one of those the client wants to have removed has been previously examined by a specialist and declared non cancerous. If you are not sure about the consent form, please feel free to use ours, it is on Voltaicplasma.com

20.0 Moles and skin lesions removal

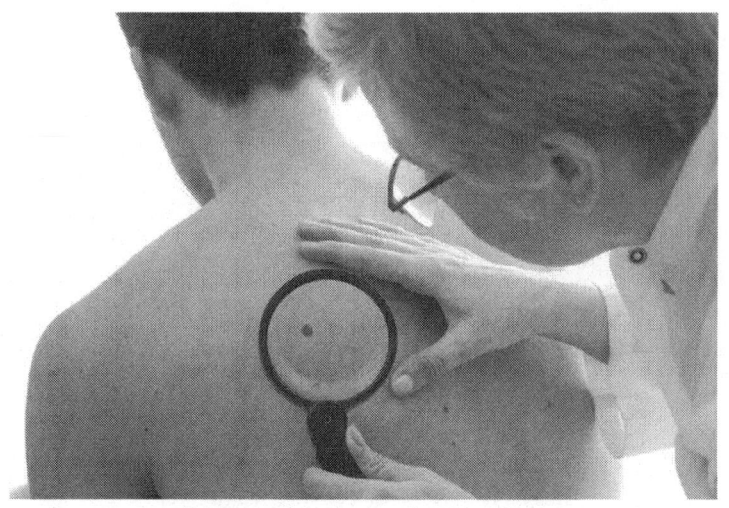

Illustration 131: Moles and Skin lesions

20.1 Manual excision using a conventional scalpel

Before considering removing a mole using any method it is essential that a proper diagnosis of the mole is carried out.

This is because if a potentially cancerous mole or birthmark is not properly removed it can potentially aggravate risks to the client. Therefore if there is the slightest concern that a mole could be dangerous, the client should be referred to a specialist. The specialist will perform a biopsy and the mole will be sent for histological examination.

This is the traditional method for removing **birthmarks. This is the best way to remove a mole or birthmark that have chances of being cancerous. The birthmark itself is removed as well as a part of the surrounding healthy skin.**

This is necessary for histological examination. The histologist needs to examine both the birthmark and the healthy skin to make sure they will able to make an appropriate diagnosis. Manual excision will almost always result in scarring, therefore it is now only used if the mole appears to be dangerous and there may be chances of further developments.

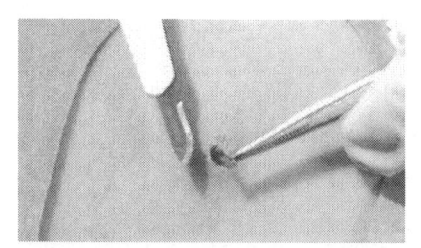

Illustration 132: This is the traditional method for removing birthmarks. This is the best way to remove a mole or birthmark that have chances of being cancerous

20.2 Mole removal using laser

The technique used to remove moles for aesthetic reasons is to ablate the skin lesion superficially. The ablation is generally carried out until the mole is "flattened". In other words, the mole is burned (or vaporized) superficially until it is level with the surrounding skin. Please note that this is a very generalised method. There are certain skin lesions like Xanthelasma, Syringoma and others that require a deep ablation to remove them completely in one session.

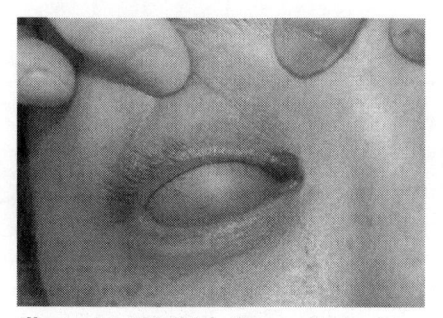

Illustration 133: Mole Removal using laser

Click here to watch video

In the video we can see an example of mole removal using a laser. This easy procedure is carried out by setting the device at a relatively high power and repeating the vaporization of the mole a number of times, until achieving the desired results. As you can see the practitioner rubs the finger on to the mole a number of times to appraise whether the mole is level with the surrounding skin. This method is used to achieve the best possible aesthetic results and minimizing the likelihood of scarring.

The technique we have seen above is oversimplified because there are several types of moles (or more in general benign skin lesions). Some moles require a deeper ablation than others. This depends on how the benign mole grows inside the skin. As we will see in removing Xanthelasma, for instance, these lesions can grow deeply inside the skin, while some others like seborrhoeic keratoses are very superficial.

www.voltaicplasma.com   Author: Andreas Russo

However, when the practitioner is not sure about the best way to remove a mole, the levelling method is preferred as this minimizes the likelihood of scarring.

20.3 Mole removal with voltaic arc or voltaic plasma

There are many ways to remove benign moles and the use of AC electrical arc is one of them. Like aesthetic lasers, voltaic arc (also referred to as plasma) allows easy removal of benign birthmarks and moles. If the mole is removed properly and the aftercare is followed, the risks of scarring are very low, however, a minor likelihood of scarring exist despite the method used and cannot be completely ruled out.

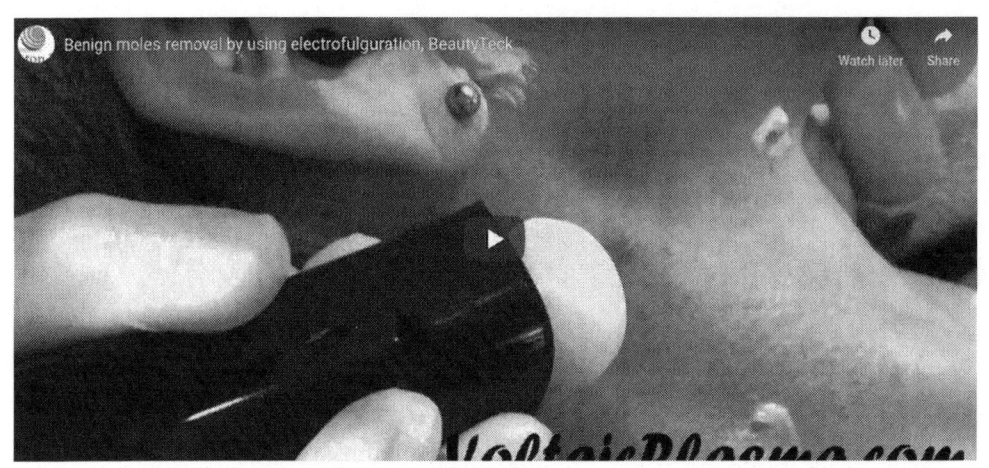

Illustration 134: Click here to watch video on Mole Removal using Plasma

This type of procedure can be performed by a healthcare professional as well as a beautician or any other appropriately trained non medical personnel as long as the mole is benign and removed for cosmetic or comfort reasons. There are several types of benign growths which are referred to as benign moles.

As a general rule *in order to minimize the risks of scarring it is recommended that the mole removed is leveled off with the surrounding skin area. Remember that no guarantee can be made of a scar-free outcome despite the method or device used to remove the benign skin lesion.*

www.voltaicplasma.com   Author: Andreas Russo

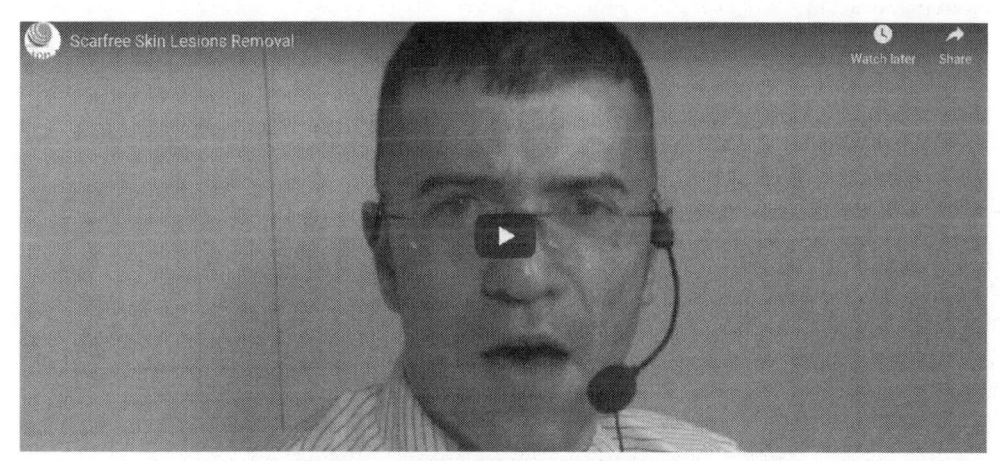

Illustration 135: Click here to watch video

Certain particular types of benign growths maybe rooted between the dermis and the epidermis and may require a specific technique to remove them in one session only. Having the knowledge of the type of benign lesion you are dealing with, will help you in the effective removal of the lesion is a single session. If the benign lesion is rooted between the dermis and epidermis, a slightly deeper ablation (or burn) may be required to remove the lesion in one session only. If these more deeply rooted moles are leveled off with the surrounding skin area, multiple sessions may be required to remove them effectively.

20.4 The techniques generally used for benign mole removal is the spray operation

Generally, moles can be effectively and quickly removed by burning them off using AC electrical arc by starting from the top and working all the way down to level them off with the surrounding skin area. Particularly thick moles maybe better removed with the device set at the maximum power level in order to remove the bulk of the mole effectively within a reasonable timeframe. Normally experienced users set the device at the top power level to coarsely remove the main bulk of the thick mole. However, when you first start using this type of device it is advisable to apply the arc at a minimum power level or generally low power settings, in order to gain confidence with this type of procedure.

Also, if you are a first time user of AC electrical arc, after every voltaic arc short spray, wipe the carbon residues away by using a cotton pad impregnated with non-flammable antiseptic to clear the carbon residues. This will allow you to get used to the amount of mole ablation possible with the device set at the predetermined power level. When the carbon residues are cleared you can see the level of ablation you have reached. You can also feel the remainder of the mole to be removed by running the tip of your finger on the mole you are removing. As long as you feel a small bump this means that you still have some work to do to level it off.

www.voltaicplasma.com   Author: Andreas Russo

Page 144

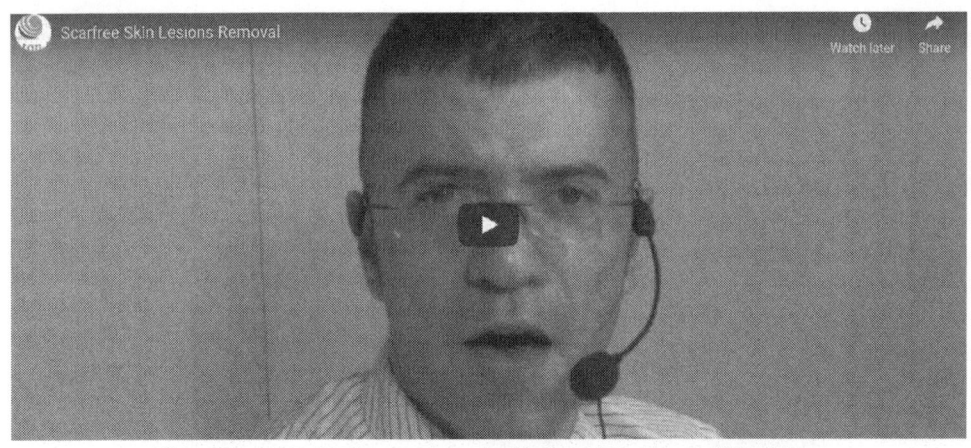

Illustration 136: Click here to watch video on Mole Removal Workshop

Start reducing the power level of the device to the minimum setting, when, after touching the mole you feel that bump is very thin and you are about to level off the mole with the surrounding skin area. This is because reducing the power level will allow a higher degree of accuracy in the ablation of the mole. The lower the power level the higher the degree of precision you will be able to operate in the leveling off of the mole. The more experience you gain the more confident you will be in the removal of the mole.

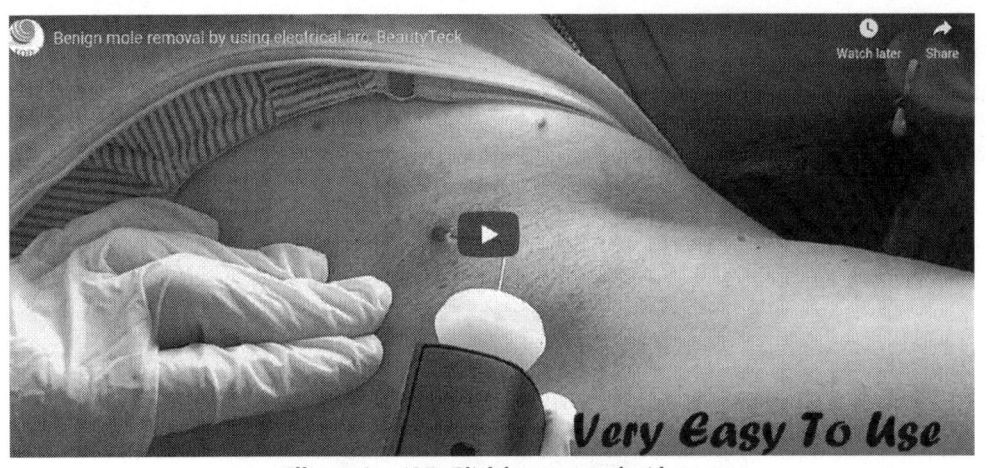

Illustration 137: Click here to watch video

When removing small and thin moles, low power levels may suffice to remove the small moles quickly. If you suspect a mole to be thin it is advisable to ablating the mole by using the lowest power level. You may also find that for small thin moles a short spraying on the top of the mole will suffice to

www.voltaicplasma.com　　　　　　　　　　　　　　　　　　Author: Andreas Russo

remove them. Always wipe off the carbon residues after every burst especially when you start removing moles using voltaic arc.

20.5 Summary

→ Make sure that the mole your client intends to have removed is a benign growth.

→ Explain the content of the consent form and have it signed by the client. Explain that there are no guarantees that a scar may not replace the mole after removal.

→ Take before pictures of the moles and store them electronically, they will turn out useful in the future.

→ Apply numbing cream on the mole. Follow the instructions of the numbing cream supplier.

→ Once the area is numb, wipe the cream residues away and start removing the mole.

→ In case of particularly thick moles, and if you are an experienced user, start burning the top of the mole with the equipment set at a top power level, to remove the bulk of the mole within a convenient time frame. Wipe off the carbon residues after each burst to appreciate the level you have reached. Repeat the process until you have almost reached the surrounding skin level. When you are close enough to levelling off the mole, reduce the power level to increase the level of precision of the ablation in order to level off the remainder of the mole with surrounding skin really well.

→ For thin moles use the device set at minimum power setting and wipe off the carbon residues after each spray burst. You may find that in some cases the thin mole is completely wiped off after a short spray burst at minimum power.

→ Apply the appropriate soothing product and antiseptic immediately after the removal.

→ Emphasizing its importance, hand out the appropriate aftercare information sheet to the Client.

→ Explicitly instruct the client not expose the area to potential infections.

→ Explicitly instruct the client to use sunscreen and avoid direct sun exposure for up to 3 months after the treatment. The sun screen must be used once the scab have fallen off of course not before.

If you want to watch examples of how moles are removed using AC electric arc please refer to the many videos on mole removal in our channel.

The latter method has been very effective, however, it is still possible to remove thick moles by applying the tip of the electrode by starting to apply the arc from the top and work all the way to the base or the benign mole.

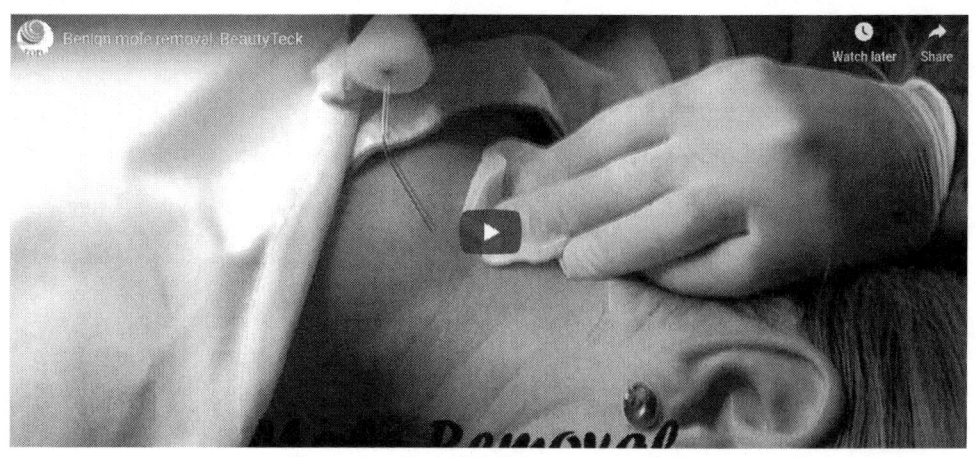

Illustration 138: Click here to watch video

21.0 Seborrheic Keratoses

Seborrheic keratoses are noncancerous (benign) skin growths that some people develop as they age. They often appear on the back or chest, but can occur on any part of the body. Seborrheic keratoses grow slowly, in groups or singly. Most people will develop at least one seborrheic keratosis during their lifetime.

Seborrheic Keratoses are completely safe, they grow superficially on the skin and they certainly do not require any intervention other than for aesthetic reasons. Seborrheic keratosis are proven to be safe therefore their removal is only for aesthetic reasons and they are not required to be removed for any medical reason whatsoever.

Because seborrheic keratoses grow more and more on the body over time they are sometimes referred to as senile warts. But they are not to be confused with warts because they have nothing to do with warts.

Removing them using plasma or fibroblast is extremely easy. You have to spray the arc on top of the keratoses and then rub off the residue with a cotton pad. If after spraying once the keratoses is difficult to remove, repeat the spraying once again and repeat rubbing the keratoses again with the cotton pad.

The results using electrical arcing are very good and usually after healing the area look as if the keratoses had never been there. Also the keratosys removal

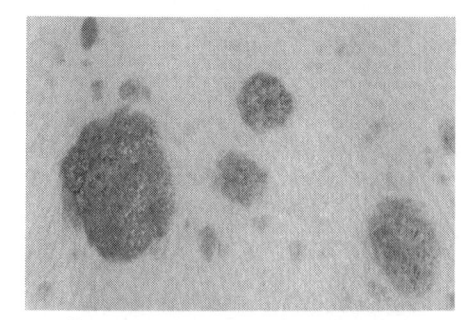

Illustration 139: Seborrheic Keratoses

Click here to watch the video

using plasma is instantaneous and the results are very good because the nature of seborrheic keratoses. Attention, because you must have an accurate diagnosis before going ahead and remove any skin lesion. If the skin lesion is not benign removing it using electrical arcing may cause issues in the future.

22.0 Syringoma

We have detailed information on syringoma on our page Syringomaremoval.com please visit this website to learn all about syringoma in details.

22.1 How to remove Syringoma using electrical arcing

Remove all makeup thoroughly and make sure the area is clean. Wipe the area you intend to treat with the appropriate nonflammable antiseptic. Once the area is clean, dry and disinfected, apply the appropriate numbing topical product for the comfort of your client only during this simple aesthetic procedure.

(For Medical practitioners only). If you are authorized to use injectable local anaesthetic you can do so for this particular aesthetic treatment, however, this is not strictly necessary and the use of an effective topical numbing product will be usually sufficient to allow you to carry out this simple aesthetic procedure in complete comfort to the client and ease to yourself.

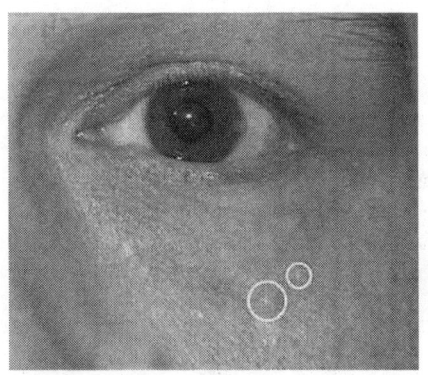

Illustration 140: Syringoma underneath the eyelid

Click here to watch video on Syringoma

For Syringoma removal it is advisable to set our electro fulguration device at a minimum power level for maximum precision of operation. If you are an experienced user you can also increase the power level slightly, however, the minimum power level is recommended as Syringoma are rarely thick.

Apply the spray mode to simply levelling the Syringoma off with the surrounding skin as shown extensively in voltaicplasma.com. Remember to wipe off the carbon residues from time to time, preferably after every spraying operation.

www.voltaicplasma.com						Author: Andreas Russo

22.2 Syringoma Recurrence

Please bear in mind that there is no currently known method to guarantee the Syringoma are removed permanently. This is because Syringoma tend to recur and therefore the effects of Syringoma removal can be only transient. This applies to any method used to remove Syringoma be it laser, electrical arcing (Electrofulguration or electrodesiccation), TCA and other cosmetic peels, including cryotherapy. This means that despite the fact that they are effectively removed completely during your professional aesthetic removal session, they can reappear a few weeks later in the same areas where they have been removed.

Unfortunately, these recurrence effects have been extensively reported by several people who have undergone various aesthetic treatments to remove them. This is due to the very persistent nature of Syringoma. Therefore it is advisable to include this information on the consent form before proceeding to treat a case of Syringoma to avoid future client disappointment.

23.0 Xanthelasma

We have detailed information on Xanthelasma on our page XanthelasmaRemoval.com please visit this website to learn all about Xanthelasma in detail.

If you are using voltaic arcing for Xanthelasma removal, you can either opt for levelling off this benign skin lesion with the surrounding skin area or you can remove also the part of the lesion which resides inside the skin. If you only level off this type of lesion, you usually require to perform a number of treatments in order to remove them completely. If you want to remove the Xanthelasma in one session you would usually need to remove the deep part of the Xanthelasma as well.

The usual question is: how do I know when to stop ablating the Xanthelasma? After wiping off the carbon residues with a cotton pad impregnated with non-flammable antiseptic if you notice that some yellow fatty residues are still present then you may want to carry on burning off the Xanthelasma until you remove all the yellow residues and there is no trace of any fatty deposits.

Be careful because if you ablate too deeply, you damage the inner part of the dermis the risks of scarring increases. Remember that there is no currently known way to remove benign lesions while guaranteeing that the final results will be scar-free. All you can do is minimize the risks of developing permanent scarring.

www.voltaicplasma.com

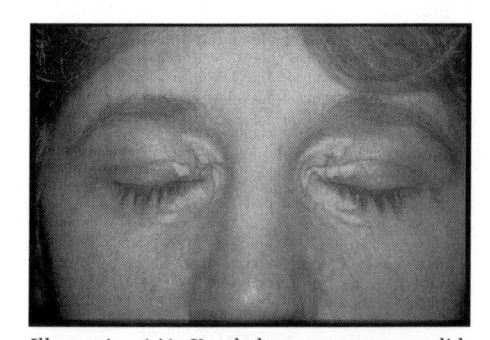

Illustration 141: Xanthelasma on upper eyelid

Click here to watch video

If removed completely, the new skin tissue grown after the part has healed, usually has a pinkish texture to it and this is normal.

The first time you attempt Xanthelasma Removal remember to be cautious and it is generally better to have the client to come back with a smaller Xanthelasma than going too deep with the removal.

The aftercare is up to your client and if infections arise after this simple aesthetic procedure, risks of permanent scarring can increase.

24.0 SkinTags Removal using Fibroblast

Skin tags are very common but harmless small, soft skin growths. They tend to occur on the eyelids, neck, armpits, groin folds, and under the breasts. One person may have anywhere from one to over 100 skin tags. Almost everyone will develop a skin tag at some point in their life. Middle-aged, adults are most prone to developing skin tags. Obesity seems to be also associated with the tendency of forming skin tags.

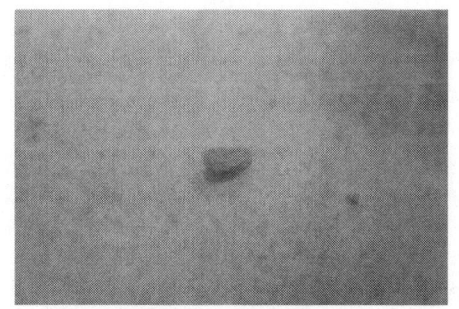

Illustration 142: Skin Tags

Click here to watch video

\Removing a skin tag does not cause more to grow and the procedures to remove them are generally easy and harmless.

When removing skin tags by using electrical arcing you have two possible approaches:

→ Apply the electric arc on top of the skin tag and work all the way down until you have almost reached the base of it (skin level). At that point, if you have not already done so, reduce the power level of the device to the minimum to allow the greatest degree of precision. Continue the carbonization of the skin tag until you have leveled it off with the surrounding skin. Remember to wipe off the carbon residues from time to time to allow you to see the level you have reached.

→ In case the skin tag you are removing is particularly large you can apply the arc onto an area of the skin tags itself close to skin level. Once the skin tag has become detached, you can then proceed to level off the remaining skin tag residues with the surrounding skin in order to accomplish good aesthetic results. The aftercare is left to your client.

Some other treatments to remove them include freezing, tying off with a thread or suture, or cutting them off.

25.0 Keloids

After the skin is injured, in certain cases the healing process can leave a raised or a depressed scar. However, not all wounds will leave a scar. Normally very superficial wounds do not leave scars, provided that the healing process is smooth and there are not significant infections. It is important to understand that generally, scars develop when a certain degree of damage to the dermis has been caused either by an injury or infection. The scar is a normal reaction to the damage caused to the dermis.

25.1 How and why does a Scar Form?

After the skin is injured, in certain cases the healing process can leave a raised or a depressed scar. However, not all wounds will leave a scar. Normally very superficial wounds do not leave scars, provided that the healing process is smooth and there are not significant infections. It is important to understand that generally, scars develop when a certain degree of damage to the dermis has been caused either by an injury or infection. The scar is a normal reaction to the damage caused to the dermis. In case of deep wounds (ie deep cuts, like those of serious accidents or surgical procedures) they usually develop into some form of scarring even if the healing process is smooth and free of infections. This is because in deep wounds the deeper part of the dermis (hypodermis) is usually affected and whenever the hypodermis is injured in some way the healing process will eventually lead to some degree of scarring, despite the way the wound has healed.

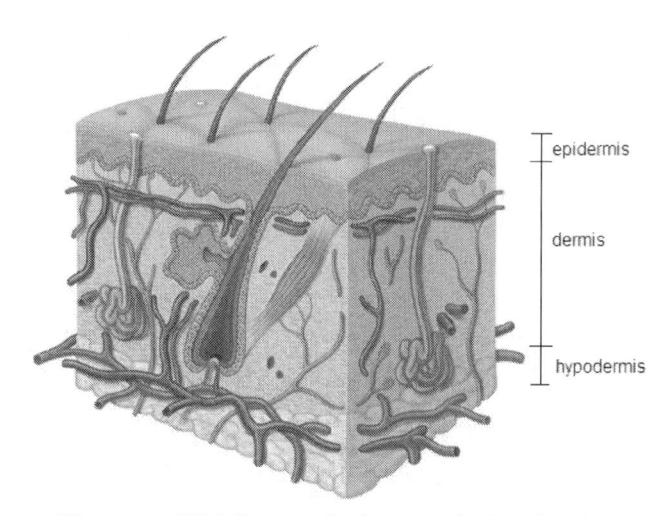

Illustration 143: Whenever the dermis or the hypodermis are affected by an injury the wound will eventually develop into a certain degree of scarring

In case the injury only involves the upper part of the dermis, if the wound heals speedily and appropriate after-care is followed then the likelihood of developing a scar decreases dramatically. On the other hand, even a superficial wound can develop into a fully fledged hypertrophic scar if infections arise and persist over a long period of time. This is because the longer the infection persists the higher the likelihood of a certain degree of damage to be caused to the dermis. Sometimes a scar is hypertrophic (thickened/raised), or atrophic (depressed), but always confined to the margin of the original wound or injury. Hypertrophic scars, initially tend to be redder and often regress spontaneously (a process which can take one year or more). Hypertrophic scars develop during the wound healing process and not only do they stop growing when the healing process is over, but also they decrease in size over time on their own accord.

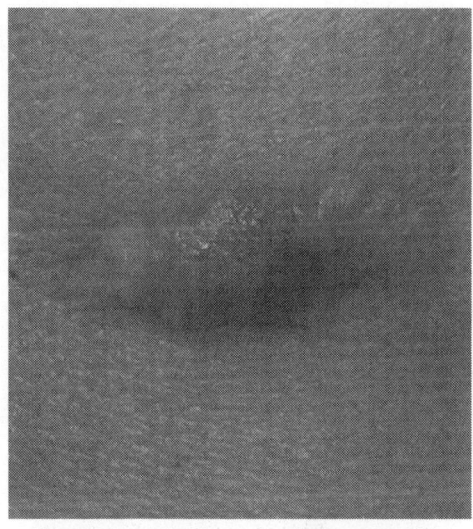

Illustration 145: Example of a Hypertrophic Scar. This picture was taken soon after the healing was over. The scar is still pinker than the rest of the skin. The Scar is also confined to the borders of the original wound.

Hypertrophic scar removal treatment, such as cortisone injections (steroids), can speed up this natural scar shrinkage process. Also, hypertrophic scar removal is relatively easy by using most ablative methods including lasers, electrical arcing, surgical excision and other methods. This is because the hypertrophic scars will not tend to grow back.

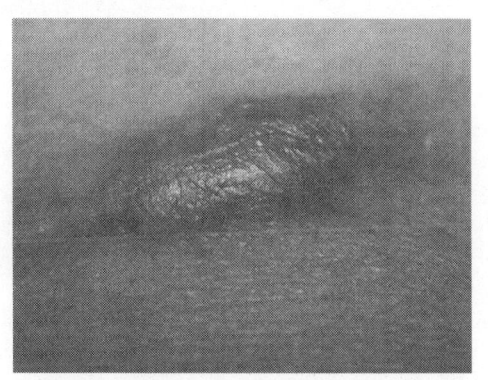

Illustration 146: Another example of a recently formed hypertrophic scar. These types of scars are very easily removed by using most ablative methods in aesthetics, including lasers and electrical arcing. They do not tend to redevelop when removed.

25.2 Keloids and the fundamental difference from hypertrophic scars

Keloids, by contrast, may start sometime after a cutaneous injury of any type including normal acne, minor burns, chickenpox, ear piercing and piercings in general, minor scratches, surgical incision, injections, tattooing, laser aesthetic treatments including skin tightening, more in general any event which will trigger the skin regeneration process.

They can also develop after some minor inflammation. Often Keloids can be mistaken for hypertrophic scars and vice versa. Keloids tend to extend beyond the wound site. This tendency to migrate into surrounding areas that weren't injured originally distinguishes Keloids from hypertrophic scars. Also, another difference between Keloids and hypertrophic scars is that Hypertrophic scars are formed during the healing process and stop developing as soon as the area has healed, on the other hand, Keloids do not stop growing when the healing process is over.
Sometimes Keloids keep growing weeks after the original injury has healed.

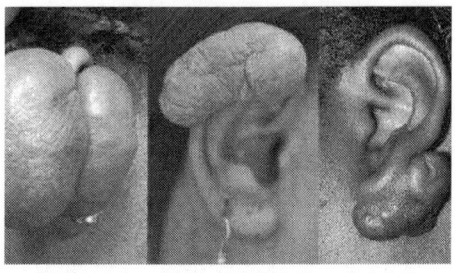

Illustration 147: One of the reasons Keloids appear often on the earlobes is due to ear piercing. This picture illustrates clearly how Keloidal formations tend to grow well beyond the original boundaries of the original injury which caused it.

Keloids "per se" are benign and non-dangerous growths, however, they can be compared to benign tumours due to their tendency to sustain growth after their initial formation. In case the growth seems disproportionate and persists over the period of several weeks leading to abnormal (irregular) shapes and disproportionate dimensions, like in case of formations displayed in Illustration 82 for example, then excision for a histological examination is recommended. This is to make sure the growth although abnormal is benign. Please bear in mind that there is no scientifically proven connection between Keloidal formations and dangerous growths.

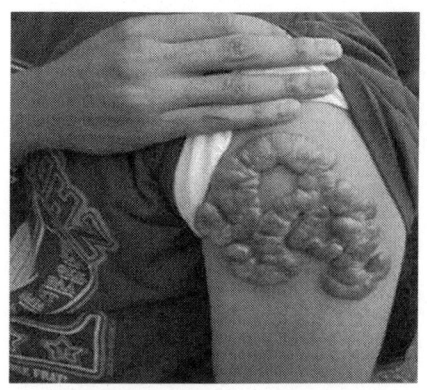

Illustration 147: A classic example of unintended Keloidal formation after a tattooing treatment.

www.voltaicplasma.com Author: Andreas Russo

The difference between a classic Keloidal formation and a Hypertrophic scar is noted by comparing the illustrartions of the hypertrophic scars and the keloids. The Keloidal formations are always clearly protruding and they do not present the normal pinkish colour of a normal Hypertrophic scar which is clearly confined within the borders of the original injury. Also it is possible to notice how the Keloidal formation is overgrowing. **In illustration 84** on the right, we can appreciate the clear Keloidal formation after heart surgery. The Keloids also formed on the suture points. The Hypertrophic scars, in contrast, are very well confined within the original boundaries of the wound that initially formed it (**See illustration 80 and 81**). Keloids affect both sexes equally, although the incidence in the young female population has been reported to be higher than in young males, probably reflecting the greater frequency of earlobe piercing among women. The frequency of Keloidal occurrence is 15 times higher in highly pigmented people (skin types 4, 5 and 6). Therefore African, Asian and Indian descendants have increased likelihood of Keloidal occurrences. It is also shown that the tendency to form Keloids is familial, therefore if one of your ancestors had this tendency then you will be more likely to form Keloids too.

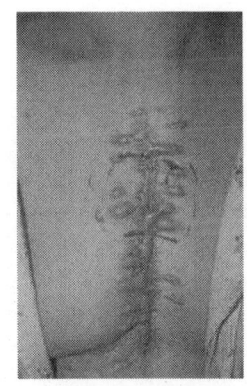

Illustration 148: Keloidal formations after heart surgery. The suture points are demarcated by the clear keloids.

25.3 Keloid removal treatments

While hypertrophic scars are very easily removed by using various ablation methods, including lasers, electrical arcing, cryotherapy, excision etc, the removal of keloidal formations can be challenging

This is because, despite the fact that they are removed using the several ablation methods currently available including surgical excision, Keloids tend to "grow back" or even expand or increase in size after their removal. Unfortunately, there is no known treatment which can scientifically guarantee Keloids will not recur after the removal.

Despite the method used to remove any Keloidal formation, if a preventative measure to avoid the

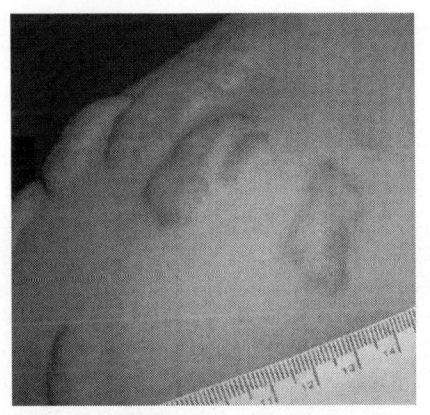

Illustration 149: Keloids on skin type 1. Keloids rarely affect lighter skin types.

While hypertrophic scars are very easily removed by using various ablation methods, including lasers, electrical arcing, cryotherapy, excision etc, the removal of keloidal formations can be challenging

www.voltaicplasma.com

Keloidal recurrence is not used the lesion will "grow back" or worse, even regrow larger. Therefore any form of ablation alone is not sufficient to remove this type of lesion, or may even be detrimental due to the natural tendency of Keloids to develop and expand after a traumatic event to the skin. The methods used to prevent the regrowth of the Keloid after their removal using ablative methods are Cortisone or Fluorouracil superficial injections, Radio Therapy and others. These regrowths preventative methods are applied soon after the Keloid removal procedure using ablative methods (ie lasers, electrical arcing, cryotherapy, surgical excision etc). This is because any ablative method inevitably causes a skin traumatic event which will, in turn, trigger the Keloidal growth. For this reason, any effective treatment has to focus on having the Keloids to stop growing back after their removal. No single regrowth preventative treatment is best for all Keloids because they may react differently to different treatments. The Keloid location, size, depth of the lesion, the age of the person, and the past response to the removal treatment may determine the best type of removal treatment.

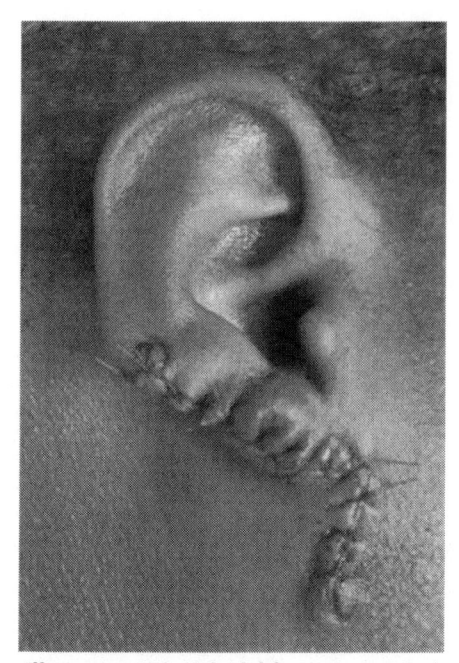

Illustration 150: Keloidal formation excised surgically. The surgical removal alone may be futile as the Keloid will tend to grow back due to the injury caused by the surgery itself. Therefore a post-surgical treatment to prevent the Keloid to recur will be necessary.

25.4 Steroids injections (or intralesional corticosteroid injections)

One of the most known and economical methods to reduce the size of Keloidal formations is the use of injectable (steroids) cortisone, directly administered into the lesion. In most cases, this alone has been shown to reduce the size of the Keloidal formations without the use of any other ablative methods. As we know ablative methods of any type bear an inherent likelihood of Keloid recurrence as well as the potential increase in the size of the Keloid itself.

Page 155

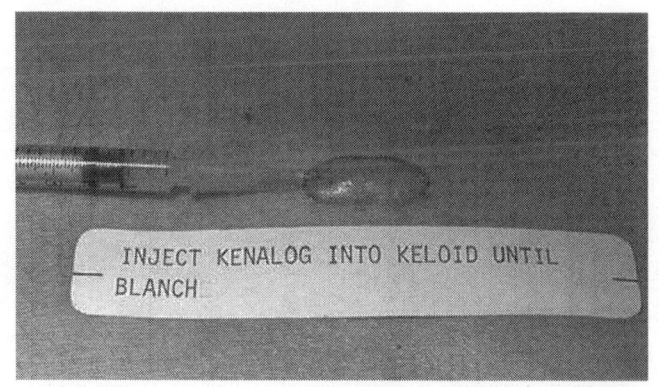

Illustration 151: "Kenalog" is a brand name for "Triamcinolone Acetonide" which is a synthetic corticosteroid used to treat various skin conditions. In this image, we can see how the needle has to be inserted into the Keloid.

Cortisone injections are administered into the Keloid at 6 weeks interval and after each session normally the Keloid will reduce progressively in size by its own accord. The advantage of using this method is primarily the wide availability of safe and suitable steroids on the market. Furthermore, the first steroid course of injections alone will provide a clear indication if the Keloid responds well to this type of treatment. The avoidance of invasive (surgical) and non-invasive (lasers or voltaic arcing) ablative treatments is a clear benefit because the skin does not require to undergo any traumatic events which could trigger a Keloidal regrowth or enlargement. This type of treatment will consist of a number of cortisone injections into the Keloids made at four to six weeks interval. This treatment on its own will suffice to reduce the Keloid in size after each course of a cortisone injection.

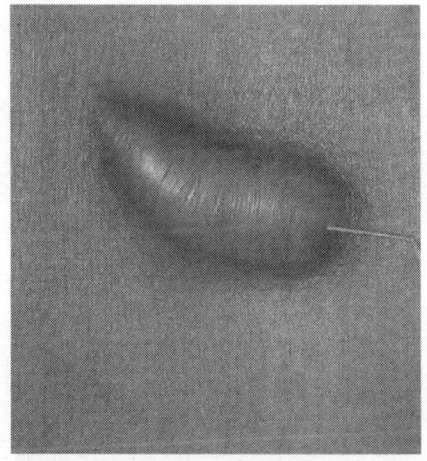

Illustration 152: Cortisone injection directly administered into the Keloidal formation.

www.voltaicplasma.com   Author: Andreas Russo

The use of cortisone injections should be the first attempt to treat Keloidal formations. It is important to emphasise that if the Keloid responds well to this treatment alone, in most cases it is not recommended to use ablative methods to fine tune the results. This is because as we know the use of any ablative treatment bears the inherent likelihood of triggering a form or recurrence. Although this treatment is not always effective it has a very high success rate and it has low risks associated with it. The results are apparent from the first course of injections as seen in the figure on the right.

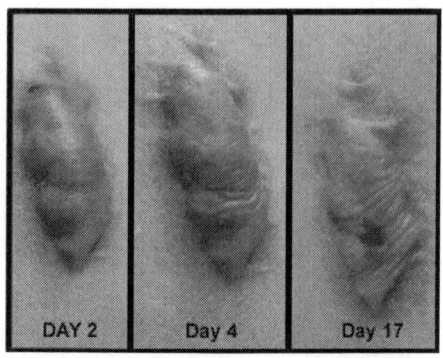

Illustration 153: This picture clearly shows the efficacy of cortisone injections into the Keloid. Ablative treatments should be avoided if the Keloid responds well to this type of treatment.

Typical drugs used for this type of procedure:

- Triamcinolone acetonide
- Hydrocortisone
- Methylprednisolone

Typical Dosage: 5-10 mg/mL for developing Keloids and 10-40 mg/mL for a pre-existing, fully mature Keloid. The larger doses are used on bulky, mature Keloids. The injections can be painful especially at high doses. Shots can be co-administered with a numbing agent (e.g., lidocaine) and/or after application of a topical numbing cream.

Possible adverse reactions can be Hypopigmentation, Hyperpigmentation, dark red blotches, or tissue atrophy. Tissue atrophy looks like indentations in the skin and can occur with large amounts of steroids and/or injection in the surrounding normal tissue.

Generally, Hypopigmentation may be reversible over time (it may take up to a year), however, tissue and fat atrophy can be permanent. Cushing's syndrome can develop if too much steroid is used.

Remember that the likelihood of side effects can be minimised but never completely avoided. Of course, if this treatment is effective, varying the dosage per session will determine the number of treatments required to achieve a satisfactory outcome. However, it is advisable to administer lower doses than normally possible and increase the number of sessions in order to minimise the likelihood of adverse reactions.

25.5 Main types of combined ablative treatments

In case intra-lesion steroid injections are not effective, then the use of ablative treatments combined with recurrence prevention treatments can be the next step forward. As stated previously the use of ablative treatments (both invasive, like surgery, and non-invasive, like laser and voltaic arcing treatments) should be avoided in the first instance due to the inherent likelihood of triggering recurrence or further growths. However, the use of Lasers and voltaic arcing coupled with steroid treatments, radiation therapy or other treatments to prevent recurrence can be very effective.

The regrowth preventative treatment is normally carried out after the Keloidal ablation has taken place. However it can be carried out even before the ablative treatment. In case the practitioner decides to use injectable steroids as a recurrence preventative measure, it is recommended to administer the steroid injections into the Keloid before the ablative treatment and then proceed to the physical removal of the Keloid by using, surgical excision, laser or the electrical arcing ablation. When using lasers or electrical arcing, the technique is simply burning the keloid to make it level with the surrounding skin as you have seen in the removal of any common mole.

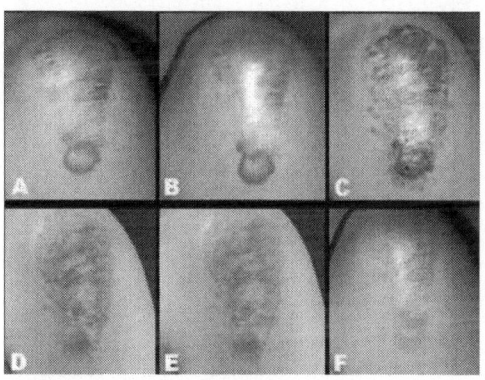

Illustration 154: The stages of Keloid removal over time. Keloids are not always straightforward to remove

At the end of the Removal treatment then another course of superficial injections should be administered to both the treated and the surrounding area to further minimise the recurrence rate.
In case of the use of radiation therapy to minimise the recurrence rate, this has to be used only at the end of the ablative treatment. The use of combined treatments bears the inherent advantage of being able to remove the Keloid within one sitting, provided that the Keloid will not recur after the healing process. Once again combined treatments should be used only as the last resort or if the client prefers it (The client should be informed about all suitable available options for Keloid removal to make an informed decision).

25.6 Types of combined ablative methods

The options of Ablative treatments suitable for Keloid removal, in case i*ntra-lesional corticosteroid injections* did not achieve the desired results, are :

- Lasers (by vaporising the Keloid) coupled with preventative measures to minimise recurrence.
- Voltaic Arcing (vaporisation) coupled with preventative measures to minimise recurrence.
- Surgical Excision coupled with preventative measures to minimise recurrence.
- Cryotherapy combined with preventative measures to minimise recurrence.
- Micro dermal abrasion combined with preventative measures to minimise recurrence.

Any ablative method on its own bear's high likelihood of triggering Keloid recurrence and therefore a form of Keloid recurrence preventative treatment should be used at least immediately after the Keloid removal. Recurrence preventative measures:

➢ The most common Keloid recurrence minimisation method is the use of corticosteroid injections after any of these types of ablative treatments. This is due to the availability, efficacy and relatively low side effects of these drugs. In most cases, the injections are administered both before the ablation treatment directly into the Keloid and after the removal treatment into the surrounding area using superficial infiltrations.

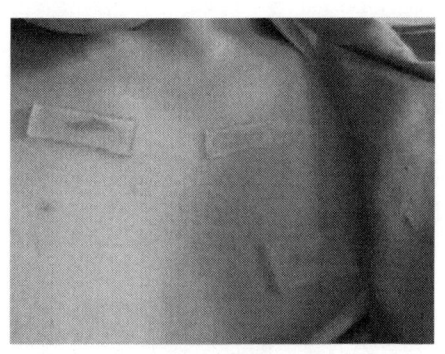

Illustration 155: Occlusion using Silicon sheets as a recurrence preventative measure after Keloid laser removal treatment.

➢ The use of Radiotherapy and other methods have been proved to be also effective.
➢ A particular study also suggests the use of Silicon Gel Sheeting up to 48 hours after an ablative treatment as a means of reducing the likelihood of recurrence. As the results are not always satisfactory this is not a first line preventative therapeutic treatment recommendable after Keloid ablative treatments. **Click Here** to learn more.

➢ Other promising Keloid recurrence preventative therapies after removal using ablative treatments include antiangiogenic factors, including vascular endothelial growth factor (VEGF) inhibitors (eg, bevacizumab), phototherapy (photodynamic therapy, UVA-1 therapy, narrowband UVB therapy), transforming growth factor (TGF)–beta3, tumor necrosis factor (TNF)-alpha inhibitors (etanercept), and recombinant human interleukin (rhIL-10), which are directed at decreasing collagen synthesis.

A useful table detailing the various type of treatments available for Keloid removal combined with regrowth prevention therapies, mentioning also the likelihood of recurrence can be found HERE .

25.7   Home Treatments

Home treatments should not involve cutting, sanding, constricting the keloids with strings or rubber bands, or using any other method that traumatizes the skin. Doing so can increase the likelihood of recurrence, infections or keloid enlargement.

Use care when attempting home remedies for Keloid removal. Safe and effective remedies to shrink Keloids include occlusion (silicone pads or gel) and/or the application of certain substances.

Please note that despite the fact that the proposed treatments are scientifically proven to improve the appearance of Keloids over time, several treatments, over a long time period are usually required in order to achieve the desired results. The duration of the treatment depends on the method used.

The following home treatments are also effective in the treatment of normal **Hypertrophic scars**. Dramatic results are only currently achievable using intra-lesional corticosteroid injections or ablative methods combined with recurrence preventative treatments.

Silicone sheeting (Simple occlusion)

Occlusion for scars treatment has been used for several years. Occlusion can be performed in several ways, one of the ways which have been widely used is the application of Silicone adhesive sheets or appropriate silicon gel. Also, silicon gel sheets have been used to prevent new Keloids from forming following an injury or surgical operations. This is a treatment that can lead to eventual improvement in the appearance of both Hypertrophic scars and Keloids.

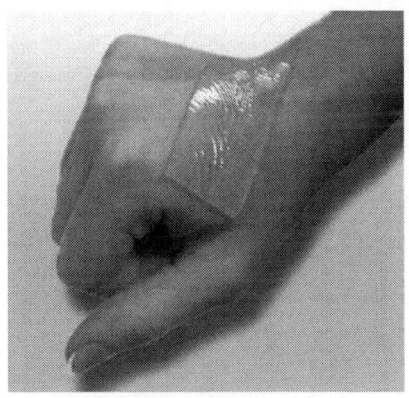

Illustration 156: Occlusion applied on Keloid sustained over months for over 10 hours a day has been shown to be effective. However, this treatment is seldom viable for most people due to the impracticality of applying occlusion over long periods of time.

However, the use of sheeting has to be endured over several months (usually over six) in order for the results to become apparent. Therefore this type of treatment although ultimately effective is unsustainable for most people as this requires forming a new daily habit which needs to be sustained over months and this is rarely accomplished. Most "ad hoc" products are silicon gel sheets, or "scar sheets" which are self-adhesive, and reusable. They are applied to existing scars and Keloids to reduce their size and appearance over time. Silicon sheets should be worn over them for at

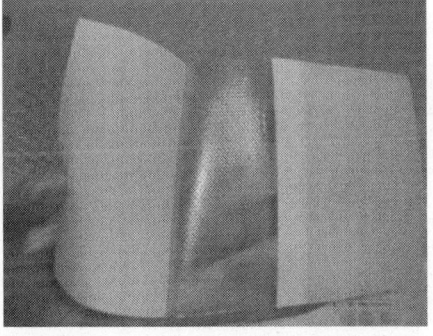

Illustration 157: Several silicon products are available on the market. They must be worn for over 10 hours a day. The treatment has to be endured for over six months in order to achieve good results.

www.voltaicplasma.com   Author: Andreas Russo

least 10 hours per day for several months in order to achieve the desired results. Silicon gel sheets are widely available on the market and can be bought at most pharmacies and many online retailers.

Vitamin E Coupled with Occlusion.

The use of topical Vitamin E based products (gel, oil, and ointments) have been shown a real efficacy in the eventual reduction in the size of the Keloid over a long period of time (several months). Therefore this solution on its own is not suitable for most people, because the use of this type of products can hardly be sustained over long periods. Likewise, as we know, the main problem with occlusion, used on its own, is the impracticality of wearing silicon sheets or gel products over long periods during the day (over 10 hours per day) and over sustained long periods of time (over 6 months). However, the combination of occlusion and the use of Vitamin E based products appears to be far more practical as the results are achieved much faster, usually within 2 months with an appropriate everyday use.

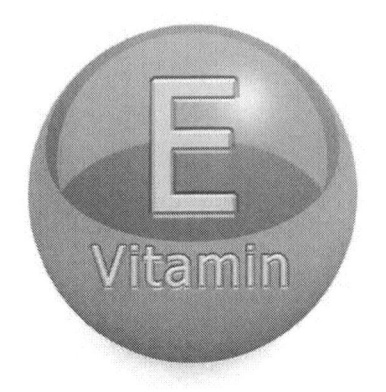

Illustration 158: It has been shown how administering Vitamin E into the Keloid or Hypertrophic scar using the right topical solutions can lead to the eventual shrinkage of the lesion

The reason for silicon occlusion to be effective in the treatment of Keloids is the "direct action on the fibroblasts and a hyperhydration of Subcutaneous tissue". This is possible because generally the use of occlusion in aesthetics is successfully used for amplifying the subcutaneous delivery of active substances. Therefore applying Vitamin E on to the Keloid coupled with the occlusion effect of silicone sheets speeds up the Keloidal shrinkage process which would otherwise be possible in a much longer period of time. To view the related scientific study showing the efficacy of Vitamin E coupled with occlusion in Hypertrophic scar and Keloid treatment please **Click Here**. Please note that results vary according to the type of topical Vitamin E based product, and the timing of occlusion carried out during the day.

25.8 Conclusions

Keloids are fundamentally different from Hypertrophic scars. Keloid removal treatment is not always simple as it is in the case of hypertrophic scars. This is because, unlike Hypertrophic scars, Keloids tend to "grow back" after any ablative treatment.

There are two main types of possible effective treatments:

1. Professional. The first line of treatment is the use of Intralesional corticosteroid injections. Failing that the preferred option is the use of ablative treatments (Physical removal of the Keloids) combined

with some other recurrence inhibition treatment. There are also several other options, however, they are not frequently used yet.

2. Home treatments. The most successful type of home treatment is the use of suitable Vitamin E topical products, combined with occlusion. If carried out appropriately, this type of treatment has been shown to reduce the size of most Keloids within 2 months.

Both professional and home treatments are effective.

Professional treatments bear the advantage of allowing the Keloid removal with high success rate within one (or multiple) sitting(s) without the client needing to wear patches on his own. The main disadvantage is the higher costs and the potential side effects.

Home treatments are effective however, this does require the sustained daily use of Vitamin E based product coupled with occlusion over an extended period of time during the day and over several weeks. The main advantage is the lower costs and the very low likelihood of side effects.

26.0 Tattoos

In this section, we will focus on understanding the physiology of tattoos. In this way, we will be better equipped to advise the clients on the various options to fade their tattoos. Also, this will help us understand how the fading techniques, currently available, work and how to use them in order to "remove", or most appropriately, "fade" them effectively according to the client's desires.

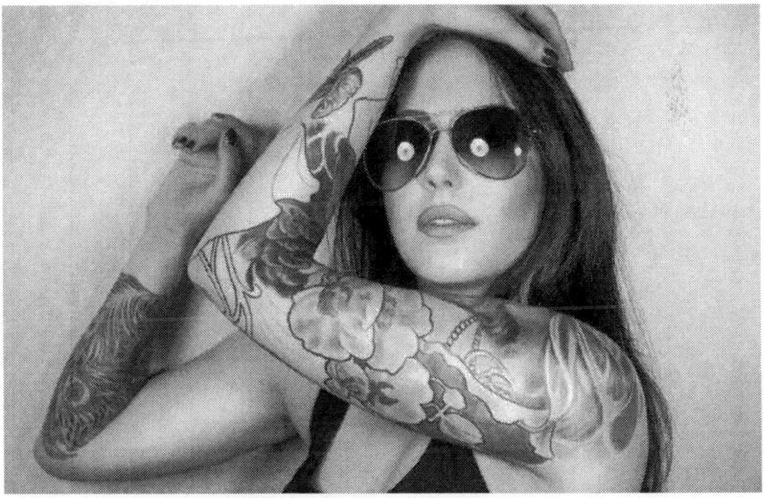

Illustration 159: Tattoo Examples

26.1 What is tattoo and an overview of its physiology

A tattoo is a skin drawing, meant to be permanently visible throughout the person's life. Tattoos historically have had various functions, mainly aesthetic and more recently they have been used for permanent make-up. In order for the tattoo to be permanent, the ink has to be injected into the dermis, this is because the pigments that only reside on the epidermis will be removed by the natural skin regeneration process. During the skin tattooing, the ink will be deposited also on the epidermis, simply by virtue of the fact that the needle is on the way to the dermis and just passing through it. As we have seen in the picture, the tattooing process consists in delivering the pigments (tattoo ink) into the dermal layer. In the process of doing so, both the epidermal and dermal layer will be modified and injured causing an open wound.

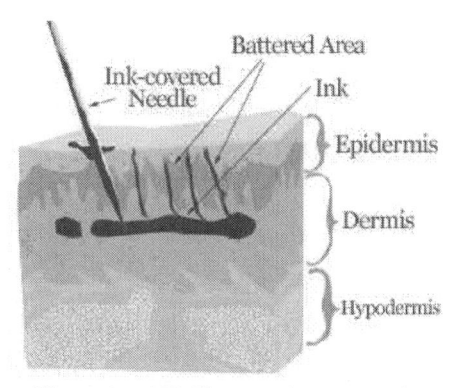

Illustration 160: The tattooing process is relatively simple. It consists in injecting the tattoo pigments into the dermal layer.

In the picture right we can see an example of how bright the finished tattoo work can be. This is because the pigments are also deposited onto the epidermis and most of the dermis is also exposed making the tattoo look at its brightest. When the area has healed completely, all the pigments deposited into the epidermis will have naturally been removed by the healing process. Therefore at that point, the pigments will not be present in the epidermal layer. The epidermal layer is transparent therefore the tattoo will still be clearly visible through it. However, the epidermal layer is not 100% transparent and it is slightly opaque.

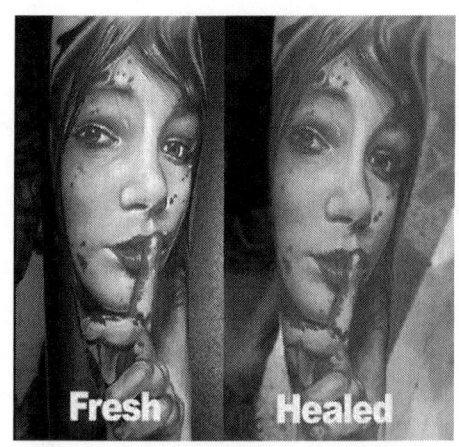

Illustration 161: Once the tattoo has healed the picture loses its original brightness. This is because the tattoo is visible through the thin epidermal layer. If the epidermal layer is removed, exposing the dermal layer, the original brightness is restored.

www.voltaicplasma.com						Author: Andreas Russo

Therefore when the tattoo has healed the original brightness is apparently lost due to the fact that it will be visible through the opaque and transparent epidermal layer. In the picture above (illustration) we can see the representative distribution of the tattoo pigments through the healing process. After the healing process, no pigmentation will be left on the epidermal layer.

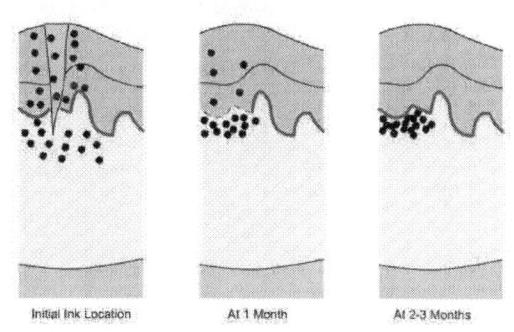

Illustration 162: When the tattoo has just been made the initial ink location is both in the epidermis and the dermis, the area is essentially an open wound. Over time the scabbing process will take care of gradually removing the residual pigments form the epidermis. In a month's time, only very few residues of ink will be left on the epidermis. Once the area has healed completely the tattoo pigmentation will only reside inside the dermis and it will be visible through the epidermis.

Therefore once the tattooed area has healed the tattoo is not as bright because the pigments have completely been removed from the epidermal layer. At that point, the tattoo on the dermal layer will only be visible through the transparent epidermal layer. Conversely, the tattoo will show its full brightness once the epidermal layer has been removed. This is normally done in the tattoo removal procedures using electrical arcing.

As we have seen because tattoos are made by injecting the pigments into the dermal layer the tattoo making process involves deliberately causing a wound to the skin. When the tattoo has just been made, the treated area is literally an open wound which is required to heal properly, in order for the tattoo work to be preserved

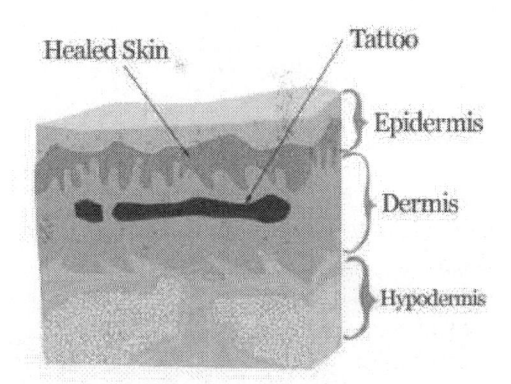

Illustration 163: In this picture, we can see where the tattoo pigments reside inside the skin once the skin has healed from the tattooing process. Although not visible from this representation, the epidermal layer is transparent, therefore allowing the tattoo to be visible.

www.voltaicplasma.com   Author: Andreas Russo

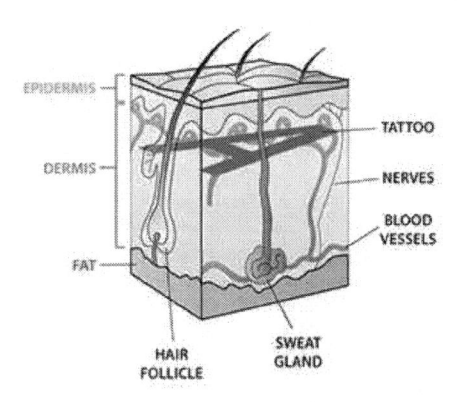

Illustration 164: 3D representation of the tattoo. Once the tattoo has healed the drawing will be visible through the epidermal layer.

Because of this, the end result of the tattooing process is not only dependent on the quality work of the tattoo artist but also reliant on the after-care routine to avoid infections and other adverse reactions. The healing process will likely last anywhere from three to four weeks, and special care will be required to be taken of the recently made new body art; this is to ensure the tattoo looks at its best once that healing process has finished.

26.2 Main risk during healing: inflammatory skin infections

A fresh tattoo is essentially an open wound, therefore it has to be treated accordingly. The main risk during the healing process of a tattoo is the likelihood of contracting an inflammatory infection of the open wound. The risk of contracting any inflammatory infection or infections in general, during the healing period, can be minimised but never completely eliminated. Infections can be contracted in several ways due to the several sources of bacteria and viruses in our everyday environment. This is because it is relatively easy for bacteria to enter the open wound of a recently drawn tattoo.

The signs of a possible infection are, oozing (a strange liquid coming out of the wound), pain, redness, swelling etc. If the infection is not treated appropriately the symptoms will worsen over time and lead to several long term undesirable effects. During the healing process, the area has to be kept infection free until the scabs have formed and fallen off by themselves. During the healing process, the client is required to make sure the area is kept clear and free from infections. Infections can be contracted during the healing process in may ways. In order to minimise these risks, the client can simply look after the tattooed part like any other open wound, using mild antiseptics and deliberately avoid those activities which will increase the likelihood of infections

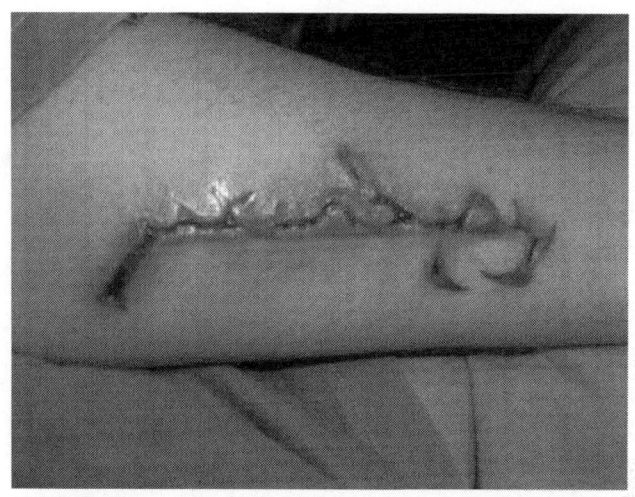

Illustration 165: This in an infection at its onset. It is noticeable how the area is red at the border of the wound caused by the tattoo work. If treated immediately this types of infection may not jeopardise the tattoo end result after healing.

In case of tattoo infections, if they are treated early on, there may not be devastating consequences for the tattoo. Therefore in case, it is suspected a tattoo is becoming infected it is best to seek medical advice immediately in order to minimise the possible detrimental effects of the infection. Usually, if the infection is treated appropriately it can be cured quickly without major consequences, therefore without compromising the final tattoo work. In the picture on the right we can see the devastating effects of the tattoo work which an infection can cause. An infection which is not properly looked after can lead to several undesired effects which could distort the tattoo work and even lead to fully fledged hypertrophic or atrophic permanent scars.

Therefore if an infection is not treated promptly, effectively and with the right products the consequences could be permanent. In the previous illustration, long-term effect of this type of infection can make the tattoo distorted and also lead to scarring.

Illustration 166: In this picture, we can see the dire immediate consequences of an infection caused by poor after-care after a normal tattooing procedure. This particular infection was being cured, however, it was still present at the time the picture was taken as proved by the redness of the borders of the affected area. The redness at the borders is an example of an infection induced inflammation.

www.voltaicplasma.com   Author: Andreas Russo

26.3   Tattoo inflammatory infections symptoms

Here are the most common symptoms of an infected tattoo. If your client is experiencing any of these, it is time to take action. Remember, if you are in doubt whether an infection is ongoing it is always advisable to consult a doctor because General Practitioners are legally qualified to diagnose infections and prescribe the medical treatment of each specific case. The tattoo artist, although will recognise an infected tattoo immediately, due to his vast experience, he may not be qualified to make a diagnosis and advise on the best medical treatment of each specific case. Legislation may vary from country to country.

- **Redness.** The area starts to redden and the redness may include the tattoo work itself and the edges too. The redness of the edges feathers out and it spreads further as the infection worsen over time if not treated properly.

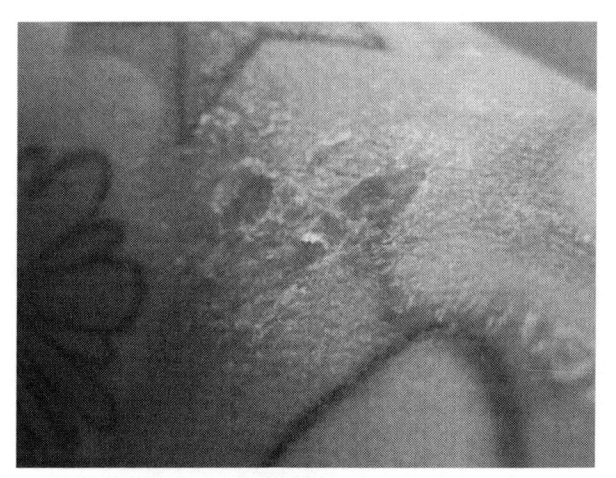

Illustration 167: Redness can be a symptom of an inflammatory infection. We can see how the inflamed area peels off

- **Swelling.** It is normal for a tattoo to swell during the first 48 hours after the tattoo as being drawn. However, if the swelling increases over three to four days instead of decreasing, or begins to extend past the tattoo, this is likely a sign of infection.

- **Heat.** An infected tattoo might feel hot to the touch. While it is normal for the tattoo to feel warm, especially during the first 48 hours, it should not feel very hot and the heat should fade away on its own accord. If it is infected, the whole tattoo and/or the area around it may feel hot to the touch, and it may also feel as if there is heat radiating from within the tattoo itself.

- **Discharge.** During the first 48 hours after the tattoo has just been drawn a slights discharge and some bleeding can occur and this is normal. However, if this continues or worsens after the first 48 hours it can be a clear sign of infection. The infected tattoo often has a slimy discharge oozing from them in various places; this may appear as a clear fluid with a golden colour or a thick yellow-green goo that sits within the tattoo. You might also see pus (white, yellow, or green).

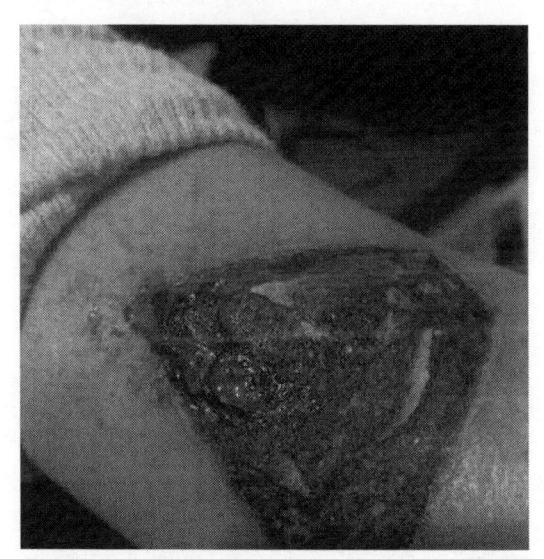

Illustration 168: Example of abnormal discharge due to infection.

- **Odour.** This a sure-fire sign that your tattoo is infected. Often the discharge from an infected tattoo will have a nasty smell or odour. The smell increases in intensity as the infection spreads or worsen.

- **Pain.** If you're experiencing mild pain that increases over the 3-5 days after your tattoo has been drawn or has sharp, shooting pains from within the tattoo itself, it is likely an infection.

- **Blistering.** Blistering may also be a sign of infection, and it can occur on top of the tattoo, manifesting as red, raised sores filled with body fluids. If your tattoo is bubbly or bright red, then this is a sign of infection. This is not to be confused with the normal swelling occurring after the first 48 hours of receiving your tattoo, any raised areas should slowly level out and decrease to the height of the surrounding (non-tattooed) skin.

- **Increased scab size.** Due to abnormal levels of discharge, the scabs on an infected tattoo may appear thick and have a yellow and green crust. This normally occurs when the infections are subsiding while the scabs are being formed. This is generally a better situation than the symptoms mentioned above.

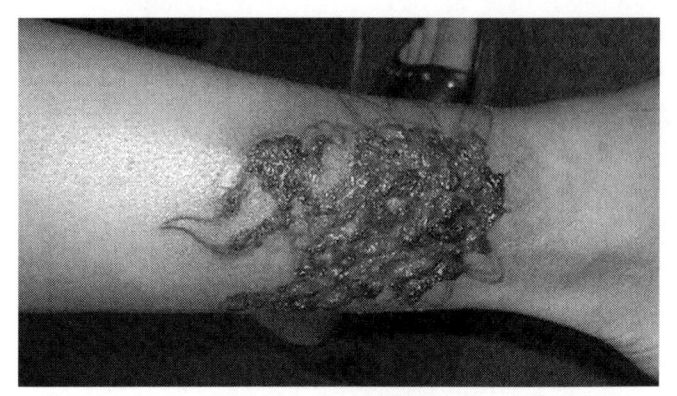

Illustration 169: The infection is subsiding. Abnormal scabbing caused by an earlier infection.

- **Fever and lethargy.** This is possible in advanced stages of infection, also this can occur if the tattoo is relatively large and infected. An infection over a large area will trigger the natural feverish body reaction, which is designed to help the body combat bacterial infections. If you have a fever or feel lethargic and these symptoms are unrelated to other illnesses, then it's likely your body is working overtime to fight the infection coming from your tattoo. If you experience any of the symptoms above, fever is one of the surest signs of infection, even if your temperature is only slightly elevated. In fact, even a slight elevated temperature can be symptomatic of serious advanced state of an inflammatory skin infection. Skin infections rarely lead to high temperature fevers.

- **Redness or streaking.** This is an extremely severe case of an advanced stage of infection. As we have seen previously, if the tattoo or the skin around it is extremely red, you likely have an infection. If you see thin red lines radiating from your tattoo, you should go to the doctor immediately as streaking can be an early sign of blood poisoning.

26.4 Introduction to the stages of the tattooing process.

As we have seen above, the tattoo is an open wound when it is just been drawn. The tattooing is a process which can last several weeks to reach its final permanent appearance. Understanding the healing stages of tattoos provides a better idea of what to expect in the days and weeks after the tattoo has been just made. The end result depends on the after-care and not only on the final tattoo work at the time it was drawn.

The tattoo healing process can be divided into three main stages:

- ✓ Stage one, healing the open wound. Most delicate part of the process, this is when an infection or diseases can be contracted through the open wound.

- ✓ Stage two, scabbing or peeling process.

- ✓ Stage three, pigments resettling.

Overall, the healing stages of tattoos stretch out over a three to four week period up to two to three months, and taking special care of the tattoo during this time is essential to preserve the wonderful work the tattoo artist has created. If you experience any symptoms beyond those mentioned here, contact your doctor (for medical advice) and the tattoo artist straight away. Although your tattoo artist cannot provide medical advice, tattoo artists are very familiar with the signs of abnormal healing and the signs of a burgeoning infection. Remember that if in doubt you should always consult your doctor.

26.5 Stage one: healing of the open wound. Soon after the tattoo has just been made

This initial stage of healing begins right after your tattoo is finished. At this point, you can consider the area, for what it is, an open wound, and it should be treated accordingly. Your tattoo artist will gently wash the area and bandage it to protect it from bacteria. Most artists recommend you keep the area covered for the first twenty- hours, although you will likely need to change the bandage because a fresh tattoo usually bleeds and can weep slightly. All fresh tattoos are temporarily bandaged to help prevent infections. This healing stage usually last about one week. If the bandage soak up too much fluid, it may wind up sticking to the newly tattooed skin, and this is definitely not good for the healing process.

Many people describe a fresh tattoo as feeling similar to a sunburn.

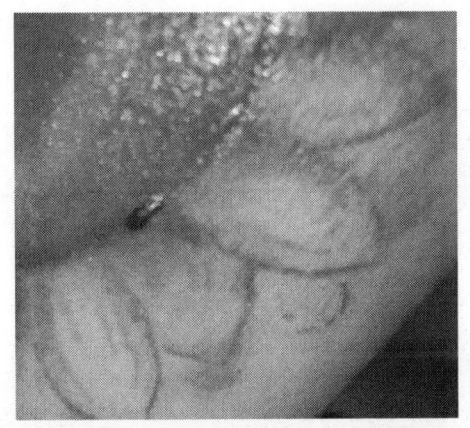

Illustration 170: Fresh tattoos can bleed and weep like any other open wound which requires healing. In this picture, we can see a fresh tattoo slightly bleeding and weeping.

The area tends to sting, and it can become inflamed, a little raised and/or swollen. This is a natural and normal reaction to the tattoo healing process. As we have seen the tattoo is an open wound caused by the injury inflicted by the tattooing procedure, and after any inflicted skin injury the skin can become inflamed and swell. This is, in fact, a normal reaction to be expected in the normal tattooing process.

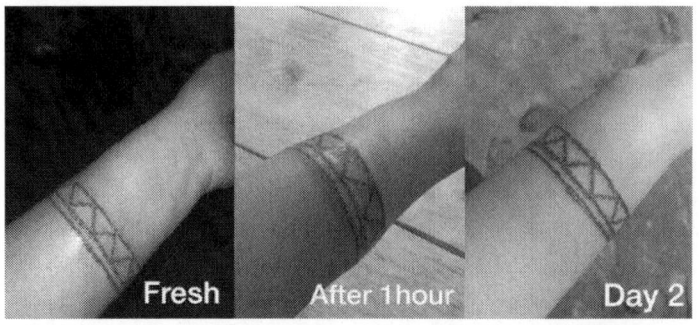

Illustration 171: This picture serves to show the immediate effects of the tattooing process. Tattooing involves not only deliberately causing a wound inside the dermis, but also impregnating the dermis with the ink necessary to make the drawing requested by the client. Sometimes swelling can be caused by both the injury caused by the tattooing needle and the dermis reaction to the new substance injected into the dermis.

Inflammation and swelling are to be expected because the tattooing process deliberately inflicts a wound (injury) into the dermis, therefore they are a normal skin reaction which often occurs soon after the tattooing. It normally begins immediately after the area has been tattooed, it lasts up to one to two days and it subsides on its own accord. Additionally, in certain cases, the swelling can be exacerbated by the individual skin reaction to the new external agent injected into the dermis (the tattoo ink colour/s). The swelling will subside on its own accord and normally two days after the treatment it will have subsided. If the swelling does not subside, this can be a clear sign of infection or some other side effect which will likely require medical attention. Scabs will begin to form over the tattooed area four to five days after the tattoo had been first made. No attempt must be made to remove them, any scabs must not be picked and should fall off by themselves.

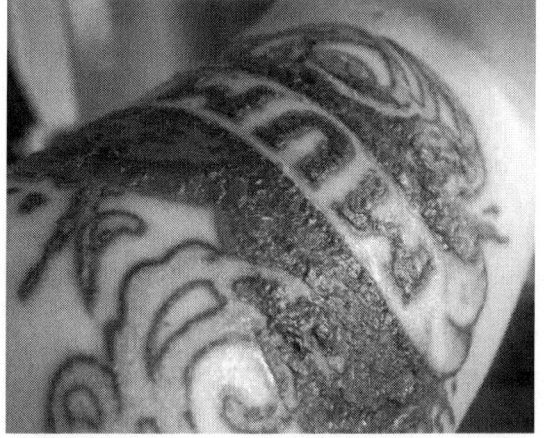

Illustration 172: The fresh tattoo is an open wound that requires healing. The scabbing process usually sets on the third or fourth day after the tattoo has been drawn, provided that the area has not become infected. During this period avoid the use of any product not expressly recommended by your tattoo artist as using unsuitable products on an open wound can cause unnecessary complications.

www.voltaicplasma.com   Author: Andreas Russo

Just gently wash the area once or twice a day with a very mild soap, pat dry with a fresh paper towel. Gently dab on a light amount of moisturising after-care lotion only if your tattoo artist recommends it.

Do not apply any creams or product on the fresh tattoo other than those expressedly recommended by the tattoo artist as applying unsuitable products on an open wound, could easily lead to unnecessary complications. After all, a fresh tattoo is an open wound which is trying to heal by its own accord.

Although people tend to heal at different rates, the first healing stage of a tattoo usually lasts about one week as long as an infection doesn't set in. Some people can experience some discomfort and even pain, in those cases the pain is more than expected, some over-the-counter pain reliever can be taken. In any case, if in doubt you can visit your doctor.

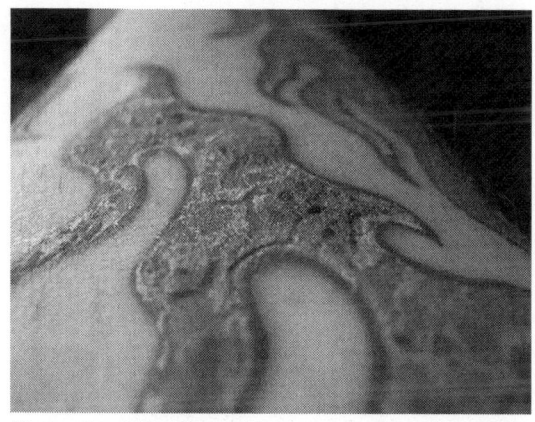

Illustration 173: The scabbing also contain some of the pigments injected during the tattoo drawing as demonstrated by this green scabbing.

26.6 Stage two: scabbing, peeling and itching

The second stage of healing usually brings the onset of scabbing, peeling and itching. After the first healing stage, the scabs are well formed and just beginning to flake off. This process will continue for about a week. The skin around the tattoo may become a bit dry. Most people experience some peeling, just as they would with a sunburn.

The client has to avoid both picking the scabs and peeling the flaky skin intentionally, doing so can jeopardise the final tattoo results. Just allow it to slough off naturally and, by all means, do not scratch your tattoo.

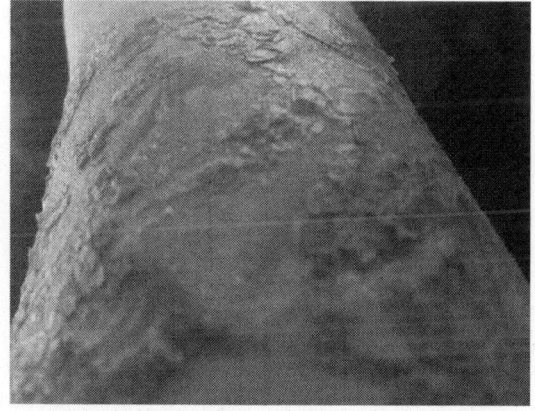

Illustration 174: Peeling effect of a tattoo after the scabbing has taken place. This process normally lasts for a week.

www.voltaicplasma.com

Author: Andreas Russo

Scratching can cause damage and ultimately spoil the look of the tattoo work by the time healing is complete. Applying more after-care lotion to the area should bring some relief to the itching, however, please note that the itching is a natural reaction of the skin to the good healing of any skin injury (including tattooing).

26.7 Stage Three

Stage three brings the final healing of the area. By this point, most or all of the scabs have fallen away from the tattoo, although the area may still be slightly dry and mildly tender. At that point, some mild itchy feeling can be still felt and the tattoo does not look as vibrant as it did when it was first finished, and this is normal. There is typically still a layer of dead skin over the tattoo at this point, this obscures it a bit, but once that layer naturally and slowly sloughs away the tattoo will look as it should. If you have managed to avoid infection and scratching, it probably looks great.

26.8 After-care during the healing recovery period.

In any case, please follow the recommendations of your own tattoo artist. If you require any medical advice consult your doctor. The after-care has to be performed by the client and consequently, the client alone assumes all responsibilities to carry it out appropriately. Always wash your hands before touching your tattoo especially while the tattoo is still an open wound (stage one)! When you get home: Remove the bandage within 2-3 hours after getting your tattoo. Re-bandage according to the instructions of your tattoo artist. On the first night, you may want to wrap your tattoo in saran wrap to prevent sticking to your bedding. Do not use any cloth bandages or pads, as the fibres of this material can adhere to your open tattoo and hinder the healing process. Wash your tattoo with an anti-bacterial liquid soap, use only the one suggested by your tattoo artist. Be gentle, do not use a wash cloth or anything that will ex-foliate your tattoo. Gently pat your tattoo dry with a clean cloth or paper towel. Do not rub, and do not use a fabric with a rough surface.

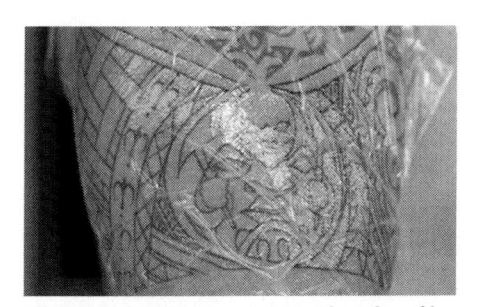

Illustration 175: Tattoo wrapped in cling film for protection. This is usually done the first night after the tattoo is done to prevent contact with the bedding. Keeping the tattoo wrapped in cling film for too long is detrimental as it creates the moist conditions for bacterial proliferation and hence infection. However, it has been found that during the first-night sleep the bandaging of the tattoo in cling film is more beneficial than detrimental.

The first 3-4 days: Apply a small amount of ointment on your tattoo as recommended by your tattoo artist. Please do not use antibiotic ointments as a means of preventing infections (this is because doing do will eventually induce a bacterial resistance to the specific antibiotic substance). Use a suitable antiseptic cream or ointment instead. Always use clean hands and do not place your fingers back into

www.voltaicplasma.com   Author: Andreas Russo

the antiseptic ointment (or cream) after touching your tattoo. Preferably you should use a clean ear bud (or similar) to place the ointment from the tab onto the tattoo, this is to minimise bacterial contamination of the ointment you are using. Make sure to rub the ointment in so that it is not shiny, or greasy– you want the thinnest amount possible. Pat off any excess ointment with a clean cloth or paper towel. Do not use petroleum jelly (Vaseline), or Bag Balm. Wash, dry and apply ointment 3-5 times daily, as needed.

Wear clean, soft clothing over your tattoo for the first 2 weeks– do not use any tight clothing, nothing abrasive or irritating (i.e. wool). For a foot tattoo: go barefoot as long as possible. If you must wear shoes, first wrap your tattoo in saran wrap, then cover with a clean cotton sock before putting on your shoe. During this period avoid sandals or flip flops to prevent damage to the tattoo. After day 4 to 5: Your tattoo should begin to scab. This is normal and a good sign! Do not pick at the scabs. Begin using a mild, white, unscented lotion, free of dyes or Perfumes. Use lotion for minimum 2 weeks, 1-2 times daily.

- Do not apply any product not explicitly recommended by your tattoo artist as doing so especially during the healing phase (stage one) of the healing process could seriously jeopardise the tattoo work.

- Do not apply petroleum based skin products to your tattoo.

- You can shower, but you may not soak your tattoo for 2 weeks. No swimming, soaking or hot tub. Avoid swimming. This is because in the swimming pool Chlorine can bleach colour and dry out the still tender skin around your tattoo. In the sea, the salty water could have undesirable effects on your tattooed area. Not hot tub.

- Do not wear tight, abrasive materials, jewellery, or shoes that rub against your tattoo.

- Do not let anyone touch your tattoo unless they wash their hands first.

- Don't soak in the tub. This can allow bacteria to penetrate the unhealed wound.

- Avoid exposing your new tattoo to direct sunlight. This can lead to fading and you could easily burn the unhealed skin.

- Do not pick at your scabs or scratch/rub your tattoo.

- Beware of gym equipment, wash it well before using it.

www.voltaicplasma.com   Author: Andreas Russo

26. 9 Adverse reactions

Even if the tattoo has been drawn correctly, using the best equipment available and the best possible quality pigmentation certain undesirable reactions can still occur. They can be minimised but never eliminated altogether.

26.10 Cancer scare due to pigments toxicity

This is a side effect which is directly dependent on the type of pigmentation used during the tattooing procedure. The best quality pigments should not lead to an increased risk of cancer throughout life. Studies to document the effect of tattoos on the body and its relationship with cancer are still ongoing however several experts are of the opinion that tattoos can increase the likelihood of developing cancer later in life depending on the type of substances used in the pigments. Where earlier tattoos were made from natural dyes, today's inks can be made from a variety of ingredients such as pigments suspended in a carrier solution for colour, of which the pigments are composed of plastics or metallic salts such as mercury sulfide, cobalt albuminate, cadmium, chromium and chromic oxides. It is also claimed that the nano particles from the tattoo ink can seep into the body's major organs.

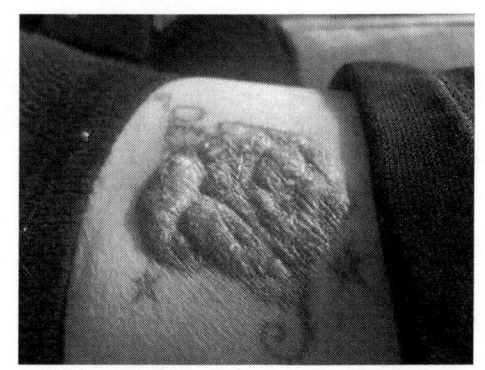

Illustration 176: Abnormal growth inside a tattoo. Cancer scares are associated with the body reaction to certain substances in the tattoo pigments.

Aluminium silicates and Barium sulphates are used to preserve some physical properties of the tattoo and ferrous oxides and titanium oxides are mixed as well for desired transparency. The toxicity of the inks, whose **chemical composition** is sometimes unknown and mostly unregulated, can travel through the bloodstream to accrue in the kidneys and the spleen. The most common health risk that you put yourself into when you get a tattoo would always be – skin cancer. Though not proven, tattoos could raise the risk of developing melanomas.

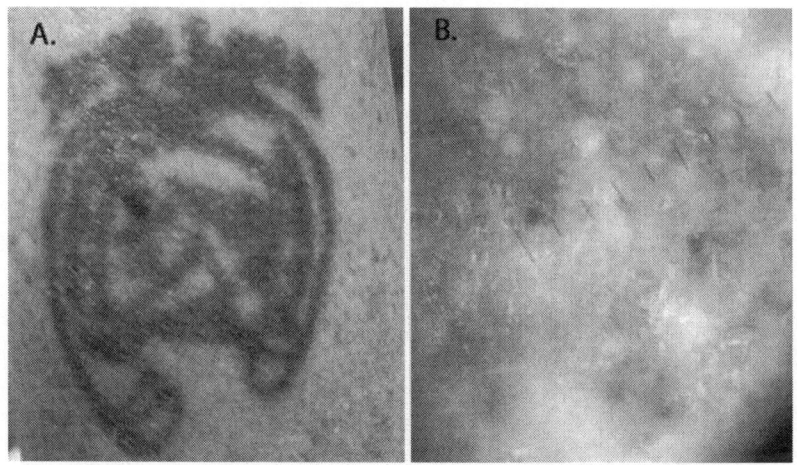

Illustration 177: Melanoma developing inside a tattoo. Sometimes these malignant growths are concealed inside the tattoo making their correct diagnosis more challenging. A direct correlation between melanoma and tattooing has not been proven to this date.

Now the actual amount and mixture of these constituents vary from tattoo parlour to tattoo parlour because it is considered a trade secret. These inks are injected below the skin layer for permanency and the toxic effect of these metals in your body, even in in small amounts, cannot be ignored. From growth retardation, mild skin irritation and to affecting the cardiovascular systems, these can all be the potential side effects of just getting a tattoo.

26.11 Viral and bacterial infections.

This is an effect merely attributable to the specific safety standards of the tattoo parlour you are using to get your tattoo done. The use of non-sterile needles during the process of tattoo application can increase the risks of contracting transfusion-transmitted diseases such as tetanus, hepatitis B and C, herpes, tetanus, staph, syphilis and HIV due to simple needles "*cross-contamination*". Hence there are several places where prospective blood donors are screened out for tattoos.

Therefore it is important that you visit an established and well-known shop which follows proper safety standards to prevent the spread of these diseases. New, sealed needles for every new tattoo, sterilizing hands and instruments regularly and using gloves are basic safety protocols every tattoo parlour is required to follow. Remember that while the tattoo is still an open wound (stage 1) although the tattoo work has been carried out in sterile conditions and there was no cross contamination you can still acquire most of the diseases mentioned above through contact of the open wound with the respective viruses and/or bacteria.

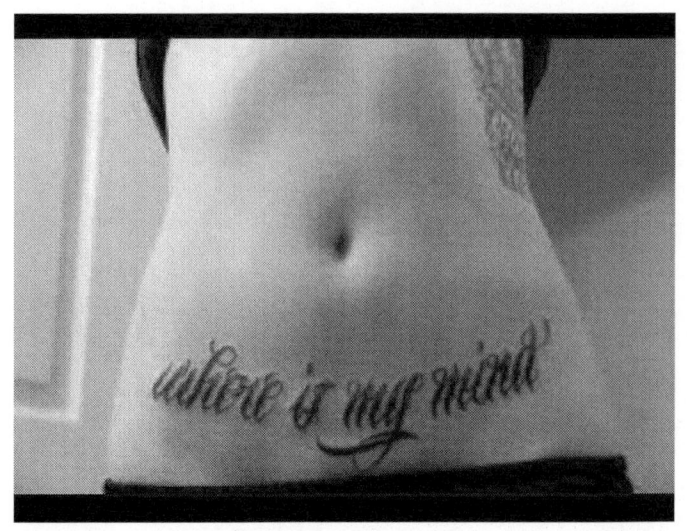

Illustration 178: Remember to choose the reputable tattoo parlours and guard the fresh tattoo against infections during the first stage of the healing period.

26.12 Keloids

People prone to developing **Keloids** should avoid undergoing any form of tattooing. Scars are bound to occur during the initial healing phase of the tattooing (stage one) if the proper care steps are not followed properly or inflammatory infections develop. **Keloids** are a type of collagen overgrowth tissue formed at the site of a wound. They are firm and rubbery and pink to purplish in colour. In contrast to scars, keloids do not shirnk with time and continue to grow. They can grow beyond the boundaries of the wounds which caused them; certain people are more prone to developing them than others depending on family history, hence they should avoid getting piercings or tattoos done.

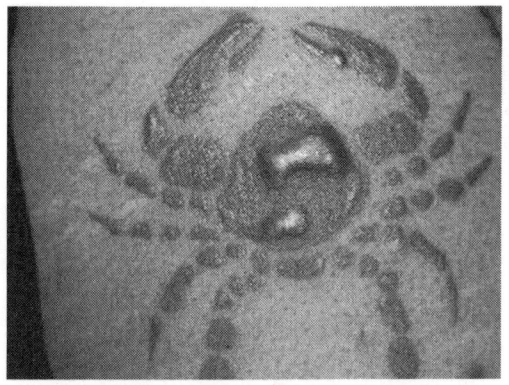

Illustration 179: . Keloidal formation caused by a simple tattooing. Every client should be warned in advance of the likelihood of developing Keloids before carrying out any tattooing.

By getting a tattoo done people with past Keloidal history, put themselves at risk of growing new **Keloids** due to the injury inflicted by the tattooing process itself. **Keloids** can develop irrespective of the way the tattoos have been drawn and the after-care carried out during the healing phase. To know more about **Keloids** please **click here** .

26.13 Allergic Reactions

Allergic Reactions to tattoos are quite common and there are different types of allergies that can be caused. Most often it is advisable to perform a patch test to determine whether your skin is too sensitive for the tattoo inks prior to actually getting it done, but it may not always be a sure way of knowing it. The main issue in order to prevent allergic reactions to tattoos is that, even if you read all ingredients stated in the pigments packaging used, no one is always aware of all his/her possible reactions to each specific agent used in the tattoo colours or their mixture.

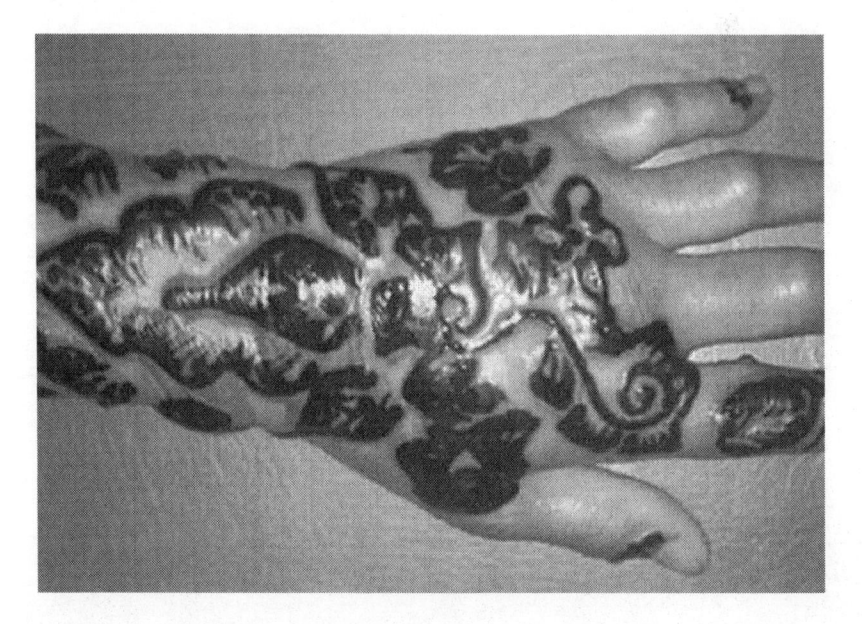

Illustration 180: Example of an allergic reaction to the tattoo pigments. Swelling occurs in the tattooed areas only

Allergic reactions have occurred with some of the many metals put into tattoo inks, nickel is one of the most common metal allergies. Others have reacted to the mercury in red cinnabar, to cobalt blue, and to cadmium sulfite when used as a yellow pigment. Some inks were found to have high levels of lead, some contained lithium, and the blue inks were full of copper. The long-term health effects of sustained allergic reactions to tattoos are still unknown due to the lack of regulation, testing, and long-term studies.

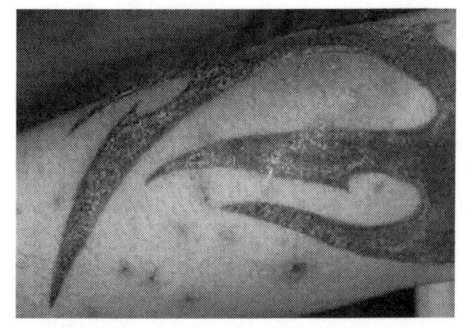

Illustration 181: Allergic reactions can display many symptoms including general redness.

Phototoxic reactions do occur, although not very common, considering the number of people who get tattoos done every year. Phototoxicity means having a reaction on exposure to sunlight. Inflammatory reactions, caused primarily by the inks, appear as swellings and red rashes.

Dermatitis caused by allergic reactions to pigments is characterized by inflamed skin rashes and by the affected area becoming scaly or flaky. These allergic reactions do not always occur immediately after the tattoo has been drawn, sometimes the effects can be delayed by months, even years. Tattoo itchiness and red bumps can be caused due to changes in weather or body temperature and often require a visit to your dermatologist.

26.14 Granulomas and lymphnodes issues

Granulomas is a collection of immune cells known as histiocytes. Granulomas form when the immune system attempts to wall off substances it perceives as foreign but is unable to eliminate. Since tattoo ink particles are foreign material, granulomas can develop around or inside the tattooed tissue. Apart from granulomas, enlargement of the lymph nodes have also been reported as a side effect of tattoos. The pigments used, leak into the bloodstream, accumulating at the lymph nodes causing painful swellings in these regions. The major cause for concern due to these inflammations is the misdiagnosis of melanoma.

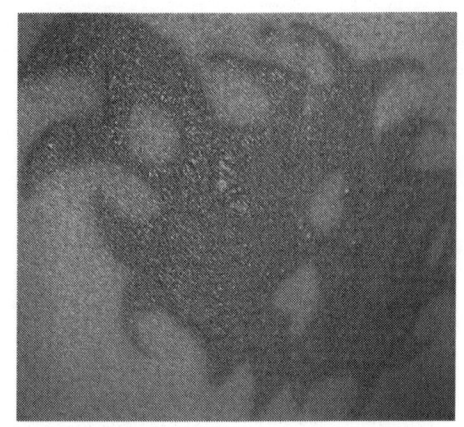

Illustration 182: Granulomas on a tattoo.

www.voltaicplasma.com　　　　　　　　　　Author: Andreas Russo

In patients with cancer risks, a Radiologist is often unable to distinguish between the ink staining in the lymph node and the abnormal tissue growth.

Other side effects of tattooing maybe:

- Haematomas. These are bruises that can occur due to the puncturing of a blood vessel during the tattooing process.
- Keratoacanthoma is a skin tumour characterized by a dome-shaped inflamed skin which gradually increases in size and its developments risks increase with tattoos.
- Hyperkeratosis. This is a condition in which is an excess growth of keratin in hair follicles are growing abnormally, This type of reaction will depend from the person and the tattoo.
- Hyperplasia can also occur, hyperplasia is an organ enlargement due to abnormal cell multiplication.

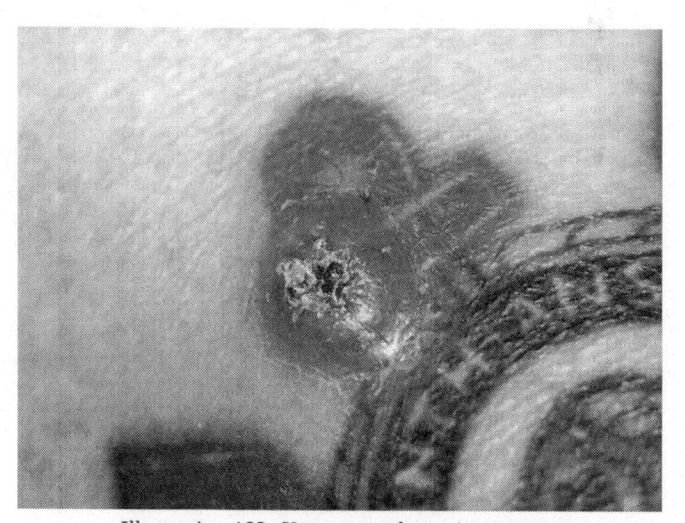

Illustration 183: Keratoacanthoma in a tattoo.

26.15 Mri errors due to tattoos

Since the inks used for tattooing contain metals, there have been complaints by people having tattoos, experiencing a burning sensation, when they are undergoing an MRI scan. Though not conclusively verified, there have been reports of the MRI image's quality getting affected by the pigments in the tattoo inks. An MRI or a magnetic resonance imaging creates pictures of the interior of the body using magnetic fields and radio frequency pulses. The concern for tattoo inks arises mainly due to the magnetic force which is extremely powerful and can affect the metal particles in the inks. Hence the MRI s done for people with tattoos requires more attention.

www.voltaicplasma.com   Author: Andreas Russo

27.0 Tattoo Removal

Here we provide an overview of the main tattoo removal treatments currently available. The EU legislation applicable and what is to be expected after this type of anesthetic treatments.

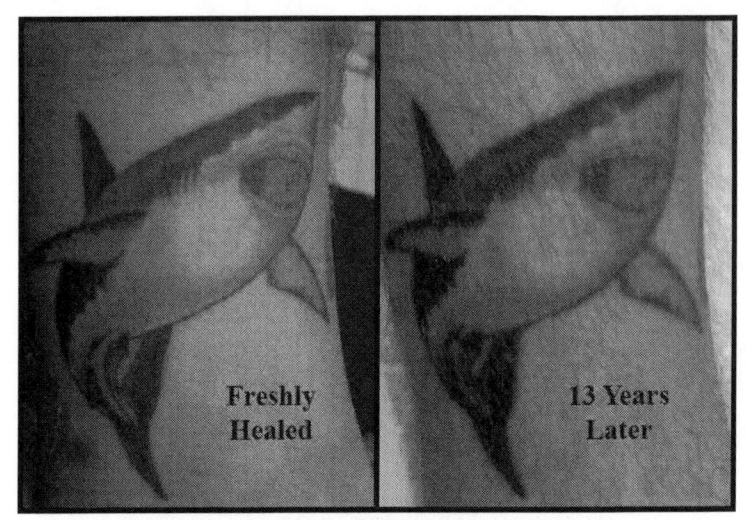

Illustration 184: Tattoo Fading Example

Terminology used, "tattoo removal" or "tattoo fading"

The procedures we are going to describe are widely referred to as "tattoo removal". This is mainly because the complete "removal" is the desired end result the clients expect from these aesthetic procedures. In reality most tattoos are very resilient, and most treatments currently available require a number of treatments in order to achieve satisfactory results whenever feasible. Because the most popular tattoo removal procedures rarely lead to the complete disappearance of the tattoo within one session we would rather refer to most types of "tattoo removal" procedures as "tattoo fading" because most of the treatments available can only realistically fade the tattoo slightly after each session instead of removing it.

www.voltaicplasma.com

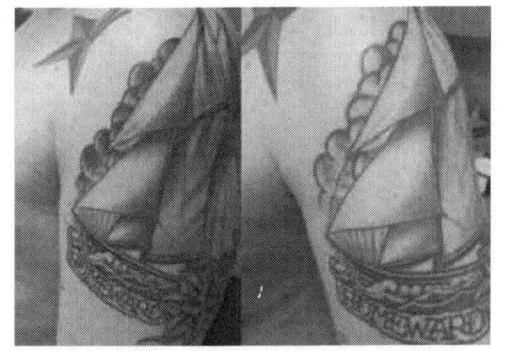

Illustration 185: Slight fading after only one mild laser treatment. Most popular "Tattoo Removal" procedures can only fade the tattoo slightly after each session.

Click here to watch video on Tattoo Removal

Author: Andreas Russo

As we will see in some cases complete removal is not feasible without leaving some scars or some sort permanent skin texture modification.

Most of the popular treatments currently available can only fade the tattoo slightly after each treatment. For this reason most procedures advertised as "tattoo removal" should be referred to as "tattoo fading" instead. **Currently only very invasive treatments can guarantee complete removal within one procedure or session only**.

However after making this clear distinction in terminology, we may refer to "tattoo fading" procedures as "tattoo removal" to align to the normal terminology used on the current aesthetic market place. Sometimes, due to the type of pigments used, it may be detrimental to try and remove the tattoo completely as doing so could require the client to undergo too many treatments. Sustained exposure to some of the most popular treatments for tattoo removal procedures (especially laser treatments) can become detrimental to the skin due to the repeated deep burns caused and therefore if the desired effects are not achieved after a few sessions then it may be advisable to discontinue the aesthetic treatments. In case where the degree of tattoo fading is too low, the likelihood of incurring into the adverse effects of these aesthetic treatments may not be worthwhile and therefore the fading treatments should discontinued or switched for others (e.g. **Tattoo Excision** or **Tattoo Cover-up**).

27.1 Legislation on tattooing and tattoo removal procedures at european level.

Tattoo drawing, although have potential side effects (including infections) and these procedures involve purposely modifying the dermis by injecting the pigments inside it, while causing an open wound, tattoos made for aesthetic and lifestyle choices are not considered to be medical applications (non medical intended uses). Tattooing procedures are currently carried out by tattoo artists who are not required to hold any formal medical qualification.

In case of tattoo removal, although when advertising, several clinics refer to them as "medical procedures" and the client is also often referred to as "patient". From a mere legislative view point tattoo fading procedures (that do not involve surgery i.e. excision) are considered aesthetic procedures. Furthermore the current interpretation of European legislation considers tattoo fading procedures as cosmetic/aesthetic applications. This is because the main reason behind a tattoo removal procedure is the fact that the client regrets their previous tattoo, and desires to either change it or remove it completely. Of course there are no medical reasons in order to have an aesthetic tattoo drawn in the first place, likewise there are no medical reasons beyond an aesthetic tattoo removal process.

For these reasons in Europe any tattoo removal procedures are widely regarded as mere aesthetic procedure. Since early 2000s, there have been several lobbying pressures in order to modify the legal status classification of tattoo fading procedures in general, in order to be regarded as medical applications (Medical Intended Uses). As we know almost any tattoo removal processes do require to inflict a burn or a purposely inflicted injury of the tattooed area in some way in order to fade or remove the pigments which reside inside the dermis. In case of tattoo fading techniques, this is done a number of times in order to accomplish the desired effects. Both tattoo parlours and clinics performing tattoo removal have to comply with local legislations, which may vary from country to country and region to region in each European country.

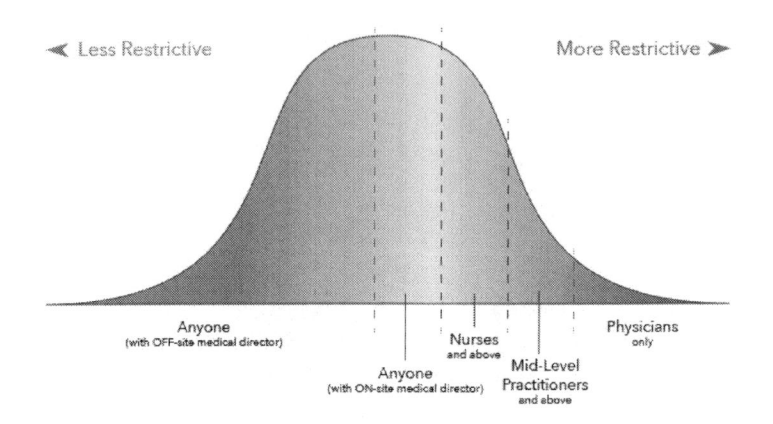

Illustration 186: Both current legislation in Europe and the UK in particular do not dictate the type of qualifications the tattooist or tattoo removal practitioner should hold to perform this procedure. Therefore, in the UK virtually anyone can start a tattoo removal business regardless of qualifications. However some insurance companies will insist the tattoo removal practitioner holds a certain level of formal qualification.

Therefore as we have seen, tattoo removal procedures are considered to be **non** medical treatments, for this reason they are not usually covered by standard health insurance policies and also they are **not** provided free of charge by the NHS.

27.2 Physiological progressive fading of permanent tattoos and the impact of tanning on their brightness

Tattoos are far more easily drawn than than being removed. This is because the pigments of permanent tattoos are made in a way so that they will withstand to the test of time. However the natural body reaction to tattoo pigments is to try to eliminate them, this normal physiological pigmentation absorption is normal and takes place very slowly. In other words, although all permanent tattoos fade over time, their fading rate is so slow that they can effectively be considered permanent.

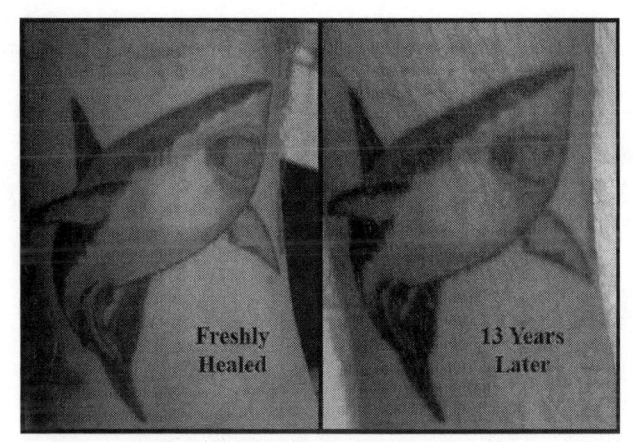

Illustration 187: Tattoo are very resilient to the test of time because they are meant to be permanent, however they do fade slightly over time on their own accord.

The rate at which the tattoo fades over time depends on a number of factors and one of them is the type of pigments used by the tattoo artist. Different type of pigments will fade at different rates and in different ways. Also sun exposure and tanning can increase the physiological fading rate. This is because the broad spectrum of sun light also includes a small proportion of infra-red light with penetrates into the skin breaking down the tattoo pigments.

In the Illustration 188 we can appreciate the deterioration of a tattoo over time. Sometimes, this natural tattoo fading is accelerated by repeated exposure to sun light (i.e. repeated tanning). It is well known that repeated intense tanning has detrimental effects on the brightness of aesthetic tattoos over time. This is because some lower wavelengths of the broad spectrum natural sun light (in particular red and infra-red) have the effect of breaking down the tattoo pigments, in a similar fashion of lasers and IPL. However the process is much slower than the degree of fading achieved with Laser or IPL treatments. In fact what we are dong with "tattoo fading" techniques is accelerating this natural tattoo fading process one way or another.

Because the tattoo pigments are meant to be permanent and they reside inside the dermis, tattoo removal procedures are normally involving a degree of dermal treatment. Because of this, "tattoo removal" or more appropriately "tattoo fading" procedure cannot be free from inherent risks.

Due to the fact that tattoos are meant to be permanent and be resilient over time, they will generally be far more difficult to remove than having them done. One session is usually sufficient to draw a beautiful medium sized tattoo, however fading it, or even removing it completely can be very challenging and sometimes not worthwhile due to the complications involved in the complete removal of particular resilient tattoos.

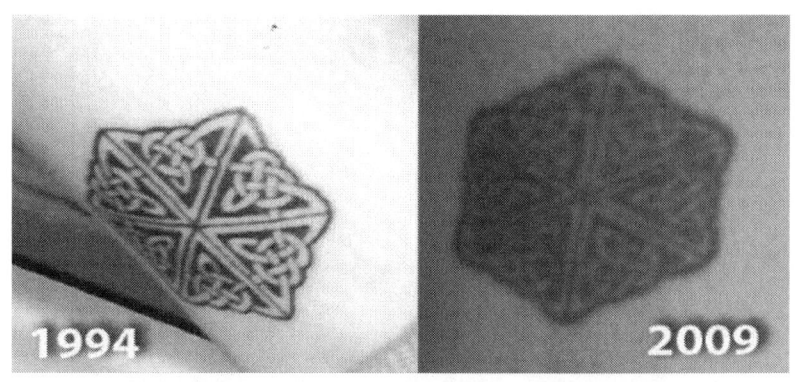

Illustration 188: The body immune system attacks the pigments and destroy them, but this process is very slow. The discolouration over time is also dependant on the type of pigmentation used. There are more and less resilient pigments. In this picture we can appreciate how the drawing blurred over time as the edges lost their sharpness over time. This type of blurring can also be experienced after tattoo fading procedures. The tattoo fading procedures are used to accelerating the natural tattoo fading process which otherwise be too slow.

27.3 Tattoo resilience and estimating the tattoo fading sessions required

One of the common questions asked by the clients is the number of tattoo fading sessions required in order to achieve their desired result (which is the complete seamless removal). It is important to manage their expectations because in many cases they do expect complete removal without leaving a trace in one or very few sessions only. In most cases there are no fading techniques currently known which will guarantee complete removal without leaving no trace.

Additionally not all tattoos present the same resilience when trying to fade them. Some types of tattoos can be easily removed in only a few easy fading sessions while others can be far more challenging and sometimes almost impossible to remove completely without leaving a scar, or some sort of trace (i.e. permanent hypo-pigmentation in case of laser removal) due to the aggressiveness of the treatment required for their complete removal. The amount of tattoo fading desired can be accomplished in two ways, either through relatively high number of mild tattoo fading treatments or through a few high intensity treatment sessions. Generally the better the pigment quality used and the better the devices used to draw the tattoos (which achieve a relative superficial pigment distribution on the dermal layer) the easier it will be to achieve the desired results while minimising the aggressiveness or intensity of the tattoo fading treatments.

On the other hand low quality pigments or even "not fit for purpose" colours can be almost impossible to remove completely using the most popular tattoo removal techniques. In some cases, the only viable option for the removal of poorly drawn tattoos (with "non fit for purpose" pigments) can be tattoo surgical excision. Also sometimes the tattoo pigments can be injected further into the dermis closer to the hypo-dermis, this can make the removal even more challenging.

LASER TATTOO REMOVAL

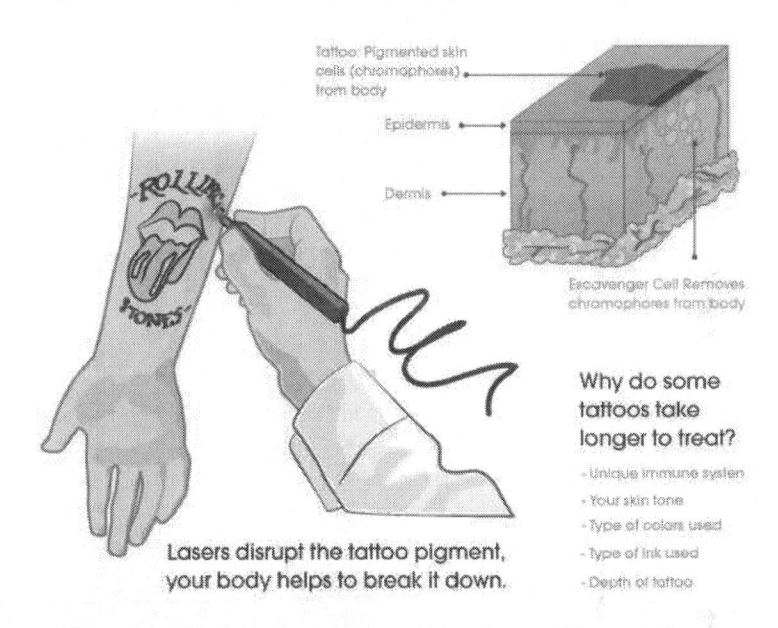

Illustration 189: Laser "tattoo removal" is only one of the several options available for tattoo fading. Although it is the most popular option not all the tattoos will fade in the same way. Please note that the deeper the positioning of the pigments inside the dermis, the more challenging the tattoo fading will be (see the section on the tattoo physiology for more information) .

Please note that the points below mainly apply to the most common tattoo fading procedures and unless stated otherwise do not refer to tattoo surgical excision. Generally the ease of removing tattoos depends on the following main factors:

> **Depth of the pigments.** The deeper the pigments inside the dermis the more challenging it will be to fade the tattoo. This applies to any tattoo fading technique. Furthermore sometimes the tattoo pigments could have been injected particularly deeply and may even be located inside or close to the hypo-dermis. In this cases it may be unrealistic to expect complete tattoo removal without leaving any trace.
> **Type of pigments.** The chemical composition determines the ease of removal. Additionally the better quality the tattoo pigments used, the easier it will be to fade them.

- **Colour of the pigments (laser tattoo fading only).** Certain wavelengths can only fade certain colours. The brighter the colours of the tattoos the more challenging they will be to fade. Conversely the darker the tattoo the easier they are to fade. The wavelength used by the laser will determine the colour it fades and the number of sessions needed. *Most other tattoo fading options are colour blind which means they fade all colours indiscriminately.*
- **Type of tattoo.** A non-professional tattoo is usually harder to fade than professional tattoos. This is because the depth of the pigments distribution may not be uniform throughout the tattoo. Therefore the tattoo may fade in different ways depending on the depth of the pigments.
- **Density and amount of the tattoo pigments.** The more dense the ink, the more layers of pigments are in the tattoo and the longer it will take to fade the tattoo. What matters is how much ink is in the skin. For example cover-up tattoos have two layers of pigmentation, therefore they will be harder to fade than normal tattoos.
- **Area covered by the tattoo.** The wider the tattoo the more fading sessions will be required to achieve the desired results. Large tattoos cannot be treated in their entirety because the risks associated to the treatment and adverse reactions would be too high in case of tattoo fading treatments which rely on burning the skin (like Lasers, electrical plasma etc). Exposing the body to extensive burns can be detrimental to the individual. This is because the potential risks and the likelihood of adverse reactions can increase dramatically proportionately with the area covered within the session. Additionally other tattoo fading treatments, which use other skin resurfacing principles, should not be used on extensive areas within one treatment, as this can increase the likelihood of their associated adverse reactions. Generally in case of large tattoos, they will be treated in smaller sections to manage the risks of the associated adverse reactions. In case of tattoo surgical excision of large tattoos, skin grafting may be necessary to replace the large area of missing skin.
- **Position of the tattoo on the body.** Some areas are not suitable for certain types of tattoo fading treatments, therefore their removal may be very challenging. These are areas subject to bending and stretching (e.g. knees, elbows, underarms etc). This applies also to those areas that are inevitably exposed to the constant rubbing of clothing (e.g. waist-line).
- **Skin tone (laser tattoo fading only).** One of the side effects peculiar to laser tattoo fading treatments is the likelihood of causing hypo-pigmentation. This is a side effect which does not generally occur after other types of tattoo fading treatments. In general the higher the treatment intensity the higher the likelihood of causing hypo-pigmentation. Conversely the lower the laser treatment intensity the lower the likelihood of hypo-pigmentation. The darker the skin tone the more the likelihood of hypo-pigmentation. Therefore when treating tattoos on dark skin tones the intensity of the treatment has to be lowered, (in order to decrease the likelihood of hypo-pigmentation) therefore increasing the number of sessions required in order to achieve a satisfactory level of tattoo fading.
- **Tattoo age (laser tattoo fading only).** The older the tattoo the more challenging it may be to fade the pigments. Conversely the fresher the tattoo the easier it may be to fade. This applies to laser tattoo removal, most other fading techniques tend to fade all tattoos approximately in the same way despite of their age.

➤ **Treatment intensity**. The treatment intensity of the particular type of tattoo fading treatment determines also the amount pigmentation fading after each session. Generally the higher the intensity the more the tattoo fades after each treatment. Conversely the milder the treatment the less the degree of tattoo fading after the treatment.

Estimating the number of sessions required in order to achieve the desired final results is often difficult if basing the opinion on the the key factors above. This is because there is seldom reliable information about the way the tattoo was originally drawn, which determines the ease of fading each particular tattoo. Often some assumptions or information about the tattoo may turn out to be incorrect. In other words, the tattoo removal practitioner may not be able to establish the reaction of the specific tattoo to the fading treatment only by looking at the tattoo or asking questions in relation to how the tattoo was drawn (there is seldom reliable information on the pigmentation distribution depth, of the chemical composition of the ink used etc).

Therefore the best option to estimate the number of sessions required in order achieve the desired results is by making an extrapolation based on the degree of tattoo fading after the initial patch testing. From this information the beauty practitioner can provide a more reliable estimation of the number of sessions required to achieve the desired results.

However, even an estimation based on the degree of fading accomplished after the tattoo patch testing may not be very accurate. How much the tattoo fades after each treatment varies from treatment to treatment. The tattoo fades most after the first few treatments, this is because the superficial pigments are the most easily removed. A relative high fading is achieved by removing the most superficial pigments. Therefore those pigments that are left after the previous tattoo fading treatment are more resilient and located deeper inside the dermis.

Therefore in certain cases where the pigments left after a number of tattoo fading treatments, are very resilient and/or located too deep inside the dermis, the amount of tattoo fading will be minor after the initial tattoo fading treatments. This is because as the tattoo fades, generally the remaining pigments are those which are the most challenging to remove. In certain cases of particular resilient pigmentation, fading the tattoo can become so arduous that further attempts to fade it can not only become futile but even potentially counter-productive as it only exposes the client to the adverse effects of the tattoo fading procedure without brining about any substantial improvements. In this case the further steps can be either surgical excision or tattoo cover-up.

27.4 Why is having a tattoo done perceived to be less risky than having it removed?

All tattoo removal options carry potential adverse reactions and any risk associated to these aesthetic procedures can be minimised however cannot be completely ruled out even following the right procedures and the after-care protocols. As we have seen, also tattooing present inherent risks, however the perceived likelihood of adverse reactions associated to their removal are generally perceived as higher.

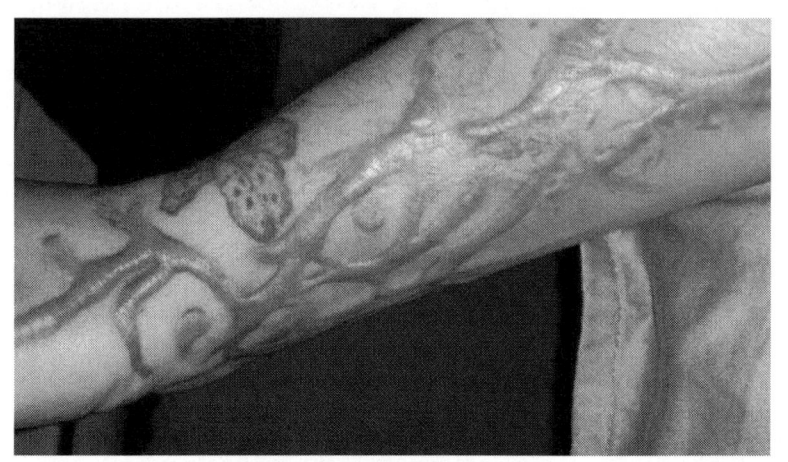

Illustration 190: Keloidal formation after tattoo removal. Some adverse reactions cannot be avoided. This is also why it is important to carry out a patch test at consultation stage.

The reason for this is very simple: although the inherent risks of both tattoo drawing and tattoo removal are very similar, tattoo removal are perceived to be riskier procedures because, unlike tattooing, several tattoo fading treatments are often required in order to achieve satisfactory results. On the other hand, the client exposes himself/herself to the inherent risks of a tattooing only once, by contrast they will require to expose themselves to the potential adverse effects several times in order to "remove" (or more appropriately fade) them. Because of this repeated exposure to the inherent adverse effects of tattoo fading treatments, the perceived associated risks are higher in tattoo removal than the tattooing process.The risks associated to each tattoo removal or fading treatment vary dramatically according to the type of fading treatments, the way the treatment was carried out (e.g. the intensity of the treatment) and especially the after-care. Therefore the client has to go through several burns or several resurfacing treatments each time being exposed to similar side effects to those of the tattoo drawing process. It is important to emphasise that most of the permanent adverse reactions to the most popular tattoo fading techniques are usually due to the client's failure to comply with the after-care procedures. To review the undesirable effects or adverse reactions to tattooin please Click Here.

27.5 Tattoo removal techniques introduction, the challenges

The request for tattoo removal is currently constantly on the increase and the prices charged for this type of aesthetic procedure are high also due to the relative complexity of the tattoo removal procedures. Additionally more and more people are are highly motivated and sometimes willing to pay almost any amount to have their tattoo removed.

www.voltaicplasma.com   Author: Andreas Russo

In the UK it is not uncommon for some tattoo removal quotes to reach 20 or 30 thousands pounds. Furthermore due to the the inherent complexity of these aesthetic treatments the tattoo removal market provides very conflicting information in connection with each type of "tattoo fading" or "tattoo removal" procedure. This is thought to be due to the several vested financial interests in "tattoo removal" procedures. Some sources point to some treatments types as being extremely risky and focus only to their potential adverse reactions of the specific type of tattoo fading treatment.

Other sources emphasise the risks of undergoing tattoo removal procedures from "non qualified" tattoo removal laser practitioners by pointing out and showing only the potential adverse effects of tattoo fading procedures. However as it is well known, all tattoo fading treatments have potential adverse reations which can be minimised but never completely eliminated. Due to these two factors (vested financial interests and the mere fact that none of the tattoo fading options currently available cannot be considered completely risk free) there are several contrasting information on the public domain suggesting one method to be more effective or safer than others.

There are several options for tattoo removal. Here we will explore the most popular ones first. Some of the most common tattoo fading treatments involve essentially skin resurfacing techniques (ie laser, plasma/electrical arcing, microdermabrasion, etc). These techniques although sometimes slowly, will lead to a certain degree of tattoo fading, however the problem with skin resurfacing in tattoo removal is that the tattoo pigments are located inside the dermis therefore the resurfacing treatment has to involve the dermal layer in order to be somewhat effective. Any skin resurfacing techniques which involves the dermal layer has intrinsic potential adverse effects including scarring. The type of skin resurfacing dictates the types and prevalence of the potential adverse reactions.

27.6 Laser tattoo fading

This is one of the most popular options available on the market. This is heavily advertised the world over and used in several cosmetic clinics. This method relies on the skin resurfacing of the dermal layer (by causing a controlled burn). Essentially the tattoo pigments as well as the dermal layer are targeted by the laser causing part of the pigments to be reabsorbed. For more information about laser tattoo removal or laser tattoo fading please Click Here.

27.7 Tattoo fading using plasma, or thermal abrasion with or without osmosis

This a technique which has been used for several years particularly in Italy and Germany and has been in use for several years in many European aesthetic clinics with very good consistent results. It combines the use of salation and thermabrasion. The thermabrasion can be carried out by using devices generating electrical arcing or certain radio frequency devices which have the same ablative (burning) effect.

Devices for this intended purpose have been on the market for the past 40 years. Today there are even several more devices on the market and this technique is increasing in popularity throughout Europe. Although very effective, this tattoo fading technique is not as popular as laser tattoo removal (fading). If carried out appropriately this tattoo fading treatment generally accomplishes a greater degree of pigmentation fading than most other techniques. For more information in connection with this type of procedure please **click here**

27.8 Tattoo surgical excision

In the video we can watch a part of the surgical procedure for tattoo excision. The practitioner removes the tattoo using a scalpel and closes the wound with stitches.

Surgical excision, also referred to as "surgical tattoo removal", is one of the most invasive options for "tattoo removal" when compared to the most popular tattoo "fading" procedures. However, this is the only procedure which can effectively be referred to as "tattoo removal". This is because only "surgical tattoo removal" can guarantee the complete removal of the unwanted tattoos within one session. All the other non surgical aesthetic treatments are mostly less invasive, however they can only fade the tattoo but seldom remove it completely within one session.

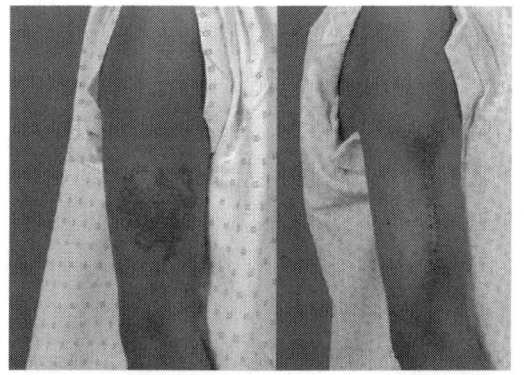

Illustration 191: Example of tattoo surgical excision. As we can see the tattoo is not in an area especially prone to stretching and bending. In this particular case the tattoo, although relatively large for an excision, is positioned on the upper arm where there is usually a certain amount of loose skin which can be removed, without causing undesirable "skin pulling" effects. We can appreciate the typical scar characteristic of a surgical excision.

Click here to watch video

www.voltaicplasma.com							Author: Andreas Russo

Before suggesting "tattoo surgical excision", the practitioner assesses the area in order to have a clear appreciation of how the part would look like if the skin where the tattoo resides were removed completely. If the "pulling effects" of the surgery is not dramatic or would not impair normal movements (hence, apart form the scar, the final result would practically look seamless), then the procedure is carried out under local anaesthetic. This is the only tattoo removal procedure which requires local anaesthetic, for all the other tattoo "fading" treatments topical numbing products usually suffice for the comfort of the client. In some cases where the tattoo covers a large area, this procedure may not be recommendable as removing large portion of the skin could be detrimental and would sometimes require subsequent skin grafting.

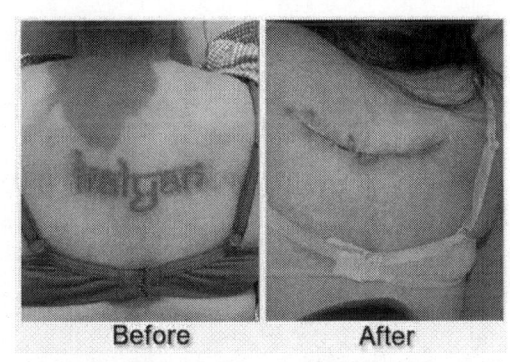

Illustration 192: The best candidates for this type of surgical procedure are relatively small tattoos, which are not located in areas particularly prone to bending and stretching. The tattoo in the picture is relatively small and not located in a critical area of the body. Surgical removal of large portions of the skin could be detrimental to the individual and should be avoided.

Not all tattoos are the best candidates for this type of procedure. If they are located on the face or areas where the skin is subject to bending and stretching (i.e. elbows, knees, shoulders etc) then this procedure may not be recommendable. Specifically, this procedure should be avoided close to the major joints were a certain degree of skin stretching is required for normal movement. The main problem with removing large tattoos using surgical excision is the fact that the skin will be "pulled" and the effects of the procedure could be clearly visible long after the removal (non seamless results).

One of the disadvantages of this type of procedure is that it will almost inevitably leave a certain degree of scarring caused by the sutures. Therefore if the tattoo is on the face, the skin constriction caused by the surgery and the scar left by the sutures do not make this type of procedure the most recommendable. Small tattoos are the best candidates for this type of procedure especially if they are located in areas where there is a relative amount of loose skin which can be removed without subsequent need for skin grafting or the skin can be removed without causing ad major "pulling" effect which could make the area look awkward.

This surgical technique proves highly effective in removing certain types of tattoos where the presence of a small scar will not bee very important.

www.voltaicplasma.com   Author: Andreas Russo

Advantages of surgical tattoo excision.
The main advantage of excision is that the tattoo will be gone immediately after the surgical procedure. This is generally the most cost effective option for smaller tattoos. This procedure although invasive, offers the clear clinical advantage of avoiding multiple exposures to burns and other intrinsic adverse effects of most common tattoo fading procedures. Because only one procedure is required for the removal of small tattoos the cost of this type of procedure is typically lower than other tattoo fading procedures.

Adverse reactions.

Adverse reactions are generally minor, but may include:

- Some degree of scarring due to the sutures is to be expected and cannot be avoided.
- Infection could occur if the area is not looked after properly.
- The skin may feel tighter for a while after the procedure due to the missing skin.
- In certain cases, where large tattoos are required to be removed using this surgical procedure, skin grafting may be necessary. The removal may not be seamless if the skin removed is relatively large (also costs could increase dramatically).

Estimated Cost:

The cost of this type of procedure is generally lower than most common tattoo fading treatments. This is mainly because the cost of tattoo fading techniques is cumulative and several treatments are required to achieve satisfactory results. In case of surgical tattoo excision of small tattoos one session will suffice to remove the tattoo. The cost for surgical tattoo removal depends on several factors:

- Country where the procedure is carried out. In certain countries the wide availability of surgeons can make this procedure more cost effective than other most popular tattoo fading treatments. Tattoo fading devices can sometimes be very costly, making the tattoo fading procedures especially "laser removal" more expensive than surgical excision.
- The size of the tattoo. The larger the tattoo the more expensive the procedure due to the likelihood of skin grafting requirement. As pointed out previously, this procedure may not be recommendable for the removal of relatively large tattoos.
- The type of anaesthesia used during the procedure. Local anaesthetic is the preferred and most cost effective option for this type of procedure. In case the surgeon opts for total general anaesthesia the procedure can be far more costly. General anaesthetic is the preferred option in case of tattoo surgical excision which also requires skin grafting. Unlike the other most common tattoo fading procedure, topical numbing products will not suffice for surgical procedures.

27.9 Tattoo fading using osmosis or salation in general

Due to its effectiveness, the basic principles of salabrasion (combination of osmosis and dermal abrasion) have been used for several hundreds years and this makes it one of the oldest form of tattoo fading procedures currently known. While the efficacy of other methods may be limited by the age of the tattoo, the pigments colours (in case of Laser tattoo fading), the type of tattoo pigments and their distributions inside the dermis, the Saline Method (Osmosis) can remove both old and new tattoos regardless of the pigments used. This method is also effective on amateur, professional grade tattoos and permanent make-up, however it cannot fade very deep pigments close to the hypo-dermis.

Additionally, since the saline method does not rely on the destruction of skin layers, the risk of scarring (although always exist and can never be ruled out) is considerably lower than more traditional methods. Finally, pain and wait time between treatments is decreased when compared to laser treatments. Where blistering is a normal inevitable adverse reaction to the burn caused by the Laser, it is not experienced after salabrasion. The evidence of the efficacy of Salation (referred to as salabrasion, or osmosis) is corroborated by fact that the degree of tattoo fading is relatively predictable and the results are repeatable. The efficacy of osmosis is also validated by various **scientific research papers** (view **further reference**) and studies carried out by radio frequency devices manufacturers.Reference.

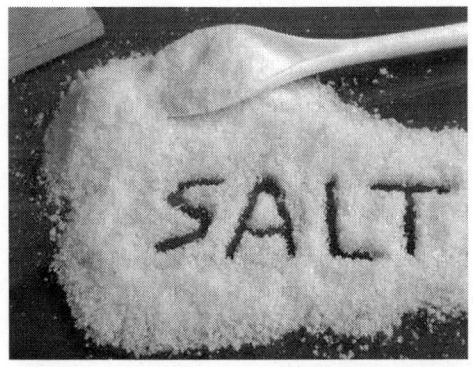

Illustration 193: Sodium Chloride (salt) induces osmosis and fades any tattoo colours very effectively (for this reason this type of aesthetic procedure is referred to as "colour blind"). Osmosis has to be combined with other types of skin abrasion treatments to be effective.

The techniques and protocols used with salation (or osmosis) have evolved throughout the years due to the different skin resurfacing devices that had been placed on the market over time or novel skin abrasion techniques. Also the fact that in Europe and in most parts of the world tattoo removal is a not a heavily regulated procedure have helped develop different protocols for this application. Osmosis (or Salabration) is a tattoo fading technique because it leads to a degree of pigmentation fading after each treatment and complete removal cannot be guaranteed within one treatment.

The main ingredient of this type of tattoo fading technique is Sodium Chloride (salt). The reason for this treatment to be effective is the fact that the osmosis induced when salt (Sodium Chloride) is placed on top of the tattoo pigments, has the direct effect of drawing not only more water molecules towards it but also the broken tattoo pigments with it.

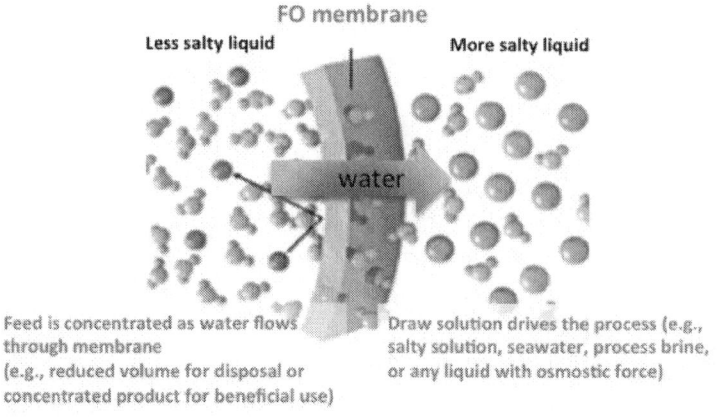

Illustration 194: This figure illustrates the general physical principle of the osmotic process. Water tends to move towards the more saline solution. With osmosis in tattoo removal the water is drawn towards the highly concentrated saline solution. This also allows the broken free tattoo colour pigments to be drawn towards the sterile saline solution or the sterile fine salt.

Applying salt on its own on a tattoo does not have the desired tattoo fading effects. This is because the **tattoo pigments are well ingrained inside the dermis** and are protected by the epidermis. Therefore merely trying to apply osmosis without another skin abrading treatment which facilitates the osmotic process is not going to produce the desired tattoo fading effects. In other words, if used on its own, the application of sodium Chloride on the surface of the tattoo has very little effects on the tattoo pigments.

For this reason this type of procedure is usually split into two parts:

Abrasion. A form or dermal abrasion is required to allow the dermis to become in contact with the sterile saline solution or fine sterile sodium chloride, this will facilitate the osmotic process to take place. Abrasion can be carried out in many different ways, the most popular techniques use mechanical means, like abrasion by using dermal abrasion devices, micro dermabrasion devices. Thermal dermabrasion by using radio frequency devices or electrical arcing devices are also used to facilitate osmotic tattoo fading.

Only these techniques are are explored here, because these are the most common methods used for this application. However abrasion can be carried out in several other ways to facilitate osmosis. Also thermal abrasion may be possible using other devices including lasers, however they will not be explored here. Local anaesthesia (which is non mandatory) is sometimes administered before the dermal abrasion treatment to avoid discomfort. Good **topical numbing products** are the preferred option for salabrasion, are more cost effective, easier to use and generally suffice for this purpose. If using dermabrasion devices the tattooed area is abraded until the area becomes red or starts to bleed slightly. Likewise if using **thermal dermabrasion** using radio frequency or **Electrical arcing-Plasma devices**, the tattooed area is treated until slight bleeding takes place.

Osmosis. The basic active substance used in Osmosis is sterile fine salt. Osmosis can be applied in different ways. Sodium Chloride can be used on its own, made into a thick paste of sterile fine salt and sterile saline solution, or as a saturated or close to saturation sterile saline solution. Sometimes bandages impregnated with highly concentrated saline solution are applied on the abraded tattoo to cause the osmotic effect. The aesthetic practitioner can choose to apply the osmotic effect on the abraded tattoo in different ways and at different intensity (by varying the timing of application) depending on the area where the tattoo is located and the desired effects.

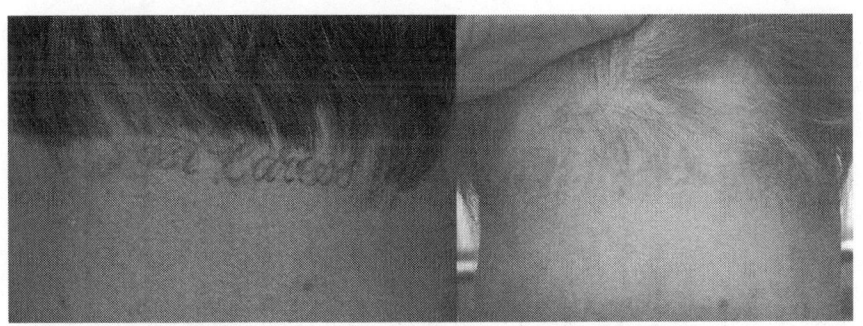

Illustration 195: Effective use of Osmosis in tattoo removal.

As stated above the osmotic effect can be carried out by applying simply sterile fine salt and bandaging the area, or by applying bandages impregnated with high concentrated sterile saline solution, or applying a dense saline paste on the abraded tattoo etc. The way osmosis is applied is often dictated by the location of the tattoo and the preference of the aesthetic practitioner. For example, when removing permanent make-up, bandaging the area or applying fine salt may not be convenient, whereas applying a thick paste for a few minutes (typically on the tattooed eyebrows) maybe the most convenient option.

The osmotic effects depend on the type of abrasion carried out before the osmosis was applied, timing of osmotic application and the type of application (i.e. whether fine sterile salt is applied, a saline paste, saline solution impregnated bandages etc). Varying one of these parameters determines the intensity of the treatment and the amount of pigmentation removal of the specific tattoo fading session.

The duration of the application will also determine the intensity of the osmotic treatment and the degree of tattoo fading. Osmosis can be applied from ten minutes to two hours depending on several factors. In order to stop the osmotic effect, the area is washed using the **appropriate antiseptic** and re-bandaged. The bandage should be removed a few hours later and the area washed again using the appropriate antiseptic and the bandaging process repeated every 5 to 6 hours for at least 24 hours.

Three to four days after the procedure scabs start to develop. The scabs must fall off on their own. Every time the area is treated there will be a degree of discolouration of the tattoo.

There are several factors that contribute to the degree of tattoo fading after each treatment using this technique:

- **Depth and type of abrasion:** Whether the abrasion is carried out mechanically, using thermal abrasion devices or radio frequency devices. The deeper the abrasion the stronger the osmotic effects. Certain types of abrasion may be more effective than others. Thermal abrasion for instance has the double effect of causing the abrasion but also breaking down some of the pigmentation due to the heat induced into the skin.

- **Timing of the osmosis application:** The longer the saline solution or the saline paste is kept on the abraded tattoo the better the osmosis effects and the more the eventual tattoo discolouration.

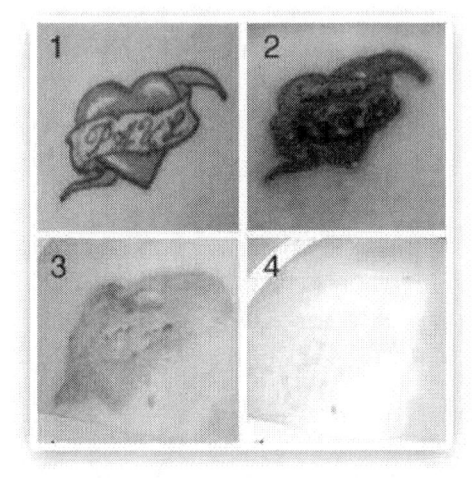

Illustration 196: Original tattoo (1), the typical scabbing on the top right(2), post treatment temporary hypertrophic formation (3), skin retuned to normal after the complete removal (4).

- **How the osmosis has been applied:** Namely it is possible to apply fine sterile salt or sterile paste or a highly concentrated saline solution. Keeping all the other parameters the same (i.e. timing of osmosis application type of and depth of abrasion etc) and changing the way the osmosis is applied, its efficacy in fading the pigments vary.

- **Depth of the tattoo pigments:** The deeper the pigments the more arduous will the complete removal be or even achieving acceptable results.

- **Type of pigments:** Like with any other tattoo fading treatment, inevitably the quality of the pigmentation determines the ease of tattoo fading.

Alternative saline treatment:

Certain aesthetic practitioners also utilise traditional tattoo equipment that is commonly used to draw the tattoo. Instead of tattoo pigmentation, a highly concentrated saline solution is injected into the tattoo. The highly concentrated sterile saline solution effectively bonds to the pigment molecules trapped deep below the superficial layers. The body naturally recognizes these bound pigment particles and pushes them up toward the surface of the skin, eventually ejecting them and causing the area to scab and the tattoo to fade.

Dermabrasion has been conceived for other aesthetic procedures, in particular for skin resurfacing used to improve the appearance of fine lines. Sometimes microdermabrasion is used for tattoo fading. There are several types of dermabrasion devices on the market.

This technique when used for tattoo fading, is also referred to as "sanding off" the tattoo. This method uses skin resurfacing in order to fade the tattoo. This aesthetic procedure can be used on its own or combined with other procedures (i.e. **_salation or osmosis_**).

On its own, this procedure focuses on stimulating the skin regeneration process by sanding off the epidermal layer, and in case of tattoo removal also the **upper part of the dermis where the tattoo resides** . This is not a very popular tattoo fading method, particularly due to its immediate gruesomeness (the treated part will in fact immediately start to bleed), the relative low degree of tattoo fading after each session and hence the fact that several treatments are required in order to to achieve the desired results, (consequently exposing the client to the intrinsic associated adverse effects of this treatment several times). Because of these reasons microdermabrasion on its own is not widely used for tattoo fading treatments. After each session scabs will form and the tattoo should have faded slightly.

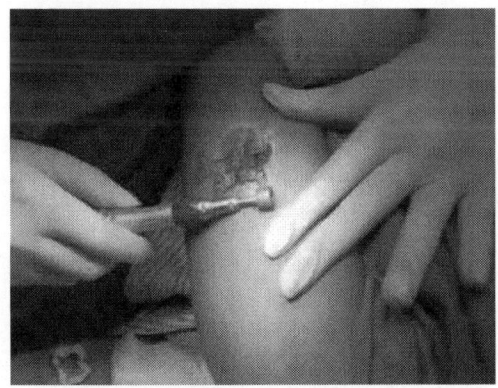

Illustration 197: Tattoo Dermabrasion

Click here to Watch video

27.10 Tattoo fading using chemical peels

Like dermabrasion, this is a technique which relies on skin resurfacing. There are several types of chemical peels that can be used for this application. The main problem, like with the use of any other skin resurfacing techniques, is that although the cosmetic peels can remove skin layers as deep as required, the pigments do not fade like the mainstream tattoo fading techniques (Plasma and osmosis, **Osmosis** on its own, **Laser**). The reason is that in order for this technique to be effective the ablation should be carried out to remove part of the dermis where the tattoo pigments reside. As we know the deeper the ablation into the dermis the more likely the risk of causing permanent hypertrophic scar formation. Also the fading results are not very consistent using this method as the ablation effects depend on the application of the particular peeling product.

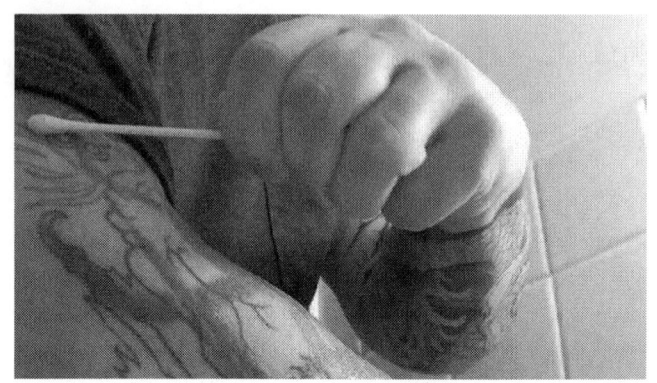

Illustration 198: TCA is one of the peels advertised for tattoo removal Click here to watch video

TCA is one of the peels advertised for tattoo removal. Also peels for tattoo fading are advertised as home tattoo removal treatments. There are several articles warning about the risks of such home treatments, referring to them as risky, however as we know all tattoo fading treatments **do all have potential adverse reactions** . It is believed this is a reaction to the low prices of these home treatments threatening the mainstream business of major cosmetic clinics. To view the video associated to this picture **click here** .

27.11 Tattoo fading using intense pulsed light (IPL)

Intense Pulsed Light devices are mostly used for permanent hair removal and they are very *rarely used for tattoo fading*. The main difference between lasers and Intense pulsed light (IPL) is that in case of lasers the device can emit one or multiple wavelenths at once, while in case of IPL the device emits a broad spectrum light. The IPL device's broad spectrum light penetrates into the skin and can fade the tattoo pigments. This is because the broad spectrum light breaks down part of the tattoo pigments. This is a similar process to **laser tattoo fading** .Intense Pulsed Light devices are mostly used for permanent epilation and they are very *rarely used for tattoo fading*.

The main difference between lasers and Intense pulsed light (IPL) is that in case of lasers the device can emit one or multiple wavelenths at once, while in case of IPL the device emits a broad spectrum light.

The IPL device's broad spectrum light which penetrates into the skin and can fade the tattoo pigments. This is because the broad spectrum light breaks down part of the tattoo pigments. This is a similar process to **laser tattoo fading** .

Before performing the IPL tattoo fading procedure, the beauty practitioner may administer a topical numbing product. A cold gel will then be placed on the area and a glass prism is applied to channel the intense light. Several treatments will follow every 3-4 weeks, all more aggressive than the first.

The skin will be pink or red after the procedure. Side effects from IPL include blistering, little bleeding, scarring, swelling and changes in pigmentation. Sunscreen with high SPF must be used on the treated area.

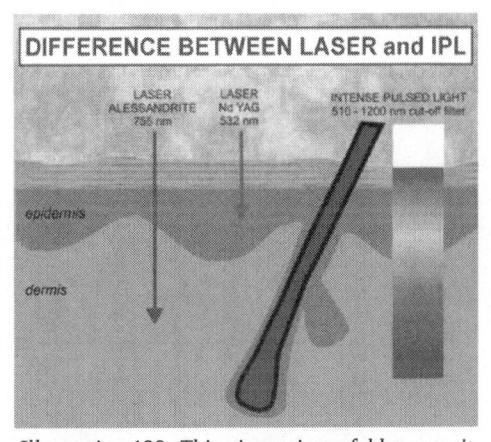

Illustration 199: This picture is useful because it illustrates how the broad spectrum light of the IPL is absorbed by the skin. The higher frequencies (represented by the yellow light) are absorbed by the most superficial layer. The lower frequencies (represented by the orange and red) penetrate into the deeper layer of the skin.

27.12 Tattoo fading using cryotherapy

Cryotherapy uses very cold temperatures to remove unwanted tissue. Like **IPL** , this is very rarely used for tattoo fading and it is not a mainstream treatment. For tattoo removal, ice crystals form on the skin with tattoo pigments, fragmenting some of them. Cryotherapy can be carried out with liquid nitrogen, carbon dioxide, argon or a combination of dimethyl ether and propane to freeze the skin. The epidermis peels and comes off; some of tattoo ink residing underneath the skin should come off as well. Several cryotherapy sessions will be necessary.

Clients may experience some pain and redness at the site, which can be attenuated by pain relieving products. Blisters go away after a few days. Small white spots may form around the area. Risks include nerve tissue damage and **scarring** .

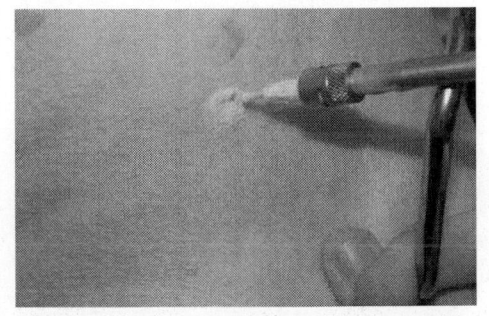

Illustration 200: Although cryotherapy is widely used for various dermatological applications expecially warts removal, it is sometimes used for tattoo removal due to its skin resurfacing effects.

www.voltaicplasma.com   Author: Andreas Russo

27.13 Tattoo removal by replacement

As we have seen the complete removal of permanent aesthetic tattoos are sometimes **very challenging**. Undergoing several tattoo fading treatments can not only be expensive but does expose the client several times to the inherent **potential adverse effects** of each particular treatment. As we know, the best degree of tattoo fading is accomplished during the first treatments, and as the tattoo fades, the pigments remaining are the most resilient. Especially those located in the deeper part of the dermis, and sometimes even inside the the hypo-dermis. Therefore once the tattoo has faded to a certain extent, in case the further fading treatments do not achieve the satisfactory tattoo fading, than alternative treatments may be more suitable. One option may be cover up.

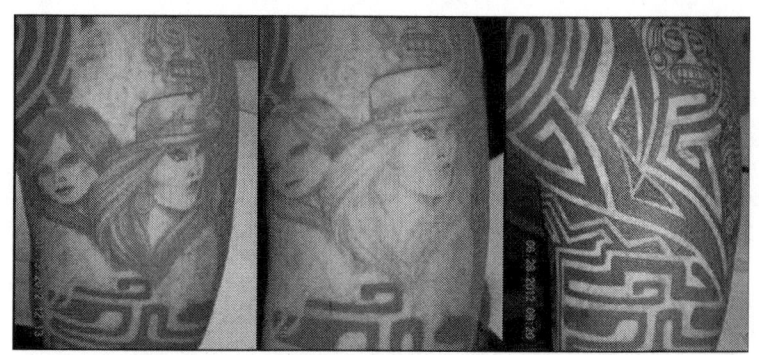

Illustration 201: In some cases the cost and the adverse reactions on the skin of tattoo fading treatment aimed at completely removing a tattoo are not worthwhile especially with laser treatments. Therefore it may be preferable to fade the tattoo as much as reasonably possible and cover it up with another. The results are quite good most of the times. In this case we can see how the tattoo fading can help cover up a previous tattoo.

Tattoo cover up can be used on an existing tattoo, without any prior fading treatment. In fact, an artfully done cover-up may render the old tattoo completely invisible, though this will depend largely on the size, style, colours and techniques used on the old tattoo and the skill of the tattoo artist. Covering up a previous tattoo requires darker tones in the new tattoo to effectively hide the older, and also can be used as soon as the fading of the particular tattoo removal treatment reduce in effectiveness (becoming not worthwhile).

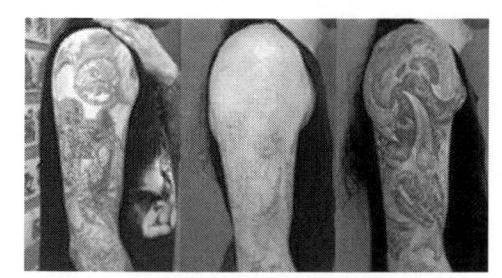

Illustration 202: Tattoo fading followed by subsequent cover-up.

www.voltaicplasma.com

Author: Andreas Russo

Generally, the main challenge of all current "tattoo removal" or better " **tattoo fading techniques** " is that, due to the inherent **physiology of aesthetic tattoos** , the pigments reside inside the dermal layer, therefore any effective treatment will inevitably affect the dermis in one way or another consequently causing a number of inherent risks including developing **scars** or other side effects. Despite the type of treatment used to fade the tattoo the inherent risks of scarring and other adverse effects can be minimised but never completely eliminated due to the very nature of these aesthetic treatments. Unfortunately, tattoo pigment targeting , there are not currently known methods that actually allow selective targeting and destruction of the tattoo pigments without also affecting the dermal layer where the tattoo resides. This is proven by the fact that the adverse reaction to the tattoo fading treatment is the same in any part of the body not covered by the tattoo. Additionally the most popular tattoo fading treatments rely on burning the skin (e.g. laser treatment, IPL, Plasma etc), therefore these treatments may carry inherent adverse effects associated to any common skin burn.

There are three types of adverse reactions:

1. The temporary adverse reactions, those which follow the treatment and cause the so called downtime (most of them will subside on their own accord),
2. Semi permanent adverse reactions
3. And permanent.

Temporary adverse reactions:

The type of temporary adverse reactions vary according to the type of tattoo fading treatment. These are inevitable due to the very nature of the treatments. Most of them will not require any treatment, as they will subside on their own accord. Some others, like inflammatory infections, will necessitate treatment.

These temporary adverse reactions are:

- Discomfort and pain during treatment.
- Frosting (laser treatments).
- Minor bleeding.
- Immediate redness and swelling.
- Blistering.
- Scabbing.
- Itching.
- Swelling and infections.

27.14 Discomfort and Pain

While a lot will depend on the individual pain threshold, it is fair to say that the majority of people undergoing the most popular tattoo fading treatments experience discomfort and pain if the appropriate numbing product is not applied on the tattoo in advance. The level of discomfort and pain also depends on where the tattoo is located and the type of tattoo fading treatment; tattoos on more fleshy areas of the body will hurt less as the flesh acts as a cushion, whereas tattoos on areas such as the wrist, feet, face and fingers could be more painful than if the tattoo were on the thigh for example!

27.15 Frosting, (during laser tattoo fading)

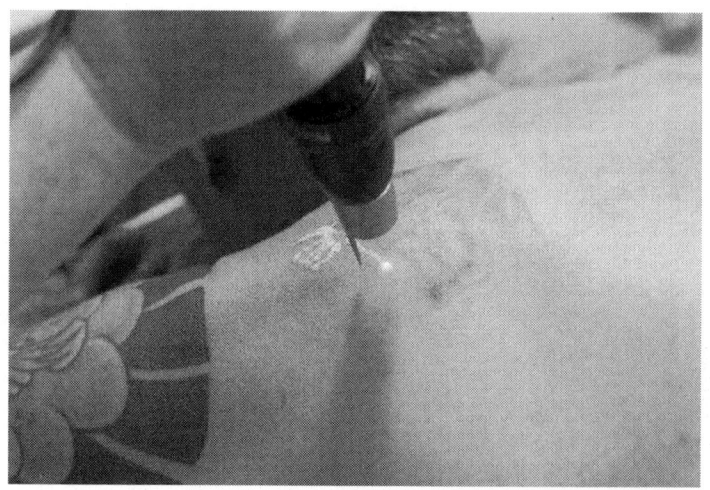

Illustration 203: Frosting caused by the the laser treatment. This is a very temporary effect. The frosting disappears on its own accord within an hour after the treatment. This is a normal skin reaction to the skin burn caused by the laser.

Frosting is a normal immediate reaction during tattoo **laser** fading treatments. The tattooed skin will naturally turn into frosty white colour. This is caused by the carbon dioxide being released as a result of laser burn which surfaces on the upper layer of the skin and usually subsides only after half an hour. The frosting is usually caused by higher laser frequencies that produce a superficial ablation of the skin. This is not normally caused by very low frequencies used in deep laser skin tightening (i.e. Fraxel laser treatments operating at over 10,000 nm). Other tattoo fading treatments do not cause frosting.

27.16 Minor bleeding

Minor bleeding is a normal reaction to most professional tattoo fading treatments. In particular Laser, Plasma and Microdermabrasion. The bleeding is caused by the breakage of the small superficial capillaries in the dermis during the aesthetic treatment. Bleeding during the most popular tattoo fading treatments is minor and lasts only a few minutes. This occurs because any tattoo fading treatment in order to be effective has to include the ablation of the dermis. However in vast majority of cases bleeding is very unlikely to ever become severe and subsides only after a few minutes.

27.17 Immediate redness and minor swelling

After the use of ablative treatments (i.e. laser, plasma, IPL), the area may turn red and become only slightly swollen a few moments and minutes after the treatment. Also this is the normal physiological immediate reaction to the skin burn caused by the particular tattoo fading treatment. The reddening and minor swelling only last a few hours and will subside on its own accord being replaced by the **blistering** (in case of **laser treatment**). This reaction is not usually experienced using other types of tattoo fading treatments.

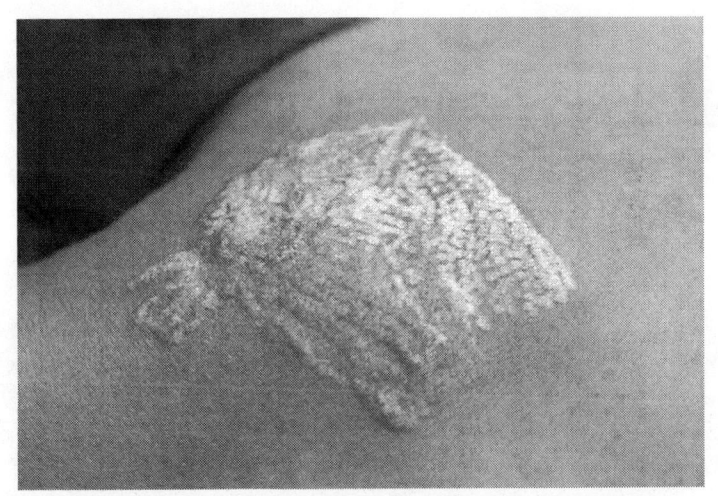

Illustration 204: Frosting, skin reddening and minor swelling immediately after a laser tattoo fading treatment. The reddening is manifested also on the surrounding area of the tattoo treated. This is a normal reaction to the burn caused by the laser tattoo fading treatment.

27.18 Blistering

Certain tattoo fading treatments like **Laser** , **Plasma** , **IPL** rely on burning the tattoo in order to help fade it. **Blistering** is a physiological reaction to any type of burns therefore any treatments which cause an intentional burn of the skin will lead to some form of blistering. The **blisters** usually start forming the day following the treatment replacing the **minor swelling and redness** caused by the skin burn. Blistering does not require any treatment and will subside on its own accord. In order to reduce the **blistering** and the downtime associated with the burn caused by the treatment, ice packing and appropriate soothing products can be used to alleviate the adverse reactions immediately after the tattoo fading treatment. Ice Packing and other soothing products should not be used after Plasma tattoo attenuation treatments. This is because there is no blistering after plasma tattoo removal fading.

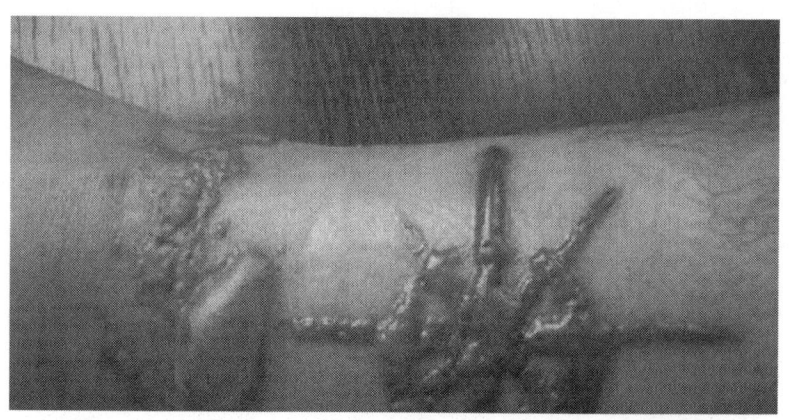

Illustration 205: Blisters after laser tattoo fading treatment. This is a physiological reaction to several laser skin treatments. The blisters must not be purposely burst.

Therefore blistering is a normal reaction and an indication that the healing process has begun. They might not look too pretty and could be tender to touch, but blisters should take between 3-14 days to heal up completely. Blisters must not be burst. Purposely bursting the blisters can interfere with the physiological healing process including increasing **the likelihood of infections** and consequently permanent **scarring** .

27.19 Scabbing

Yet another sign that the tattoo removal is working and healing is taking place. Scabbing is a typical part of the healing process after certain types of tattoo fading procedures. The scabbing process starts to develop two to three days after tattoo fading procedures using plasma (voltaic arcing), **osmosis** and **micro dermabrasion** . Scabs often contain fragmented ink particles. When the scabs fall off, the top layer of the ink will come off with it. Picking at or peeling off the scabs can increase the risk of scarring, so however tempting, it must be avoided. A lot will depend on the size, type, intensity of the treatment and location of the tattoo, however most scabs will fall off on their own accord within two weeks, provided there is no inflammatory infection under-way.

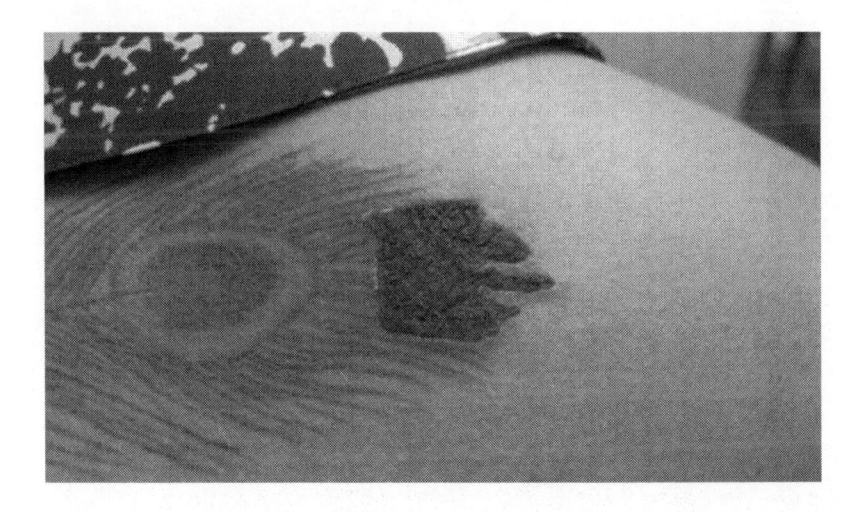

Illustration 206: Scabbing after a tattoo fading treatment patch testing. The scabs must not be picked and will fall off on their own accord a few days after the treatment.

27.20 Itching

This should be seen as a good sign, as the immune system kicks in and starts to heal the affected area, also this is a sign that there is no ongoing infection. An itching sensation is common, but just like any other type of skin irritation, the client must not scratch the treated area. Scratching could impact on the effectiveness of the removal and more importantly break the skin and cause a wound, which could increase the likelihood of infection and scarring. Generally, the client should not apply creams or lotions on the treated area. However in case the itching becomes unbearable the client should seek medical advice.

27.21 Swelling and infections

Our body's natural defence system will react to things like illness or infection in a number of different ways. But while swelling usually occurs after being bitten by an insect or other inflammatory causes, it can also happen after undergoing tattoo fading treatments especially due to infections. Inflammatory infections can be easily contracted during the healing process due to the fact that the area is an open wound and like any other wound is exposed to several types of bacteria which cause infections.

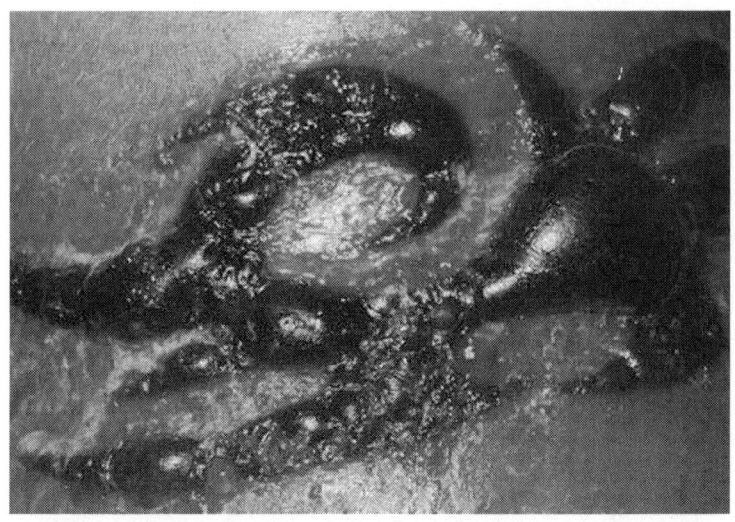

Illustration 207: Inflammatory infections can be contracted during the healing process. This can happen after any type of tattoo fading treatment. Infections can also cause some degree of swelling.

Inflammatory infections are the main cause of permanent adverse reactions like scarring and permanent change in skin texture. After laser tattoo removal it is very important not to burst the blisters (which form a couple of days after the treatment) because this causes an open wound and puts the client at an increased exposure to infections. Usually the risks of inflammatory infections diminish as soon as the **scabs begin to form** . The risks of infections can be minimised but never completely avoided. The bast way to minimise the likelihood of contracting an inflammatory infection during the healing process it to keep the area clean and use the appropriate **antiseptic products** at regular intervals.

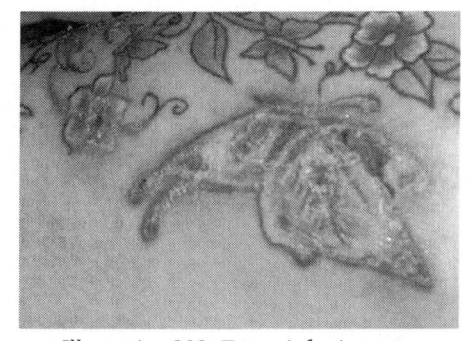

Illustration 208: Tattoo infections can manifest in several ways. Sometimes redness is a sign of the onset of an infection. Inflammatory infections are the primary cause of permanent scarring, permanent change in skin texture and other permanent adverse reactions.

www.voltaicplasma.com   Author: Andreas Russo

27.22 Permanent and semi-permanent adverse reactions

Semi permanent adverse reactions. The most common semi permanent adverse reactions is a temporary change in skin texture. This is a normal reaction to the skin regeneration process of skin resurfacing treatments. As it is well known, after skin resurfacing treatments the new skin has a *pinkish colour* and a slight different texture to the rest of the skin. The pinkish colour is due to the lack of pigmentation of the new skin. Over time the skin texture blends in with the rest of the skin and new pigments will form. This applies to all the tattoo fading techniques discussed in this web page including laser tattoo fading. In other cases, in particular, with the use of Osmosis the common semi-permanent adverse reaction in those cases, especially where an infection has taken place, is a often *temporary* raised scar. This *temporary* raised scar usually lasts two to three months and in most cases this will subside over time and the area will blend with the surrounding skin.

27.23 Permanent adverse reactions

The types of permanent adverse reactions can be: **Scarring (or permanent change in skin texture)**, **Keloidal formations**, **hyper-pigmentation** and hypo-pigmentation (The latter is an adverse reaction associated with laser treatments only) . These types of permanent adverse effects can occur despite the type of tattoo fading treatment carried out. In any case the likelihood of these inherent adverse effects can be minimised but never completely eliminated.

27.24 Scarring

Permanent scarring is an inherent risk of any type of tattoo fading treatments, it can be minimised but never completely excluded. Rarely permanent scarring occurs due to the tattoo fading treatment alone. Permanent scarring is often caused by the damage inflicted by the infections contracted during the healing stage. Also in case of laser tattoo fading treatments the **normal blisters** must not be purposely burst as this also can increase the likelihood of complications especially infections. If the tattoo fading treatment lead to scabbing, the scabs must not be picked and must fall off on their own. If scarring does occur, it is not usually very noticeable and can be minimised with **Vitamin E oil or over the counter silicone patches** .

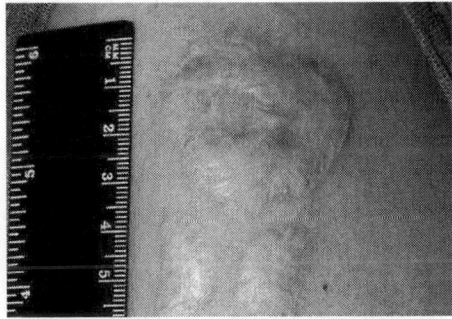

Illustration 209: The inherent risks of developing permanent change in skin texture or scarring, can be minimised but never eliminated due to the very nature of the tattoo fading treatments currently available. Risks of scarring are dramatically increased if an infection is contracted during the healing process.

www.voltaicplasma.com

Author: Andreas Russo

The risks of permanent scarring can never be completely eliminated, even if the tattoo fading procedure is carried out appropriately and the client follows the after-care instructions rigorously. This is because certain individuals are particularly prone to to developing some sort of scarring or permanent difference in skin texture. This is one of the reasons to carry out a patch test at consultation stage. Also some individuals may be prone to developing **keloids** and some may not even be aware of this predisposition.

27.25 Hyper-pigmentation

Any tattoo fading treatment relies on a form of skin resurfacing, that may be done by means of burning the skin using **lasers**, **electrical arcing**, **chemical peels** etc. Whenever the skin is starting its physiological regeneration process and it is exposed to UV light sources, both natural or artificial, the normal skin reaction can be a hyper-pigmentation. This type of hyper-pigmentation is possible, not only following tattoo fading treatments but also, after any other type of skin resurfacing including cosmetic peels. Therefore cosmetic tattoos and permanent make-up may darken following tattoo fading treatments. Although further resurfacing treatments can fade the hyper-pigmentation away, hyper-pigmentation can be very challenging to resolve at times.

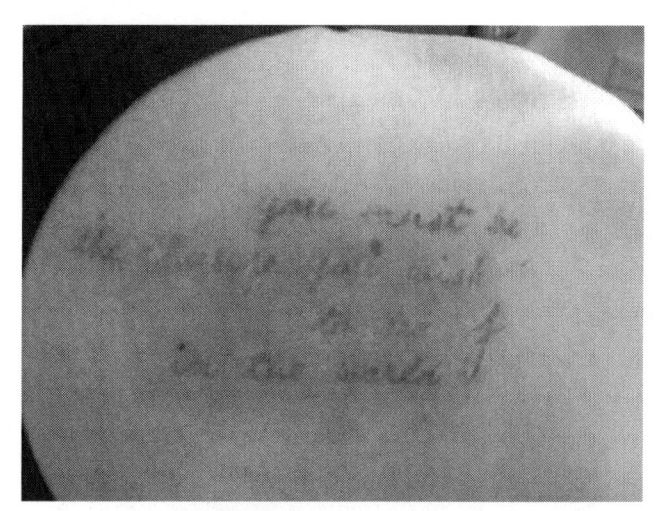

Illustration 210: Hyper-pigmentation is an adverse reaction possible following any type of tattoo fading treatment. The likelihood of this occurrence increases if the person exposes the treated area to UV sources and sunlight in general.

Hyper-pigmentation unfortunately is an inherent risk of any type of skin resurfacing treatment, therefore it can be minimised but never completely ruled out after tattoo fading treatments. The best way to minimise the likelihood of hyper-pigmentation is to avoid sun exposure including any source of UV light. The use of total sunscreen up to two months after the healing process should be mandatory.

Please note that sun and UV light exposure must be avoided even while using total sun screen up to two months after the last treatment.

27.26 Hypopigmentation

Hypo-pigmentation is a common adverse reaction to aesthetic laser treatments in general (including laser skin tightening, laser skin resurfacing etc). The potential risks of this permanent change in texture and colour can be minimised but never excluded after laser aesthetic treatments. Hypo-pigmentation is particularly common in darker skin tones (six, five and four) however it has been reported on lighter skin types (including one and two). This type of adverse reaction is prevalent only after tattoo laser fading treatments and they are very rare after other types of tattoo fading treatments.

Hyper-pigmentation is where over production of pigmentation occurs during the healing process, conversely hypo-pigmentation is where the skin's normal pigmentation has been removed and new melanin cannot either permanently or temporarily be produced. Hence the hypo-pigmentation effect can be permanent or semi-permanent.

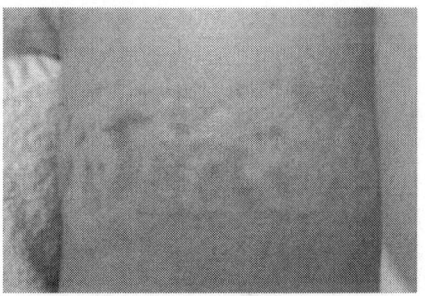

Illustration 211 Hypo-pigmentation after laser tattoo removal. Hypo-pigmentation is a particular common adverse reaction to Laser aesthetic treatments in general. They are particularly common on the darker skin types (five and six) however they have also been been reported on lighter skin types (including one and two)

It can sometimes take months or even years for your skin's pigment to appear normal again. For some people, the skin texture may never be the same. As a result of hypo-pigmentation, lighter patches of skin will be visible where the tattoo once was and on the area of the skin treated by the laser. However, in most cases hypo-pigmentation is bound to be more tolerable than the unwanted tattoo.

27.27 Conclusions

Most of the tattoo **fading treatments are currently marketed as tattoo removal treatments** . To date, the only procedure which can be correctly addressed as tattoo removal is **Surgical Excision** . Only **tattoo surgical excision** can guarantee the complete removal within one sessions only, the other techniques can fade the tattoo, however complete disappearance within one session cannot be guaranteed. In the vast majority of cases several sessions are required in order to achieve a satisfactory tattoo fading. Sometimes, the complete seamless (scar-free) removal of tattoos is not always possible using any conventional tattoo fading techniques currently available. In these cases **tattoo cover-up** may be a good option after fading the tattoo as much as possible using most tattoo fading technique available.

Clients are keen to have an estimation of the number of treatments required to achieve their desired results . The number of sessions required can vary from as few as one in case of permanent make-up removal and can even require up to 10 or more sessions in case of resilient tattoos. The number of sessions required also depends the type of tattoo fading treatment as well as the intensity of the treatment. In order to make a realistic estimation, a patch test should be carried out to extrapolate this information from the degree of tattoo fading accomplished after the patch testing. Patch testing also reveals if the client can be susceptible to any particular type of inherent permanent adverse reactions to the particular tattoo fading procedure.

Although laser tattoo fading currently is the most popular "tattoo removal" procedure, there are also several other effective tattoo fading treatments available (i.e. Plasma, Plasma and Osmosis, Osmosis associated with other dermabasion treatments, microdermabrasion, IPL, Chemical peels, Croytherapy etc). Despite the method used to fade the tattoos, in case after a number of tattoo fading sessions, the degree of tattoo fading is only minimal, tattoo removal by replacement may be the best option.

28.0 Laser Tattoo Removal

Laser tattoo removal. It is highly advisable to read the general section on tattoo removal before studying this section focusing on laser tattoo fading.

28.1 Why are lasers so popular in tattoo fading treatments

Lasers have been used for this aesthetic application over several years. Tattoo fading lasers are very easy to use and the intensity of the treatment is not dependent on the way the device is used during the treatment itself. This is because as we will see the intensity of the treatment is largely determined by the setting of the device and not by the way the laser is operated. This makes laser tattoo fading devices relatively easyto use. There is little error related to the way the laser is then used during the treatment. The only mistake which can be made is overlapping the lasers burst on the tattoo while operating the device. However, this is very easily avoided as the operator can appreciate the **frosting** caused by the laser and avoid treating the area again.

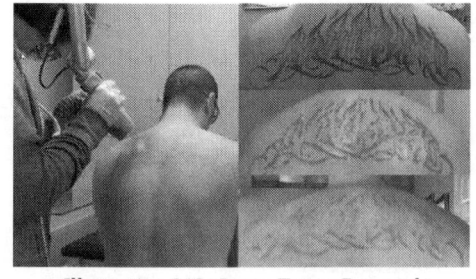

Illustration 212: Laser Tattoo Removal

www.voltaicplasma.com Author: Andreas Russo

These aesthetic treatments only last a few minutes, are straightforward to perform and the price per minute for this type of treatment is relatively high. Therefore very profitable to the cosmetic clinics performing them. This is because the duration of the treatment *per set* is very brief and the price charged for treatment is relatively high (because the clientèle is usually highly motivated to have their tattoo faded or removed). Also, several numbers of treatments are required to achieve satisfactory results making the cumulative total amount charged relatively high. Both the ever increased demand and the profitability of these treatments to clinics have made laser tattoo fading treatments the most popular aesthetic treatment for this application.

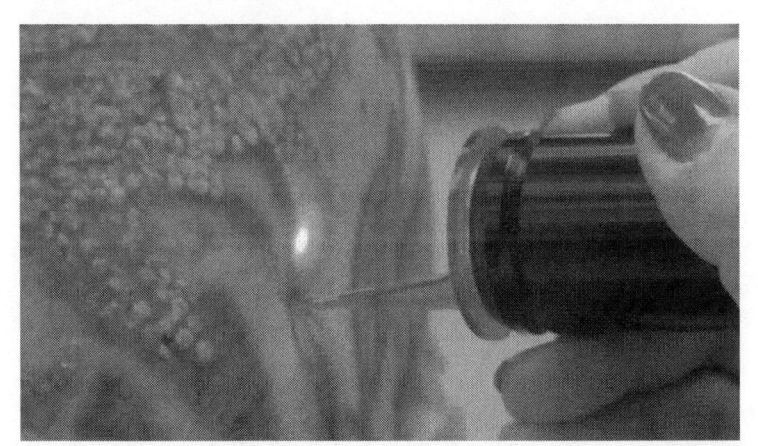

Illustration 213: Laser tattoo fading treatments are widely advertised as tattoo removal treatments. They are the most popular method to fade tattoos in most western countries

The fading results are relatively easily recognised after the first few sessions when the least resilient colours have faded most. Furthermore, the common perception that the use of lasers in aesthetics "utilises the latest cutting-edge technology" therefore safe and effective has contributed to the rise in popularity of this type of treatment.

28.2 An overview of laser's physics and basic principles of operation in aesthetics

The main characteristic of lasers is their capability of emitting a coherent light source at a predetermined frequency (or wavelength). Lasers can also emit a number of different frequencies. The difference between sunlight, including most other artificial light sources and lasers, is that lasers can only emit light at predefined discrete wavelengths. Most lasers can only operate at one predetermined frequency at a time which is set by the laser operator. Lasers are also designed to emit a discrete number of frequencies at a time (multi-frequency/wavelength lasers). The wavelength can be one or multiple but a laser can never emit broadband light energy like most other artificial light sources and other aesthetic devices (e.g. **IPL devices**).

Multi-frequency lasers are also used for tattoo fading and are advertised as very effective tattoo removal devices. This is because the combination of different wavelengths can bring better fading due to the different penetration of each wavelength and the different effect of each wavelength on each tattoo colour. However, in any case, the main difference between lasers and most other natural or artificial light sources is that the lasers, although can emit a different number of frequencies at a time, cannot emit broadband light. Due to this peculiarity of lasers and the different way each wavelength gets absorbed by the skin, lasers have a broad array of applications in skin treatments. Different wavelengths are absorbed differently by the skin and different penetration of the skin lead to different results and hence different applications are aesthetics.

The depth of the light penetration into the skin is mainly determined by the frequency emitted. The higher the frequency the more superficial the effect of the laser on the skin and the less the light will penetrate inside the skin. Conversely, the lower the frequency the more deeply the light will penetrate inside the skin.

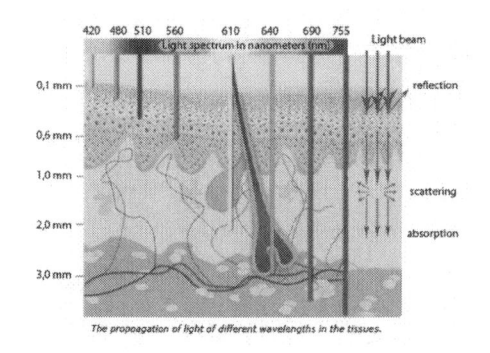

Illustration 214: his figure illustrates the way light propagates inside the skin. The shorter wavelengths (blue-green) have only a superficial ablation effect, while the longer wavelengths (red and infra-red) penetrate more deeply into the skin. The higher the wavelength (the lower the frequency) the deeper the penetration of the specific wavelength. This is one of the reasons for the high versatility of lasers. This physical phenomenon allows lasers to have several applications in aesthetics, for example, they are used in skin resurfacing, permanent hair removal, tattoo removal etc. The type of treatment is mainly determined by the frequency, the light intensity and other factors. The above wavelengths are those which produce the typical frosting effects during laser tattoo fading and other laser aesthetic treatments.

Illustration 214 shows how different wavelengths get absorbed by the skin. Generally, the higher the frequency (lower wavelength) the more superficial the effect of the light onto the skin. Higher frequencies light energy to have a relatively low rate of penetration and its action is relatively superficial. Conversely the lower the frequency (higher wavelength) the deeper the penetration of the light radiation into the skin. Therefore in order to accomplish the desired results the appropriate wavelength can be used for any given type of desired aesthetic result.

The difference in the way any given wavelength propagates inside the skin makes lasers extremely useful and versatile devices. This is because in most cases the user can simply change the nature of the aesthetic treatment by varying the wavelength of the device along with other parameters. For example in order to perform a very superficial ablation (e.g. removing superficial skin imperfections, moles, birthmarks, benign lesions or performing a very superficial skin peels) the wavelength used is relatively high (over 420 nm/blue or violet). At these high frequencies, the burning, as well as the skin resurfacing effects, are very superficial. For example, if lasers are used for permanent epilation (permanent hair removal) the degree of light penetration required is a level deeper (orange). This is because in permanent hair removal the laser has to destroy the hair follicle rooted in the dermis. Therefore the laser light has to affect the deeper parts of the dermis where the root of the hair follicle resides. Therefore the wavelength used is lower (in the region of 600 nm or over).

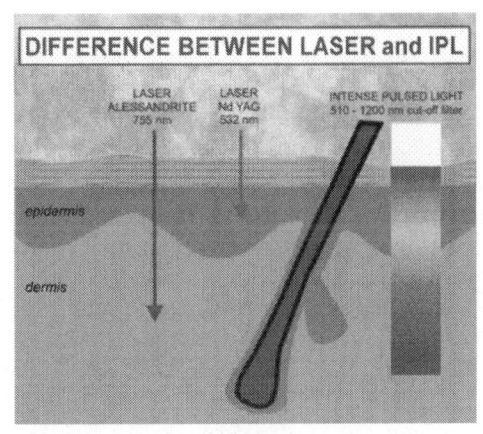

Illustration 215: In here, we can appreciate the main difference between lasers (a monochromatic or discrete multi-chromatic light source) and IPL devices (Intense Pulsed Light) generating a broadband light source which has a multi-level capanility of penetration into the skin. The main application of IPL devices is permanent hair removal

In case the aesthetic treatment demands a deeper level of penetration, then the radiation (light) frequency is lowered. Although lasers can be used for permanent hair removal the devices widely used for this application are IPLs.

Likewise in case of deep skin resurfacing and laser skin tightening, we are trying to heat up the dermis in order to trigger collagen regeneration. In these cases we are looking for deep penetration effects, hence the wavelength chosen can be over 700 nm (red or infra-red). It should be very clear now why Lasers are so versatile, and hence used in several skin applications and aesthetic treatments. This is because by varying the wavelength/s emitted along with other few parameters the nature of the treatments changes dramatically.

However, this is an oversimplified description of the way laser light penetrates into the skin. There are several other parameters which play a role in the effect of light energy into the skin. One of them is the diameter of the light beam used. Generally the larger the diameter of the light beam the deeper the penetration into the skin conversely the smaller the diameter the more superficial the penetration.

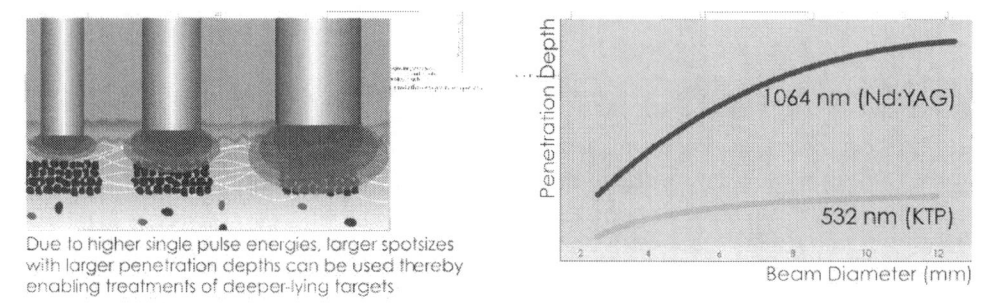

Due to higher single pulse energies, larger spotsizes with larger penetration depths can be used thereby enabling treatments of deeper-lying targets

Fig.3 Depth of penetration and efficacy depends on spot size

Illustration 216: Depth of Pentration and application depends on spot size

The above graph shows how this phenomenon varies with the wavelength used. The red line shows how lower frequencies (1064nm) can penetrate more deeply by increasing the light beam diameter. The yellow line (532nm) shows how the higher the frequencies have less degree of increase in penetration while increasing the diameter.

Therefore the spot size, or the width of the laser beam, affects the treatment. The light is optically scattered in the skin, like automobile headlights in fog. Larger spot sizes slightly increase the effective penetration depth of the laser light, thus enabling more effective targeting of deeper tattoo pigments. Larger spot sizes also increase the treatment intensity and help achieve the desired tattoo fading effects faster.

Additionally, the skin heating (or skin burning effect) produced by the laser, is related to a number of parameters generally not directly correlated with the depth of laser light penetration.

The treatment intensity of the laser is usually calibrated in two main ways, by:

1. regulating the intensity of the light emission as well as the impulse of the laser while visually appreciating the " **frosting** " effects (method used in most aesthetic applications including tattoo fading called Q-Switching),

2. only setting the intensity and the impulse of the light emission on the device (this is typical of deep skin tightening laser treatments where the " **frosting** " effects are not visible). This is the case where the frequency of the laser is very low hence the light penetration into the skin is so deep that it is not possible to appreciate the burning effect of the laser visually.

www.voltaicplasma.com   Author: Andreas Russo

28.3 Visually appreciating the ablation effects of the q-switched laser

This method relies on varying the intensity of the lighting emission and duration of the pulse (see **Q-Switching**) while having a visual appreciation of the immediate effects of the laser ablation (" **laser frosting** "). It is important to realise that the intensity of the treatment is mainly determined by the setting of the device and the visual appreciation is mainly used to make sure the treatment effects are not accidentally exacerbated by overlapping the laser ablation. This method is normally used for removal of benign moles, correction of skin imperfections, superficial laser skin resurfacing treatments as well as laser tattoo removal. The laser operator controls the ablation effects in two ways, both by varying the settings of the device and visually by appreciating the **frosting effects** on the skin.

An example of appreciating visually the immediate ablation effects caused by the aesthetic treatment during skin resurfacing is shown in the following video. The frosting effect is immediate and it provides the operator with an appreciation of the treatment intensity performed on the client. The user can control the intensity of the light beam by varying the settings of the laser device as well as having a direct visual appreciation of the immediate effects the laser has on the skin.

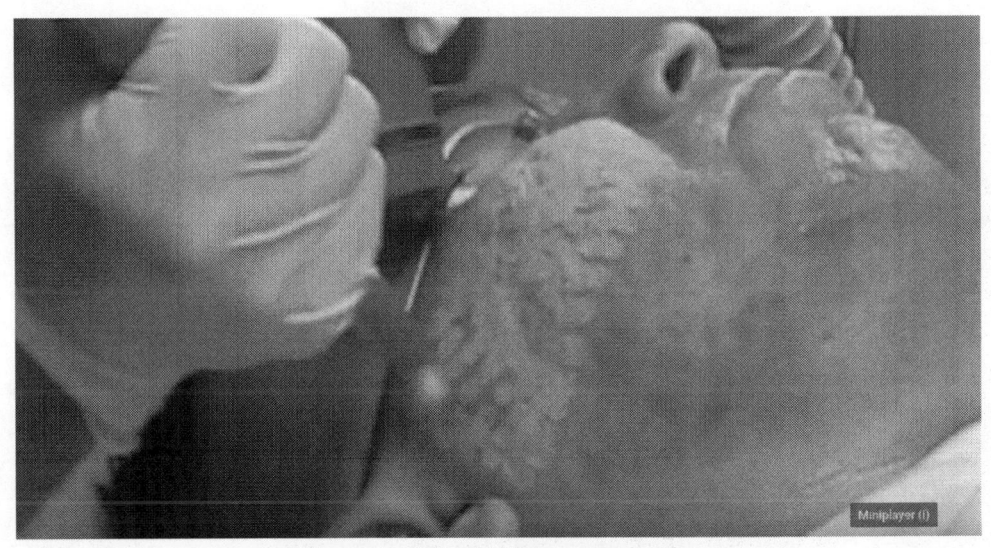

Illustration 217: Click here to watch video

Also, another example of where the intensity of the treatment is also appreciated visually by the operator during the treatment is the classic laser moles removal. In the video below we can appreciate how the treatment is directly controlled by the operator by repeating the laser ablation during the mole removal procedure.

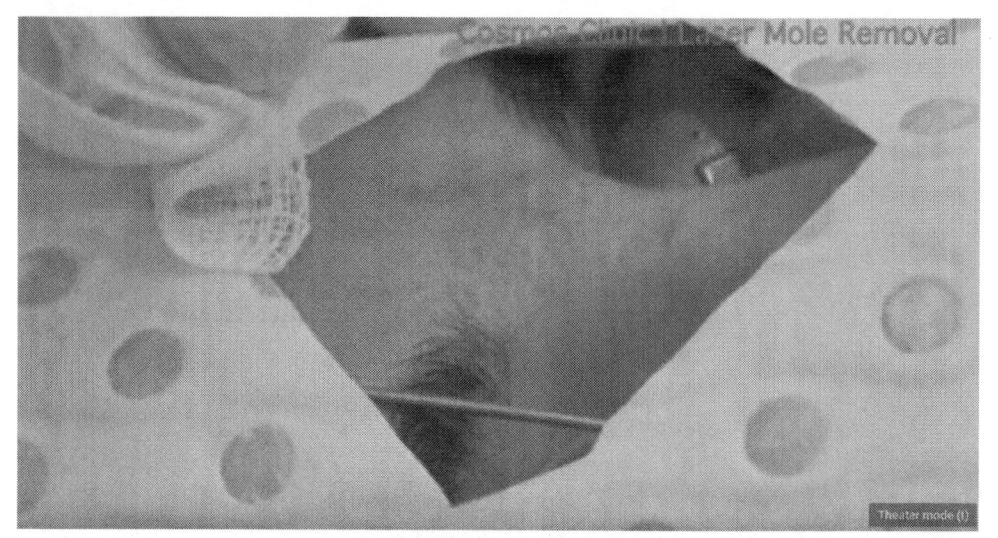

Illustration 218: Click here to watch video

28.4 Varying the timing of the light emission without frosting effects

On the other hand, when the laser ablation or the heating effect is required to be performed deeply into the skin, the operator has no way of visually appreciating the immediate ablation (burning) effects on the skin. For example, in deep laser skin tightening, the effects of the skin treatment are not immediately visible (with frosting or other immediate visible skin reactions), therefore the treatment has to be calibrated only according to previous experience.

The treatment intensity is determined by setting the light intensity and duration of the laser pulse. The longer the duration of the laser pulse the higher the intensity of the treatment, conversely the shorter the pulse the lower the treatment intensity. In these types of laser skin treatments, the effects of the treatment (redness and swelling) only become visible one or two days following the aesthetic procedure. In these cases, the treatment intensity is only predetermined by calibrating certain settings of the laser device itself.

As an example of low frequency and deep penetration treatment is the use of a deep laser for skin resurfacing. In the video below we can see an example of deep Laser skin tightening treatment. This is a typical example when the intensity of the treatment is set by regulating certain parameters and there is no direct immediate appreciation of the effects of the laser on the skin.

www.voltaicplasma.com   Author: Andreas Russo

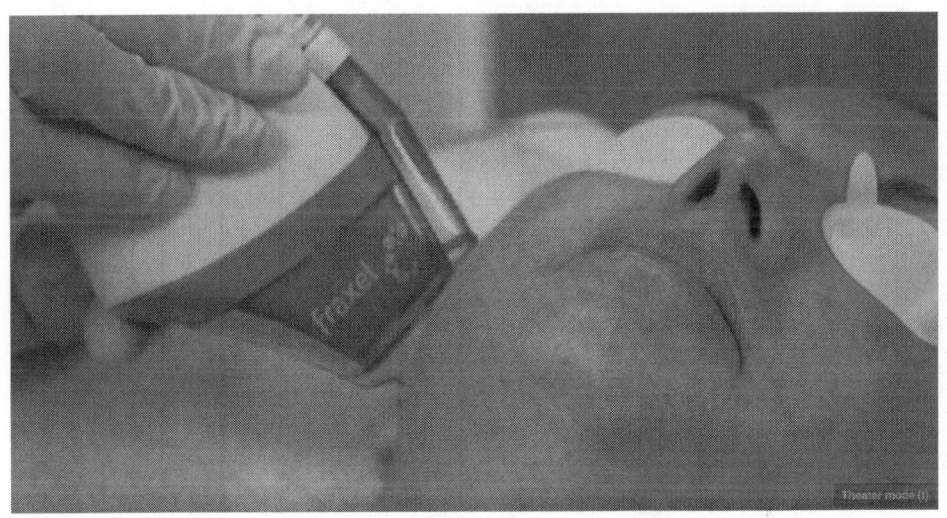

Illustration 219: Click here to watch video

28.5 The physics of laser tattoo removal

Laser tattoo removal or more appropriately laser "tattoo fading" work by causing a controlled skin burn in order to fade the tattoo pigments. As we know the tattoo pigments are located inside the dermis. Therefore in order to fade aesthetic tattoos using lasers or any other method a degree of dermal ablation will be inevitably required.

If you are familiar with superficial laser skin resurfacing and the basic principles of laser skin tightening, you will notice the similarities with laser tattoo removal procedures. Like in laser skin resurfacing and laser skin tightening, the laser causes an intentional dermal burn. The main difference in tattoo fading is that the laser device is calibrated in a slightly different way and generally the intensity of the treatment is higher than normal laser skin resurfacing.

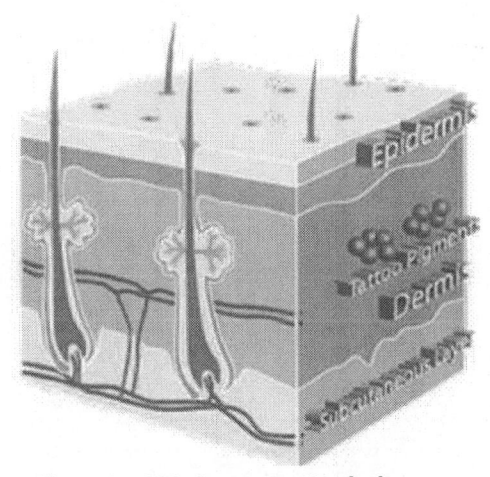

Illustration 220: As seen previously the tattoo pigments are located inside the dermis (for more information click here). Hence in order to reach the tattoo pigments and fade the tattoo, a degree of dermal ablation will be necessary regardless of the method used to fade the tattoo, including laser treatments.

www.voltaicplasma.com

In laser skin resurfacing (or laser skin tightening) the laser has to heat up the dermis, the same principle applies to laser tattoo fading. It is the heat (or burn) caused by the laser light that triggers the skin resurfacing and skin tightening. In a similar fashion, the laser treatment speeds up the absorption of the tattoo pigments in stages, both by breaking down some of the pigments and by triggering the skin regeneration caused by the dermal burn inflicted by the laser.

Similarly to laser skin tightening, during the tattoo fading treatment, the laser causes a dermal ablation which triggers the dermal skin regeneration process, also partly scattering the tattoo pigments. After each treatment, part of the pigments tends to be reabsorbed by the immune system. Some manufacturers advertise selective ablation (burn) targeting of the tattoo pigments, however in any case the laser energy is absorbed by the skin as a whole and not only the tattoo pigments. This is demonstrated by the fact that the skin burn is generated anywhere the laser light is applied and not only on the tattooed area. In case of laser tattoo fading the skin burn is generalised across the treated area as demonstrated by the blistering which forms one or two days after the laser ablation. Unfortunately, there is no currently known tattoo removal or tattoo fading treatment which can selectively target the

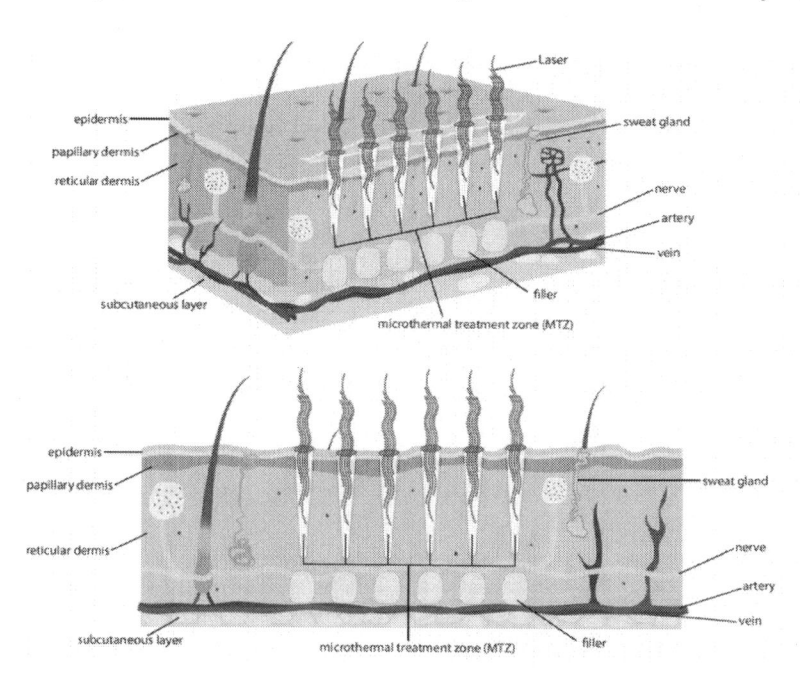

Illustration 221: The physics that apply to laser skin resurfacing also apply to laser tattoo fading. As we see in this simplified representation of laser skin resurfacing, the laser light penetrates into the dermis. It is the heat (or burn) caused by the laser light that triggers the skin regeneration and skin tightening.

tattoo pigments during laser treatments. In other words, there is no aesthetic treatment capable of selectively destroying the tattoo pigments alone without also affecting the dermis in one way or another.

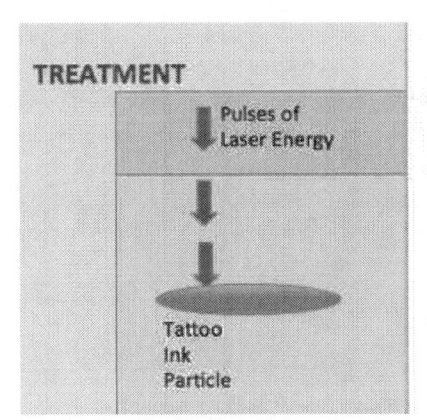

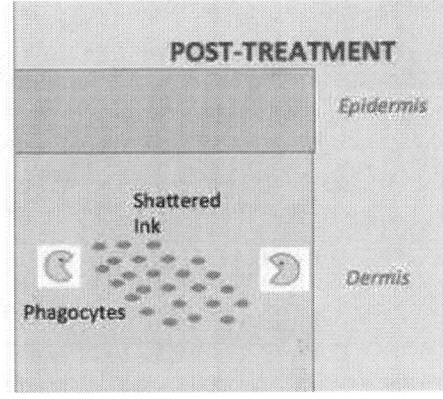

Illustration 222: This figure illustrates the basic principle of laser tattoo fading. This is an oversimplified model to illustrate the basic working principle of laser tattoo fading. Part of the light is absorbed by the tattoo pigments and they are partly broken down. The scattered ink is absorbed by the immune system. Not all tattoo ink can be broken down by the laser during the treatment, only a part of the tattoo is absorbed after each session.

The Right hand side figure is another oversimplified representation of the laser tattoo fading process because not all wavelengths are absorbed by the dermis at the same depth and in the same way. Lasers can only emit a discrete (finite) number of wavelengths and **each wavelength gets absorbed differently by the skin** . The deeper the tattoo pigments the harder it will be to break them down without causing some degree of thermal dermal permanent damage (**hence permanent adverse effects**). This is because in case of very deep pigmentation, most of the laser energy is absorbed by the epidermis and the upper part of the dermis and only a smaller proportion of light is absorbed by the tattoo pigments. Only red and infra-red wavelengths can reach the lower part of the dermis,

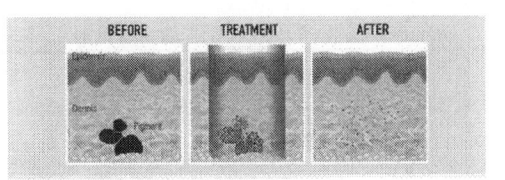

Illustration 223: This is another representation of laser tattoo fading or laser skin resurfacing. We also refer to this process as laser skin resurfacing and this is also a representation of the way the laser light penetrates into the skin for laser skin resurfacing and laser skin tightening. On the left, we can see the tattoo pigments, in the middle an oversimplified representation of the laser tattoo fading treatment. On the right, we can see a representation of the "scattered'" pigments. This is an over simplified representation also because, as we know, lasers can only very seldom scatter all the tattoo pigments within one session especially if the pigments are located particularly deeply inside the dermis.

www.voltaicplasma.com

Author: Andreas Russo

however even their energy will be partially absorbed by the upper dermis and only a fraction of it will reach the deeper dermis and hence the deep pigments. Normally these wavelengths (red and infrared) are used for deep laser skin resurfacing, laser skin tightening and permanent hair removal.

Below we have yet another representation of laser tattoo pigments fragmentation. Once again this is another oversimplified representation of the complete fragmentation of all tattoo, which is usually unrealistic within one session. As we already know only part of the tattoo is fragmented and absorbed slightly. Hence not all tattoo pigments are reabsorbed after one tattoo fading session. Moreover, not all wavelengths are absorbed by the tattoo pigments and the tattoo fading mostly relies on the skin resurfacing effect to speed up the natural absorption process. Additionally, **some tattoo pigment colours do not easily absorb a particular laser wavelength**, therefore, being difficult to fade using laser treatments.

In illustration 224, the tattoo pigments are represented as being evenly located in the upper part of the dermis. This is an oversimplified representation of the tattoo pigments distribution. The tattoo pigments are seldom evenly distributed inside the dermis at the same depth. In reality, they are often found and distributed at different depths inside the dermis. Some part of the tattoo may have deeper or shallower pigments distribution depending on how the tattoo was drawn at the time and the type of pigments used.

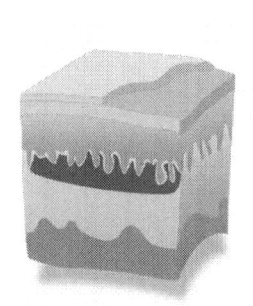

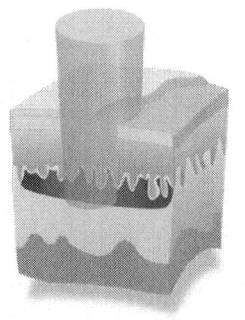

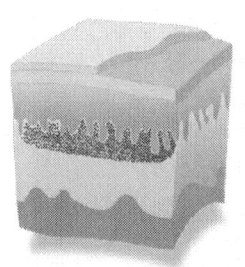

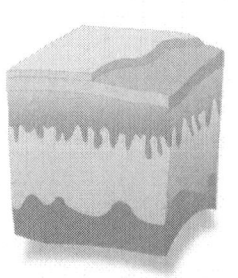

Illustration 224: Oversimplified representation of laser pigmentation scattering. Rarely all pigments are scattered all at once. Although this is a rare occurrence, it can happen in case of fading dark colours and in high-quality tattoos like permanent make-up. Also, the distribution of the tattoo pigments is seldom uniform and can be uneven. Also, bear in mind that this is an oversimplified representation of the way laser treatments work for tattoo fading. Not only the tattoo pigments are affected by the laser, but also the skin undergoes a certain degree of burn caused by the laser treatment.

www.voltaicplasma.com   Author: Andreas Russo

The basic principle of laser tattoo fading is that the deep skin resurfacing caused by the laser forces some of the pigments to be reabsorbed by the immune system. This pigmentation absorption is a natural effect which occurs regardless over time. The deep intense burn caused by the laser speeds up the **natural tattoo pigmentation fading** . However as seen previously, this process is speeded up by tattoo fading procedures in general and in particular laser tattoo fading.

Tattoo laser fading treatments are an example of where the overall treatment intensity is mainly determined by varying the settings of the laser device. Although the user can intentionally increase the burn inflicted by overlapping the ablation spots while performing the treatment, the overall intensity is generally determined by the setting of the device. This is done by controlling the light emission using very short pulses (Q-Switching). This is one of the reasons for the feeling of being "hit by a strong elastic band" experienced by those who undergo laser fading treatments.

28.6 Q-Switching Lasers

The main principle of operation of tattoo fading lasers is represented in the figure below. These laser devices utilise the "Q-Switching" method to generate an extremely short but highly intense coherent light pulse (generally in the order of nanoseconds). This light impulse is usually several orders of magnitude larger in intensity than lasers generating a constant output.

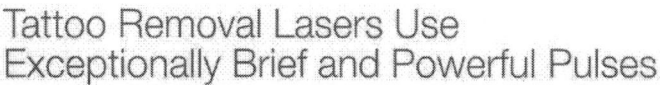

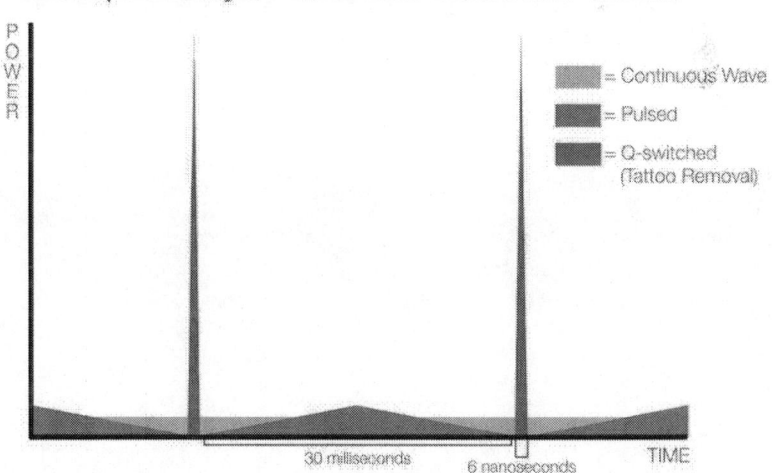

Illustration 225: Q-switching laser

The **Q-Switching** is the most used laser arrangement for tattoo fading. As seen in the figure the power is extremely high for a very short duration (nano or pico seconds). This ensures that the intensity of the treatment is mainly determined by the way the device is set by the user and not by the way the hand-piece is used during the treatment. Pulse-width or pulse duration is a critical laser parameter. All Q-switched lasers have appropriate pulse durations for tattoo removal.

While using **Q-Switching** lasers, once the tattoo fading laser has been set up by the user, the operator needs only to make sure the spots do not overlap in order not to unintentionally doubling the burn inflicted on the same area. However this is quite easily avoided becuase every time the light hits the skin it leaves a clear "frosting" spot. In this way the laser treatment intensity is mainly controlled by the setting of the device and there is minimal margin of error during the treatment itself.

In the video below we can see an example of a classic Q-Switched laser for tattoo fading treatment. As we can see there is the usual frosting characteristic of the laser tattoo fading. This frosting immediate reaction to the burn inflicted on to the skin caused by all laser tattoo fading devices.

As we have seen the main principle of operation of tattoo fading devices is Q-Switching . As we can see in the figure below there are several types of Q-Switching devices used for tattoo fading, the lasers can be made to use Ruby, Alexandrite, YAG, or KTP. The material used in the core of the laser has only the effect to determine the main operational frequency of the Q-Switched laser. As we will see one of the main downsides to laser tattoo fading is the fact that lases cannot fade all colours in the same way. Some colours are almost impractical to be faded by lasers (especially certain green tones and very bright pigments).

Q-switched Laser	Wavelength	Pulse Duration	Tattoo Colors
Ruby	694 nm	< 40 ns	black, blue, green
Alexandrite	755 nm	50 ns - 100 ns	black, blue, green
Nd:YAG	1064 nm	< 10 ns	black, blue
KTP	532 nm	< 10 ns	red, orange, yellow, brown

Illustration 226: In this table, we can see the main four frequencies used in laser tattoo fading devices. All tattoo fading devices use the Q-Switching method. Some frequencies can target some tattoo colours only. On the right, we can see the types of colours targeted by each frequency.

Some tattoo fading lasers are advertised as being capable of removing all colours and in one treatment only. These are lasers which combine more than one wavelength. The most common all-in-one tattoo removal lasers combine the four frequencies seen in the table above. However, despite the claims made by the manufacturers, unfortunately, **laser tattoo fading treatment is fundamentally colour selective** . This means that some colours are faded more than others. Most other tattoo fading treatments are colour blind, this means that they fade all colours indiscriminately. Some latest lasers are advertised to produce a high-intensity pulse lasting few picoseconds, however, no independent investigation on the actual way they operate, their true efficacy has been done.

28.7 Laser colour sensitivity

As we have seen most tattoo fading treatments, other than laser tattoo fading devices, are colour blind. Colour blind means that these treatments tend to fade all tattoo colour pigments indiscriminately.

Unfortunately, in case of laser tattoo fading, different tattoo colours fade at different rates. Some colours are not easily absorbed and do not fade significantly after laser treatments, especially certain tones like green and bright colours.

The below graph shows an *estimation* of the degree of *relative* light absorption of the tattoo pigments at each wavelength. This has not to be confused with the amount of pigmentation fading after each tattoo removal session. This is because although the light radiation may be absorbed by the particular pigments this does not necessarily translate into a proportional fading of the specific colour pigments.

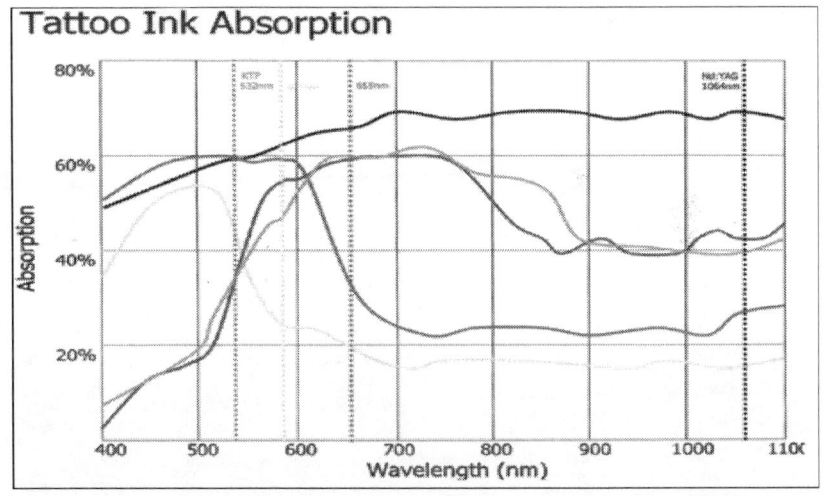

Illustration 227: Tattoo ink absorption. The relative light absorption of each tattoo colour is dependant on the specific wavelength of the light that hits the pigment. The graph shows the relative absorption of each fundamental colour versus the wavelength.

The below graph serves to show the fact that the inherent physics of light absorption of the tattoo pigments renders the laser treatment outcome inherently dependant on both the wavelength used and the tattoo colours.

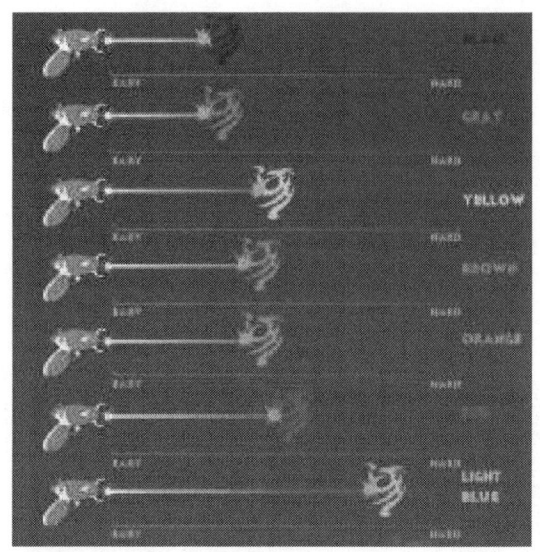

Illustration 228: The figure is an oversimplification of the real effectiveness of tattoo colour fading due to laser treatment. The darker colours are the easiest to fade using lasers.

Illustration 229 is meant to provide a rough idea of the challenges faced in fading certain colours versus others using tattoo fading lasers. As we can see the colour green is not even mentioned in this representative chart. This is because as it is well known in the industry lasers have little or no impact on the green tattoo colours. This does not apply to all tattoo fading treatments, in fact, this limitation only applies to laser tattoo fading. Due to the very nature of lasers, unfortunately, certain wavelengths are more effective on certain tattoo colours and cannot fade others. The easiest tattoo pigments colours to fade are black or dark colours in general, while bright and particularly certain tones of green pigments are the most difficult to fade. Generally the brighter the colours the harder they are to fade using lasers, conversely the darker they are the easier they are to fade using lasers. Sometimes green and bright colours will be far easier to cover up or remove using other treatments rather than persisting in the use of laser fading treatments, which have certain potential permanent adverse reactions.

www.voltaicplasma.com   Author: Andreas Russo

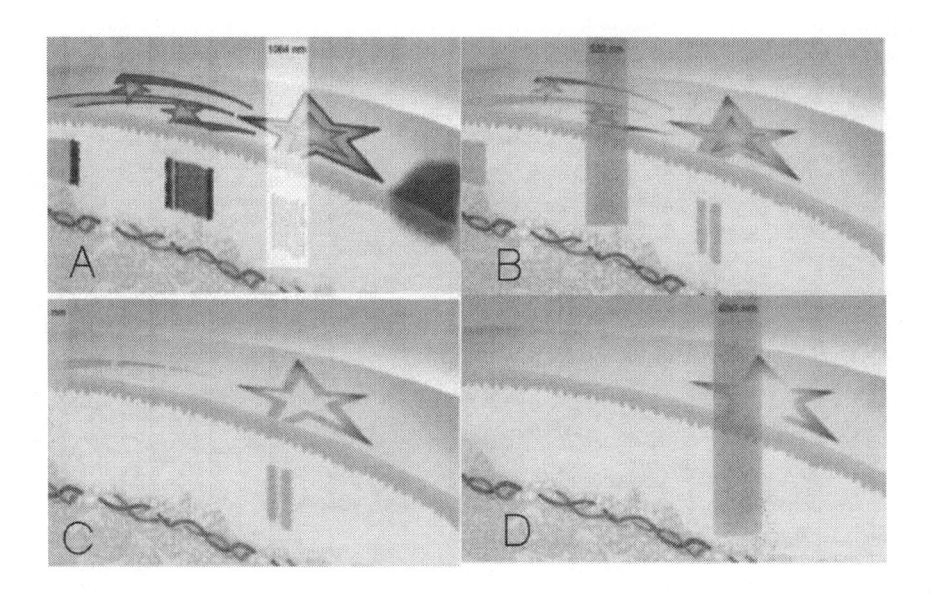

llustration 229: This figure is used only to illustrate what colours are the easiest and most difficult to fade using lasers. (A) represents the initial tattoo, (B) the initial fading of the tattoo after a few sessions, (C) the results after several sessions (where green and bright colours are left), (D) the most difficult colour to be faded is usually left last. Green is the most challenging colour to fade using lasers.

Illustration 229 shows how the first colours to be faded are black and dark tones. As we see in B, the easiest colours to be attenuated are the darkest, the brightest are usually left after the first few treatments. In C (after further tattoo fading treatments) the colours left are the brightest and green. Lastly, as seen in D, normally green is the most resilient tattoo pigment with laser tattoo fading. The colour green is so resilient to lasers that it is sometimes considered not feasibly faded using lasers. However, there are manufacturers claiming that their new devices are capable of fading bright and all colours indiscriminately incuding green. These claims have not been independently verified.

The Ilustration 230 below shows a practical example of laser tattoo fading and it demonstrates what we have said earlier, i.e. different colours fade at different rates. The type of tattoo shown is particularly colourful therefore it may be particularly challenging to fade using lasers. On the left, we can see this colourful tattoo at the beginning of the laser removal treatment. As seen on the right the tattoo has faded only slightly after a few lasers sessions, however, the brightest colours are the most resilient while the darkest ones including red have faded most.

www.voltaicplasma.com   Author: Andreas Russo

Page 226

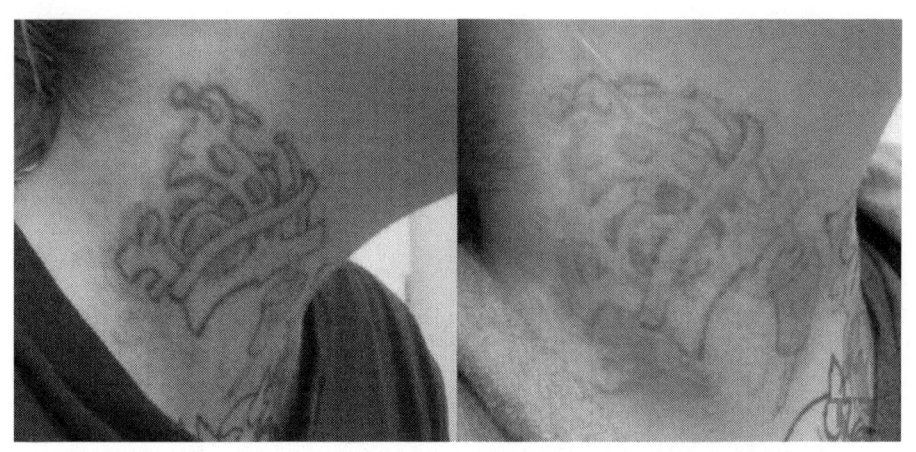

Illustration 230: Lasers are colour sensitive. This is a practical example showing how different colours fade at different rates when using tattoo fading lasers. Certain colours fade more than others. As a rule of thumb, with laser tattoo removal the hardest colours to fade are the brightest and especially green. Yellow and brightest colours are still present. The darkest colours have mostly all faded. Also, it is noticeable the colour scattering caused by the laser treatment.

In particular, illustration 231 provides an estimation of the efficacy of two particular wavelengths in fading certain tattoo colours. Please bear in mind that this figure is only a rough representation which serves to illustrate the dependency of the wavelength with the efficacy of each specific tattoo colour. However, actual results may vary from the graph above because generally, the efficacy of lasers are good on dark tones despite the wavelength. The purpose of the figure above is to show how the fading efficacy on individual tattoo colour is fundamentally dependent on the wavelength used. Different wavelengths fade pigment colours differently. As we can see from the graph, the hardest colours to fade are green, yellow and the brightest tones in general.

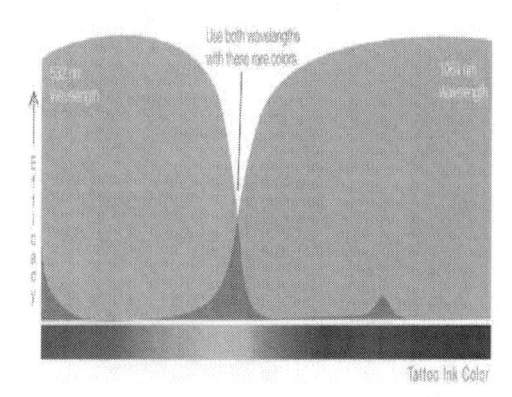

Illustration 231: This figure illustrates the efficacy of two wavelengths on laser tattoo fading of certain colours. As we know not all colours fade in the same way after laser treatments. This representative graph shows there is an efficacy drop at the yellow-green colour. As it is well known these are the most difficult colours to be faded using laser tattoo removal.

www.voltaicplasma.com

Although there are other tattoo fading treatments which are colour blind, the resilience of green and bright colours have been addressed for years in laser tattoo fading treatments.

Efficacy of Nd:YAG Laser Wavelengths

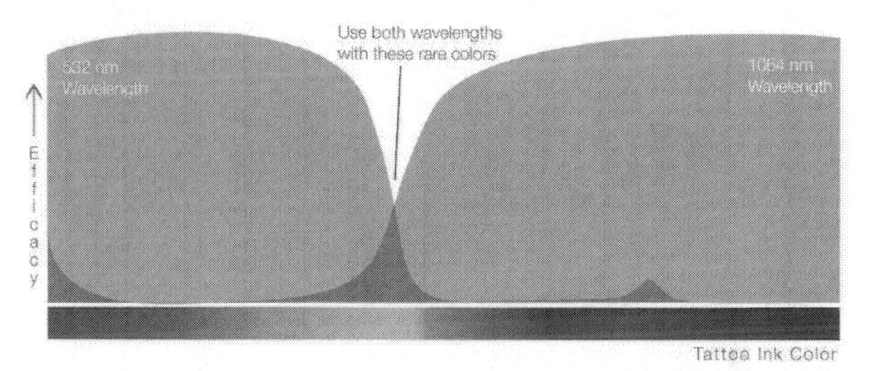

Illustration 232: This graph shows an estimation of the efficacy of each wavelength on tattoo individual colours. In order to increase the efficacy of lasers on particularly bright colours and green, other wavelengths have been introduced. This graph, in particular, shows how light radiation at 694nm has an increased efficacy on bright colours and green. Please note that despite the research and the numerous trials to increase the efficacy of fading green and bright pigments they are still challenging using lasers. These colours can be faded using alternative tattoo fading treatments which are not colour sensitive.

Certain colours have proved more difficult to remove than others. In particular, this occurs when the tattoo is treated with an inappropriate wavelength. It has been shown that green ink tattoos somehow respond to treatments with 755 nm light and also to 694nm, 650nm and 1064nm. Some manufacturers have come up with multi-frequency lasers and their treatment intensity levels are particularly high compared to mono-frequency Q-Switched lasers. The result is that often, due to the high intensity of the multi-wavelength laser treatment most of the pigments fade dramatically, however, due to the deeper skin burn caused by the laser, there is usually an increased likelihood of undesired

www.voltaicplasma.com

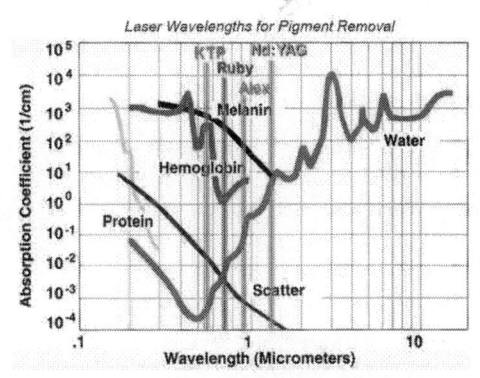

Illustration 233: Wavelengths vs absorption coefficient. This logarithmic graph provides further evidence of the colour sensitivity of lasers. A higher absorption coefficient does not necessarily translate in a proportional pigmentation fading rate.

permanent adverse effects like hypo-pigmentation, permanent change in skin texture and permanent scars.

- Q-Switched Alexandrite and Ruby operating at 755 nm and 694 nm. The weakest of all the Q-Switched devices, they generate an orange/red light which is highly absorbed by green and dark tattoo pigments. However, the alexandrite laser colour is slightly less absorbed by melanin, so Alexandrite laser has a slightly lower incidence of unwanted pigmentary changes than a ruby laser. This laser (Alexandrite) was reported to have some moderate effects on green tattoos, but because of its weaker peak power, it works only moderately well on black and blue ink. It does not work at all (or very minimally) on red, orange, yellow, brown, etc. This laser wavelength (755 nm) is also available in picosecond pulses (instead of the ordinary nanosecond) with unverified claims that it removes ink faster.

- Q-switched Nd:YAG: 1064 nm. This laser creates a near-infrared light (invisible to humans) which is also poorly absorbed by melanin, making this the only laser suitable for darker skin. This laser wavelength is also absorbed by all dark tattoo pigments and is the safest wavelength to use on the skin due to the low melanin absorption and low haemoglobin absorption. This is the wavelength of choice for tattoo removal in darker skin types and for black ink. Dye modules are available for some lasers to convert 532 nm to 650 nm or 585 nm light which allows one laser system to treat multicolour tattoo inks. The role of dye lasers in tattoo removal is discussed in detail in other literature.

28.8 Introduction to tattoo fading treatments transient adverse reactions

As we know tattoo fading lasers are colour sensitive while **other tattoo fading treatments are colours blind**. There have been several claims of outstanding effectiveness on all tattoo colours made by certain tattoo fading laser manufacturers, however, the inherent physics of lasers has its own limitations which appear hard to be overcome.

Temporary adverse reactions typical to laser tattoo fading treatments are several, however, these are only transient (temporary).

These temporary adverse reactions are:

◆ **Pain**: caused by the treatment.
◆ **Bleeding**: which can occur during the treatment itself. This is only minor and it subsides almost immediately on its own accord.
◆ **Frosting**: This is typical of tattoo laser treatments only. No other tattoo fading treatments present similar reactions other than cryotherapy, which is seldom used for this application. In the case or cryotherapy, the frosting is caused by the induced freezing of the skin.

- **Blistering**: Blistering is inevitable after tattoo fading laser treatments, it can only be somewhat minimised performing low-intensity treatments and with the use of potent topical soothing products immediately after the procedure.
- Associated to the blistering is the **discomfort** during healing. The level of discomfort depends on the intensity of the treatment, the sensitivity of the individual, and whether or not an appropriate soothing product was used. It is indeed the level of discomfort experienced during the treatment and during the days following the treatments associated with the relatively low rate of tattoo fading which sometimes discourage people from undergoing further treatments.
- **Transient textural changes:** are occasionally noted but often resolve within a few months on their own accord; however, permanent textural changes and scarring can also occur. If a client is prone to pigmentary or textural changes, longer treatment intervals are recommended.
- Occasionally, "**paradoxical darkening**" of a tattoo may occur, when a treated tattoo becomes darker instead of lighter. This occurs most often with white ink, flesh tones, pink, and some cosmetic make-up tattoos.

- A local **infection** is always possible. The likelihood of this occurrence can be minimised by following the appropriate aftercare, especially avoiding puncturing or bursting the blisters.
- **Photoallergic reactions:** Local allergic responses to tattoo pigments have been reported. Allergic reactions to tattoo pigment scattering after Q-switched laser treatment are also possible because lasers by mobilizing the ink may trigger a systemic allergic response. Rarely, when yellow cadmium sulfide is used to "brighten" the red or yellow portion of a tattoo, a photoallergic reaction may occur. The reaction is also common with red ink, which may contain cinnabar (mercuric sulphide). Erythema, eachting sensation, and even inflamed nodules, verrucose papules, or granulomas may occur. The reaction is usually confined to the site of the red/yellow ink. Oral antihistamines and anti-inflammatory steroids have been used to treat allergic reactions to tattoo ink also after photoallergic reactions to laser fading treatments.

28.9 Pain during the laser treatment

One of the challenges of laser tattoo fading is the pain and discomfort during the treatment itself. Laser tattoo fading treatments are uncomfortable - many people say that laser treatment is worse than getting the tattoo on. While the tattooing soreness is normally bearable, laser tattoo fading treatment is often reported to be unbearable. The pain is often described to be similar to that of hot oil poured on the skin (caused by the deep burn inflicted during the treatment), or a "snap" from an elastic band (caused by the high energy impulse generated by the **Q-Switched** laser). Depending on the person's individual pain threshold, some people can have the treatment done without using any form of numbing product, while others prefer to undergo the treatment using a topical anaesthetic (numbing cream). Please note that the use of local injectable anaesthetic is not required for this type of treatment because there are **appropriate topical over the counter numbing products** or effective topical products specially made for this and other aesthetic applications, which normally allow a pain-free treatment. Different numbing products have different efficacy and modality of application (follow the specific manufactuer's instructions). Hence local injectable anaesthetics are not required for this type of aesthetic procedure.

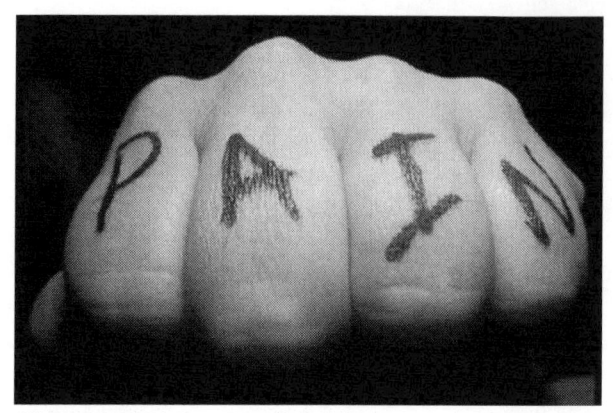

Illustration 234: Laser tattoo fading treatments are inevitably painful. This is caused by the deep burn-induced during the laser treatment.

28.10 Bleeding

Bleeding is a common immediate consequence of laser tattoo fading treatments.

This is because the laser's high power impulses have to cause an ablation inside the dermis in order to be effective. A large number of capillaries are normally present inside the dermis, and the ablating power of the laser at the dermal level has the direct effect of breaking some of those capillaries hence causing some minor immediate bleeding. This is generally a very normal reaction and should not be interpreted as a sign of direct unintended harm caused by the treatment, but as a normal direct consequence of the treatment itself due to its very nature.

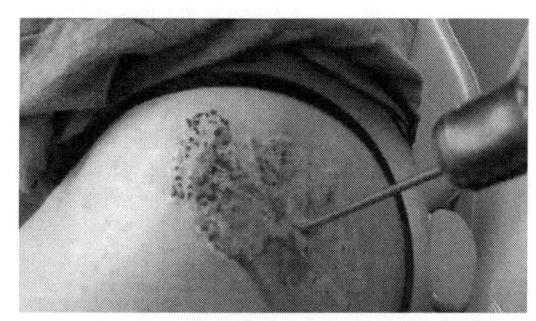

Illustration 235: Bleeding is a common and immediate reaction to most laser tattoo removal treatments.

The degree of bleeding depends on the wavelengths used, the power level used by the impulse of the **Q-Switching** laser and the individual's level of vascularisation of the treated area. Some areas may be more vascularised than others.

In any case, the bleeding is only minor, as the vessels broken during the laser treatment are only superficial capillaries. This minor bleeding stops a few minutes after the treatment. Also because of the likelihood of minor bleeding, one the of the recommendation made by the tattoo removal clinics is not to take aspirin or blood thinning drugs before tattoo fading treatments (just to avoid slightly more prolonged bleeding).

28.11 Discomfort, blistering and normal skin reactions throughout the healing process

Laser tattoo fading procedures are quite painful, unfortunately, the pain and discomfort do not end there. While, as we have just seen the pain during the treatment is an easily solved problem with the use of appropriate topical numbing products, unfortunately, any laser treatment purposely inflicts a deep burn into the skin in order to fade the tattoo. Because of this skin burn, a direct consequence of every tattoo fading treatment is a fully fledged purposely inflicted burn injury which requires healing time. This burn is merely caused by the physics of the laser itself, although it can be somewhat attenuated, it cannot be avoided by varying the laser functioning parameters, by altering the laser design or modifying the treatment modality.

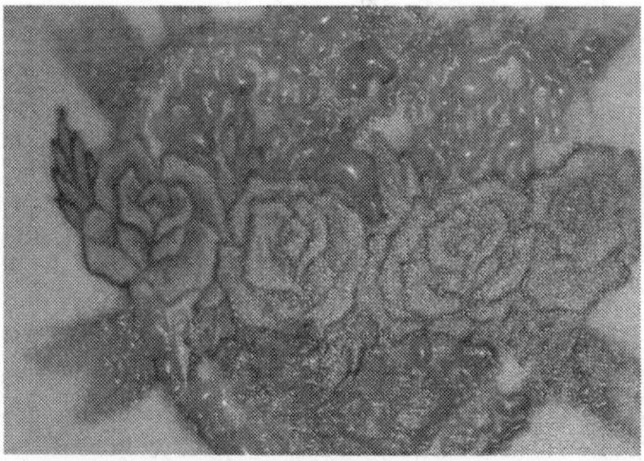

Illustration 236: Blistering is a normal reaction to laser tattoo fading treatments. Blistering can be minimised but never completely avoided. This is due to the very nature of the laser tattoo fading treatment which inherently inflicts a burn onto the skin in order to fade the tattoo.

Depending on the area covered by the treatment and the intensity of the treatment, the extent of the skin burn caused by the laser can be significant at times. Having a relatively large and deep skin burn can be a very unpleasant and uncomfortable experience during the healing process. Like most skin burns, the direct effect of the laser tattoo fading treatments is blistering. The discomfort usually peaks when the blistering have fully formed.

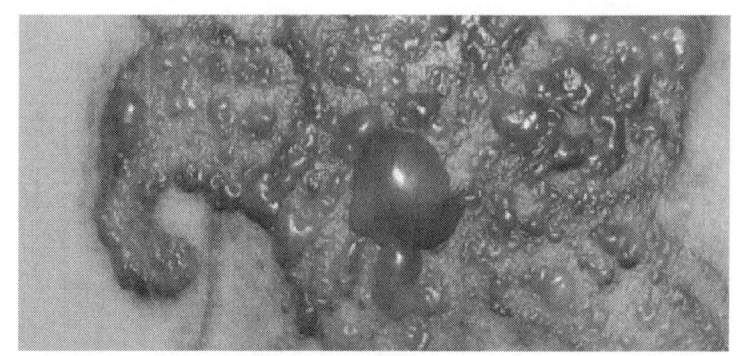

Illustration 237: Example of moderate blistering after a mild tattoo laser treatment. The skin reacts to the tattoo fading treatment as it would after any other skin burn. Blistering is one of the ways the skin reacts to deep and intense laser skin burns.

Like any other skin burn, the discomfort lasts as long as the burn is still healing. The discomfort usually starts to subside on its own accord as the blisters heal, however, some degree of discomfort can persist even after the blisters have subsided and the treated tattoo has healed completely. In certain cases, the part may feel tender to the touch and over sensitive for several weeks, even after the blisters have subsided and the part has healed completely.

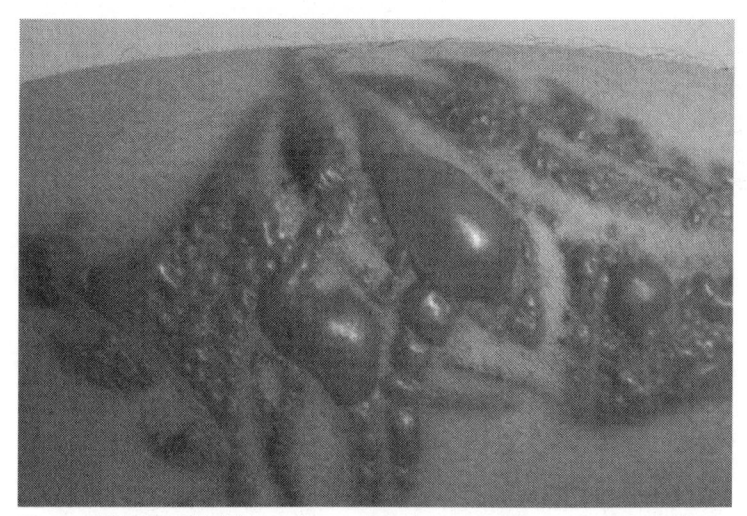

Illustration 238: The blisters increase in size proportionately with the laser treatment intensity. The higher the intensity the larger the blisters and the more the discomfort levels experienced during the healing process.

One of the reasons for not treating wide tattoos all at once is to make the clients return for further treatments. The wider the area treated using lasers or the higher the intensity of the treatment, the larger the area subject to the skin burn, the higher the discomfort and pain experienced during the healing process. Additionally causing a skin burn over a relatively large area may have side effects like lethargy and other feverish-like symptoms which physiologically occur after large skin burns.

Very often, the overall unpleasant experience sometimes deters the clients (incorrectly referred to as patients) from undergoing all the treatments required in order to completely remove or close to completely removing the tattoos.

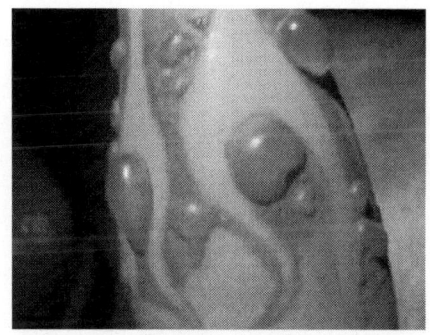

Illustration 239: Relatively large blisters caused by a laser high-intensity treatment. The higher the intensity treatment the larger the blisters and the more uncomfortable the healing process.

Sometimes, due to the discomfort levels, most people prefer to undergo the minimum number of laser tattoo fading treatments required, and then opting for tattoo cover-up as soon as the tattoo pigmentation has faded enough to make it a feasible option.

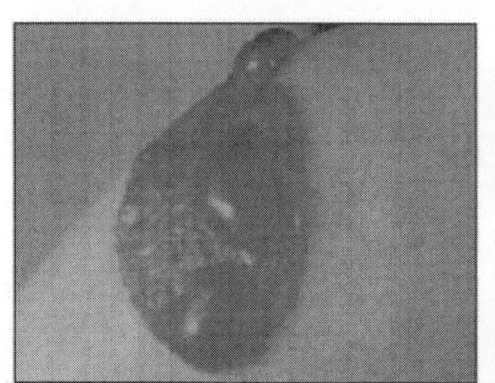

FIGURE 1A. Tense bulla formation on the arm 24 hours after Q-switched laser treatment to the area

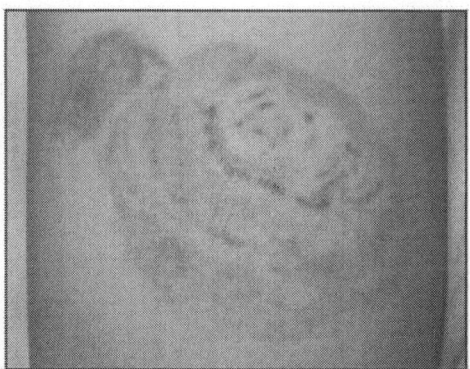

FIGURE 1B. Well-healed treatment area

after lasers treatments can be minimised but never completely avoided due to the inherent physics of the laser tattoo fading treatment.

The amount and size of blistering developed during the healing process depends on the intensity of the laser treatment. The higher the treatment intensity the larger the blisters and the longer it will take for the area to recover, conversely the milder the treatment the smaller the blistering and the faster the recovery process.

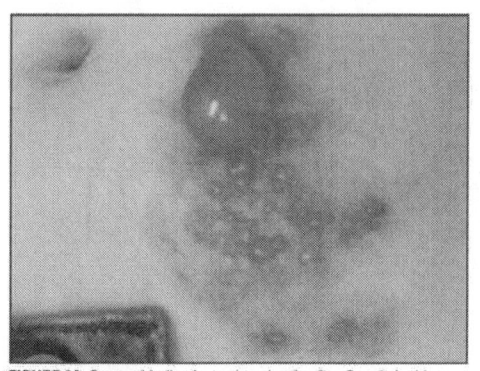

FIGURE 3A. Grouped bullae formation shortly after Q-switched laser treatment to the area

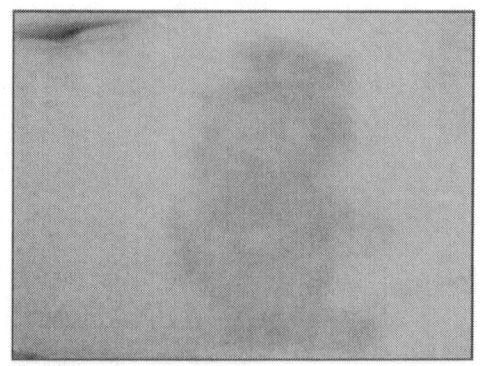

FIGURE 3B. Well-healed treatment area

If the burn inflicted by the laser treatment is not too intense the area can heal normally and the tattoo will have faded slightly after the recovery period. In case of very high-intensity treatments the burn inflicted by the laser may as well remove most of all the tattoo pigments, however, the blistering will be very large and the <u>likelihood of permanent adverse reactions due to the treatment</u> increases dramatically.

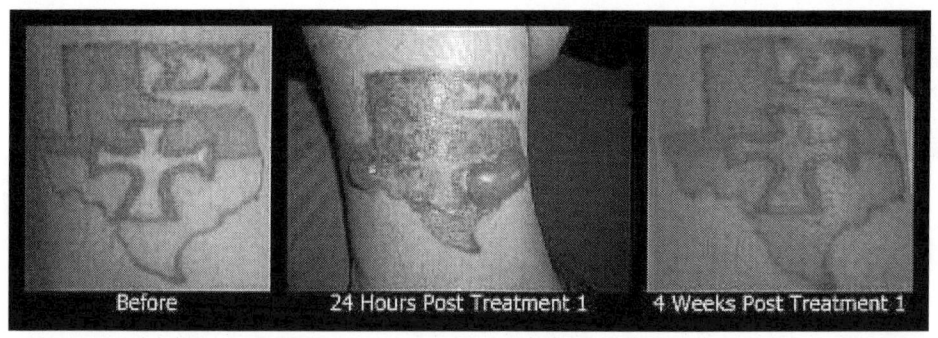

Illustration 240: A typical example of before picture, during the blistering and after the area has recovered from the burn caused by the Laser.

The blisters start to form 24 hours after the treatment, peak two to three days after the treatment and will gradually subside by their own accord.

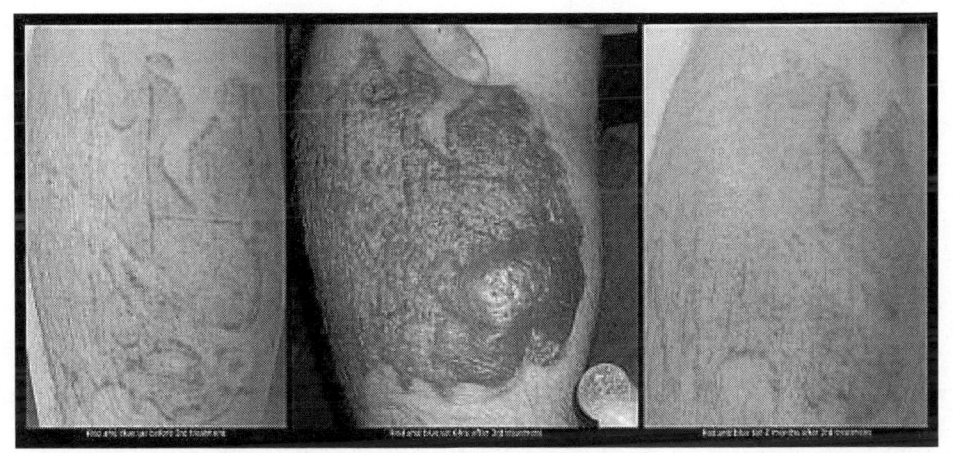

Illustration 241: A further example of tattoo fading blistering after laser tattoo fading treatment.

It is important not to interfere with the healing process of the blisters. In particular, the blisters must not be burst or pierced intentionally to avoid an increased likelihood of infections and other adverse reactions. For more information about the appropriate after-care for the blisters caused by the laser tattoo removal treatment please watch the video below.

28.12 The number of laser treatments required and the kirby-desai scale

Uninformed clients sometimes expect that their unwanted tattoos will be completely removed within one session and with seamless results. This is very rarely possible using lasers tattoo fading treatments. Once the clients are informed about the real results of this type of aesthetic treatment, the first questions they will ask are the number of sessions required and how much it will cost them to achieve the best tattoo fading results. Ultimately, these two questions are inextricably linked. The total cost of the laser removal treatment will be the number of sessions times the cost per session.

No matter what their qualifications or their expertise, no aesthetic practitioner can predict for certain exactly how many sessions it will take to achieve the clients' desired results. Because there are several factors that will determine the number of sessions required. Before a patch testing is carried out, all an experienced tattoo removal practitioner can do is provide an educated estimation. Anyone who claims to provide the exact number of treatments for a complete and seamless tattoo removal is probably trying to sell something based on false promises.

Complete laser tattoo removal often requires numerous treatment sessions, typically spaced **at least seven weeks apart**. Treating more frequently than seven weeks increases the likelihood of adverse effects and does not necessarily increase the rate of ink absorption. Anecdotal reports of treatments sessions spaced less than seven weeks (four weeks) lead to more scarring and hypo-pigmentation and could increase liability for clinicians (especially in case an appropriate consent form is not in place). At each session, only a fraction of the tattoo pigments is effectively fragmented and faded over the following weeks. Remaining large particles of tattoo pigment are then targeted at subsequent treatment sessions, causing further tattoo fading. The number of sessions and spacing between treatments depends on various parameters, including the area of the body treated and skin colour. Tattoos located on the extremities, such as the ankle, generally take longest. Aesthetic practitioners may recommend that clients wait many months between treatments to facilitate ink resolution and minimise the likelihood of unwanted adverse effects.

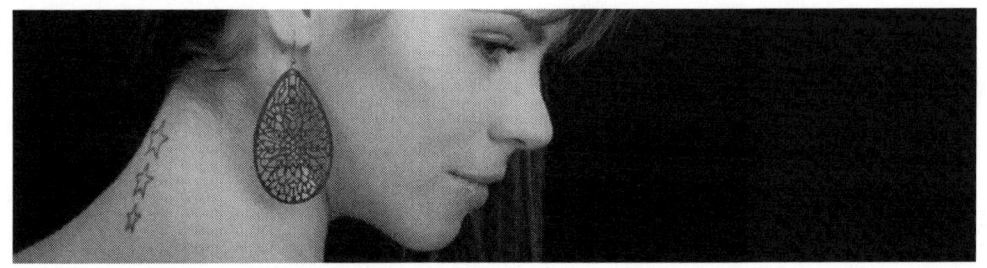

Illustration 242: Tattoo example

In the vast majority of cases, satisfactory results are achieved after several sessions and the results are seldom seamless. In general, the number of sessions required to achieve satisfactory fading results can vary from 6 to 15 depending on several factors. Some tattoos can be particularly easily removed and completely seamless removal can be achieved in one or two sessions (this is generally the case of certain high-quality **permanent make up** tattoos), however, this is not the norm. Most tattoos can be extremely resilient and it may be even impractical or not advisable to try and achieve complete removal. Some laser tattoo removal manufacturers claim their latest devices remove all tattoos within one session without adverse permanent reactions, these claims are unverified.

While certain tattoos are easily removed in few sessions (especially permanent makeup), despite the claims made by laser manufacturers, there is no evidence that all tattoos can be removed within one treatment without leaving a visible scar, hypo-pigmentation or another type of permanent skin texture change. Seamless complete tattoo removal is more the exception than the norm, especially due to the way tattoos have been originally drawn. In case of particularly resilient tattoo pigments, a certain degree of tattoo fading will be regarded as a good result because complete removal without leaving any scar or permanent skin texture change may be unlikely.

So, what are the most important factors in determining the number of sessions especially in laser tattoo fading procedures? Most of the factors have already been covered in details in the general tattoo fading section. it is advisable that you review these points before continuing reading. To review these points please **CLICK HERE**. Some of the points below are particularly typical to laser tattoo fading treatments only:

- **The intensity of the treatments:** Like any other type of tattoo fading procedure the higher the intensity of the treatment the more the degree of tattoo fading after each session and therefore the fewer sessions required to achieve satisfactory fading. On the other hand the higher the intensity of the treatment the higher the likelihood of permanent undesired adverse effects like hypo-pigmentation, permanent change in skin texture and scarring. Conversely, the milder the treatment intensity the less the tattoo fades after each treatment and therefore more sessions will be required.
- **The number of wavelengths used by the device.** This is peculiar to laser tattoo fading treatments only. As we know, lasers are devices that can emit a discrete number of wavelengths at a time (either one, two, three etc). Some manufacturers have devised multi-frequency lasers which can emit a number of different frequencies all at once. This is in an effort to eliminate all or most tattoo colours as quickly as possible. Multi-wavelengths tattoo fading lasers have a generally natural tendency to fade the tattoos more than mono wavelengths frequency lasers. This is because the more the wavelengths used by the laser, the higher the treatment intensity and the more the tattoo will fade after each session. As the intensity of the treatment increases so the inherent likelihood of permanent adverse reactions increases. Conversely, mono wavelengths (or mono-frequency lasers) will fade the tattoo to a lesser extent after each treatment.
- **Tattoo colours:** As it is well known, unlike other tattoo fading treatments, lasers fade colours at different rates and some colours can be particularly challenging to be faded. Therefore more colourful and bright tattoos are the more challenging to fade. Whereas darker tattoos may require fewer treatments to achieve satisfactory fading.
- **Skin tone:** The darker skin tones are more prone to develop hypo-pigmentation after laser treatments. For this reason, the darker the skin tone the milder the laser treatment is required to be in order to try and avoid hypo-pigmentation. Hypo-pigmentation is the only reason to tune down the intensity of the laser treatment. Other types of fading treatments do not usually display this type of adverse reaction. For this reason darker skin tones may benefit from other types of tattoo fading treatments which do not lead to hypo-pigmentation.
- Sometimes estimations based only on previous experience can be completely unreliable. The best way to estimate the number of sessions required in order to achieve the desired results is an extrapolation after appreciating the results of a patch test or an extrapolation after appreciating the first session's results. This is because every tattoo is different and there is seldom little background information about the tattoo itself and the way it was originally made.

There are several factors which determine the number of sessions required in order to achieve the desired results. Factors influencing this include skin type, location, colour, amount of ink, scarring or tissue change, tattoo layering etc. Since the number of laser tattoo sessions required to achieve the desired results is a frequently asked question, a predictive scale, the "Kirby-Desai Scale", was developed by Dr Will Kirby and Dr Alpesh Desai. They were dermatologists specializing in tattoo removal techniques. This scale assesses the number of treatments necessary for laser tattoo removal, provided that the practitioner is using a Q-switched Nd: YAG with six weeks between treatments.

Kirby-Desai Tattoo Removal Scale

SKIN TYPE
- I — Always Burns & Never Tans — ☐ 1 point
- II — Burns Easily & Tans Minimally — ☐ 2 points
- III — Sometimes Burns & Slowly Tans — ☐ 3 points
- IV — Burns Minimally & Usually Tans — ☐ 4 points
- V — Rarely Burns & Tans Well — ☐ 5 points
- VI — Never Burns & Always Tans — ☐ 6 points

LOCATION
- Head/Neck/Face — ☐ 1 point
- Upper Trunk/Shoulder — ☐ 2 points
- Lower Trunk/Upper Leg — ☐ 3 points
- Lower Arm/Leg — ☐ 4 points
- Wrist/Hand/Ankle/Foot — ☐ 5 points

AMOUNT OF INK
- Amateur — ☐ 1 point
- Minimal — ☐ 2 points
- Moderate — ☐ 3 points
- Significant — ☐ 4 points

LAYERING
- No — ☐ 0 points
- Yes — ☐ 2 points

SCARRING & TISSUE CHANGES
- No Scar — ☐ 0 points
- Minimal Scarring — ☐ 1 point
- Moderate Scarring — ☐ 3 points
- Significant Scarring — ☐ 5 points
- Note: Pre-existing scar tissue will remain after treatment.

COLORS
- Black Only — ☐ 1 point
- Mostly Black w/Some Red — ☐ 2 points
- Mostly Black & Red w/ Other Colors — ☐ 3 points
- Multiple Colors — ☐ 4 points
- Note: Some colors such as blue, green, aqua, purple, pink, orange, brown and yellow may never go away.
- Note: White, pink and peach colors may turn dark following treatment.

Estimated Number of Treatments Required to Achieve Goal:

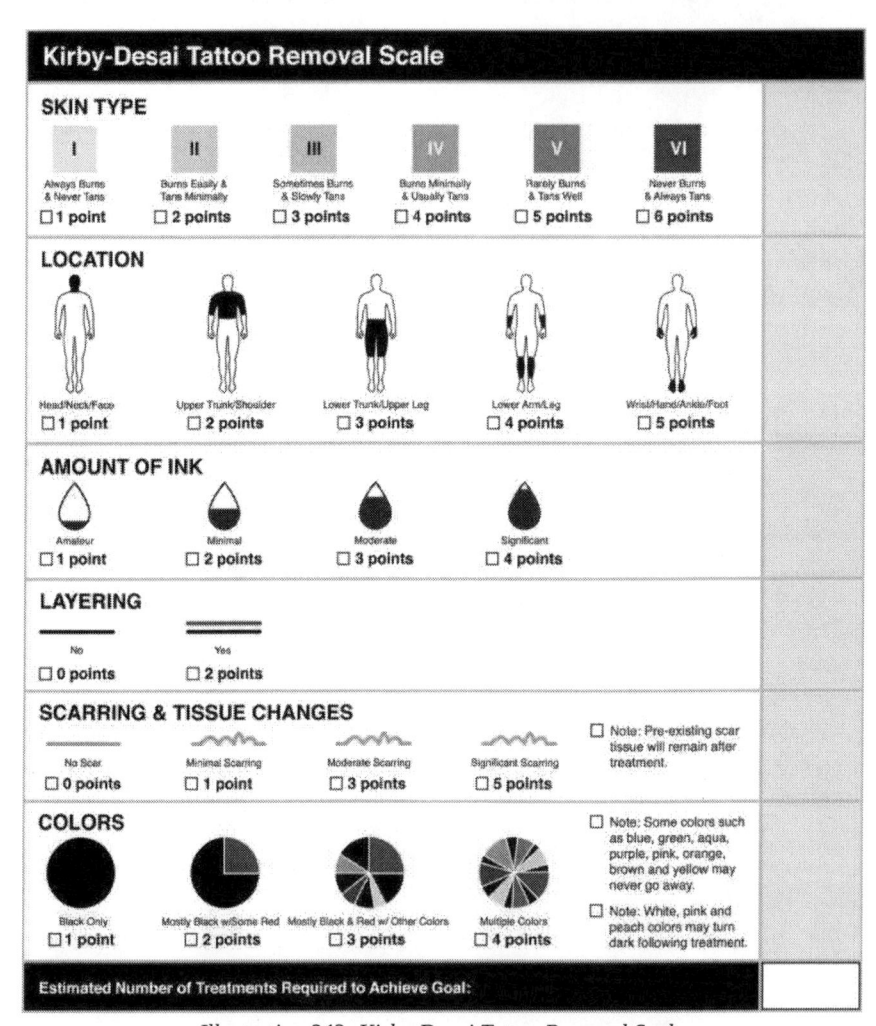

Illustration 243: Kirby-Desai Tattoo Removal Scale

The Kirby-Desai Scale assigns numerical values to six parameters: skin type, location, colour, amount of ink, scarring or tissue change, and layering. Parameter scores are then added to yield a combined score that will show the estimated number of treatments needed for satisfactory tattoo fading. Some recommend that the Kirby-Desai scale is used by all laser practitioners prior to starting tattoo removal treatment to help estimate the number of treatments required for tattoo removal and as a predictor of the success of the laser tattoo removal treatments. Prior to 2009, clinicians had no scientific basis (other than patch testing) by which to estimate the number of treatments needed to remove a tattoo and the use of this scale is now standard practice in laser tattoo removal.

The video below serves to provide an example of the real fading results achievable after mild laser tattoo fading treatments. This video can serve to manage the clients' expectations when first undergoing tattoo fading treatments. Watch Our Video on Laser Tattoo Remoal

28.13 Realstic results of laser tattoo fading

At first sight, most laser tattoo removal advertisements seem to promise seamless total tattoo fading results. Marketers should not be blamed for this initial misconception about laser tattoo removal procedures, because this is what attract people in the first place. Marketing the real results and the real expectations from the laser treatments would not be very effective and could deter people from inquiring about the treatment to start with. Unfortunately, marketing campaigns focusing on the real results are not very effective in the commercial world, especially when at first sight all the major clinics suggest seamless removal results. Therefore the common initial expectation of the uninformed client is the complete and seamless removal of their tattoos within one easy session. However, as we know, this is seldom the reality of laser tattoo removal treatments results as also demonstrated by the terms of business presented prior to the treatments.

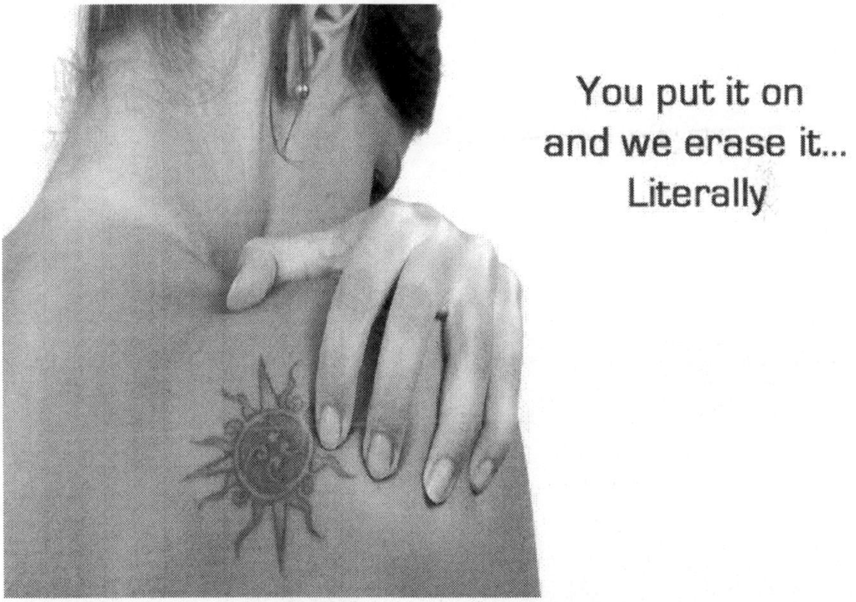

Illustration 244: Example of common tattoo removal advert. These are designed to capture the audience attention, however, these claims cannot reflect what it is currently possible to accomplish in reality.

www.voltaicplasma.comAuthor: Andreas Russo

As a matter of fact, there are currently no laser tattoo removal devices or techniques which can guarantee consistent seamless results. It is sometimes possible to remove certain types of tattoos using lasers within one or very few sessions, however this is the exception and not the norm; also very high-intensity treatments make tattoo fading possible for most tattoos in very few sessions however this does increase the likelihood of causing intense skin burns which will lead to permanent very visible adverse reactions (mainly scars, hypo-pigmentation and permanent skin texture change).

When the pigments are located too deeply into the dermis or in case of multi-layered tattoos seamless removal may be highly unlikely in any case. This is because the ablation has to be carried out so deeply inside the dermis in order to remove all the pigmentation that the likelihood of permanent adverse reactions is very high. Usually, these types of tattoos can be faded to a certain extent, however complete seamless disappearance is very unlikely. More generally as a rule of thumb, **the higher the points on the Kirby-Desai** scale the more **unlikely** a complete seamless removal will be. Conversely, the lower the points the more likely a seamless removal will be. An example of low points tattoo is permanent make-up, usually removed within one or two sessions.

As we know, laser tattoo fading treatments consist in inflicting a skin burn on the tattooed area in order to scatter the colour pigments. The skin does not react well both in the short and long-term to skin burns. Therefore, due to the very nature of this type of aesthetic treatment, tattoo removal seamless results are more the exception than the rule.

Aware of the high likelihood of permanent adverse reactions to the laser treatment, very few cosmetic clinics are willing to guarantee seamless results, despite the claims (implicit or explicit) made during the advertising campaigns. This is because experienced aesthetic practitioners are very well aware of the nature of laser treatments as well as what it is to be expected from this type of tattoo fading treatments. The real expected results also emerge in the informed consent forms, which clinics use in order to minimise their potential liabilities due to the permanent real adverse reactions. Often there may be skin texture change which can be permanent, hypo-pigmentation, colour scattering, a trace of the previous pigmentation or the tattoo will not be completely removed as it may be impractical to do so without leaving a scar tissue.

The client should be made aware of what is to be expected from tattoo laser fading treatments. Some of the permanent adverse reactions to laser tattoo fading treatments are:

- ✓ Hypo-pigmentation: **Hypo-pigmentation** associated with some sort of skin texture change is the most common permanent long-term adverse effect to burns caused by lasers. It does not usually occur after other tattoo fading treatments. Hypo-pigmentation associated with some sort of skin texture change is the most common permanent long-term adverse reaction to burns caused by lasers. The likelihood of hyperpigmentation is exacerbated in dark skin types, and this is the reason for many mild treatments to be used on dark skin tones. Some clinics even prefer to avoid laser treatments on skin type 4, 5 and 6.

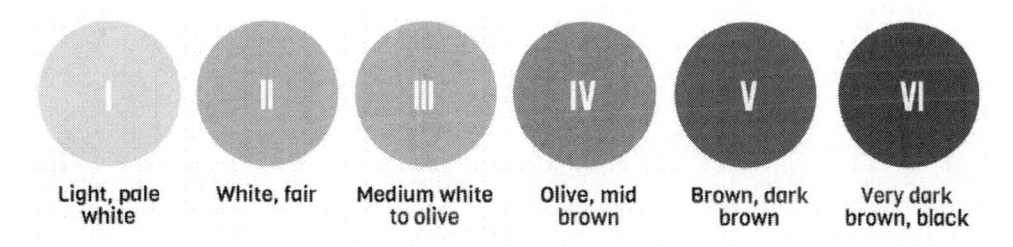

I	II	III	IV	V	VI
Light, pale white	White, fair	Medium white to olive	Olive, mid brown	Brown, dark brown	Very dark brown, black

Illustration 245: Skin types

Aesthetic cosmetic laser treatment is sometimes avoided on skin types 4, 5 and 6 altogether to due to the likelihood of hypopigmentation. Those clinics which would perform laser treatments on these darker skin tones perform very mild treatments, in order to minimise the likelihood of hypo-pigmentation.

Especially in darker skin tones, the likelihood of hypo-pigmentation is so high that some cosmetic clinics do not suggest laser treatments at all. In case of dark skin, the aesthetic practitioner may still inform the clients of the inherent potential adverse reactions (especially hypo-pigmentation) and if the clients agree they perform the least invasive laser treatment to minimise the risks of hypo-pigmentation even if the number of treatments required to achieve the desired results increases dramatically (sometimes exceeding 2o treatments in case of resilient tattoos). Hypo-pigmentation is very likely to occur especially after intense multi-wavelengths or very high-intensity treatments. It can sometimes be temporary, however, it is mostly permanent. Many people prefer to have hypo-pigmentation rather keeping their unwanted tattoo. Hypo-pigmentation is sometimes resolved with permanent camouflage make-up (another form of tattooing).

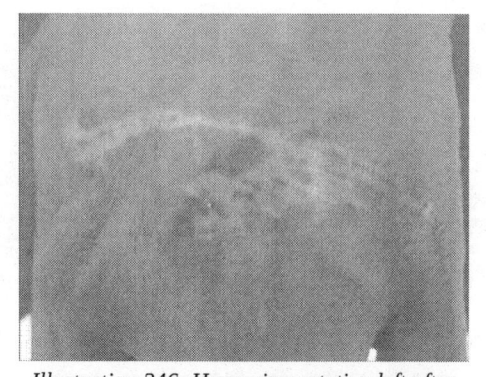

Illustration 246: Hypo-pigmentation left after tattoo fading treatment. Some blue pigments are still present. Most hypo-pigmentation are permanent, however, this type of hypopigmentation will fade slightly over time. On the other hand, the skin texture will unlikely completely blend with the rest of the skin.

✓ **Hyperpigmentation:** This can occur because the tattoo fading treatment also triggers skin regeneration. As it is well known, exposure to sunlight without sun protection can cause hyperpigmentation. In certain cases, some light tattoo colours such as yellow or white can

- become dark. This paradoxical darkening can lead to an aesthetic change. These colours can be removed with further laser sessions.
- **Permanent skin texture change:** This occurs especially after intense laser treatments. This is a common adverse reaction to laser tattoo fading treatments and can also occur after other types of tattoo fading treatments.
- **Can cause scars especially hypertrophic:** The likelihood of hypertrophic scars development is exacerbated by high-intensity treatments using multi-wavelengths lasers. However, the main cause of permanent scarring is poor after-care or predisposition to scarring. This type of adverse reactions can occur after any type of tattoo fading treatments.
- **Keloid formation:** This can also occur after any other type of tattoo fading treatment.
- Incomplete, even impossible, elimination of all traces of tattoo ink. Polychrome tattoos, in particular, pastel colour, yellow and dense or deep tattoo pigmentation are particularly hard to be faded completely. A phantom tattoo (residual traces) can be observed at the end of the course of several treatments.
- **Phototoxicity of certain types of tattoo pigments:** Some tattoo pigments contain metals that could theoretically break down into toxic chemicals inside the body when exposed to light (including that of lasers). This has not yet been reported in vivo but has been shown in laboratory tests.

The higher the intensity of the treatment the more the tattoo pigmentation is scattered by the treatment, however the more the likelihood of developing adverse permanent adverse reactions due to the deep burn caused by the high-intensity laser treatment. Conversely, the milder the treatment, the milder the burn inflicted, the less the pigmentation scattered and the lower the likelihood of developing permanent adverse reactions after each individual treatment. For this reason, most cosmetic clinics prefer to split the removal treatment into several low-intensity treatments. Not only does this minimise the inherent likelihood of developing adverse reactions but it also increases the overall price of the tattoo fading treatment due to the increased cumulative cost of several sessions.

It has to be reminded that although mild treatments minimise the likelihood of adverse reactions, due to the cumulative skin damages caused by the laser burns also a high number of laser treatments can lead to adverse effects. In other words, the cumulative damage of several relatively mild laser burns can cause similar adverse permanent reactions to one or few intense laser treatments.

Please note that any permanent adverse reaction can occur regardless of the way the treatment has been performed. Sometimes even one relatively mild laser treatment can trigger one or more adverse reactions. Unfortunately, there is not currently known tattoo fading treatment capable of guaranteeing seamless tattoo removal.

28.14 Hypo-pigmentation examples

In this section, we are going to see some real results of laser tattoo fading (removal) procedures. Of course in some cases where the tattoo has a low score in the Kirby-Desai scale the results can be seamless, however, this is not the reality of most tattoo fading treatments, especially those who have a high Kirby-Desai score. The more challenging the tattoo to remove, the more likely the removal of the tattoo pigments will come at the price of some type of adverse reaction. We mainly present those results which display hypo-pigmentation because this is the most common permanent adverse reaction to laser tattoo removal treatments. Not all laser fading procedures will present adverse reactions and some tattoos can be removed seamlessly, however, this is only the case of high-quality tattoos, and those tattoos with a low score of the Kirby-Desai scale.

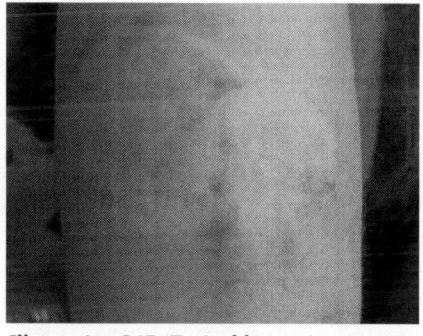

Illustration 247: Typical hypo-pigmentation and change in skin texture after intense laser treatment. Hypo-pigmentation is an adverse reaction only peculiar to laser treatments, so far it has not been reported after any other type of tattoo fading treatment.

Hypo-pigmentation is usually permanent however slowly gets better over time. Normal pink hypo-pigmented skin is found after the normal healing of most wounds. The type of permanent hypo-pigmentation caused by laser treatments should not be confused with the normal temporary lack of melanin after a normal wound heal. This is because unfortunately, laser treatments seem to have the inherent tendency of either permanently destroying the melanocytes or somehow permanently inhibit the natural production of melanin.

As seen in the figure on the right, lack of melanin can occur in random patches on the area treated by the laser. The higher the intensity of the treatment, the higher the likelihood of this type of adverse effect.

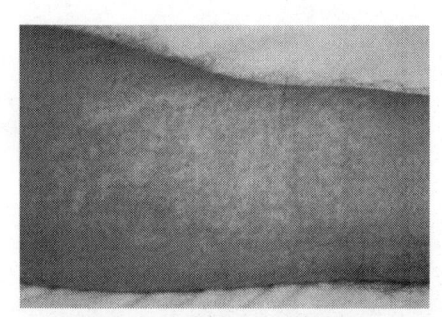

Illustration 248: Scattered hypo-pigmentation caused by laser treatment. Typically, this is an inherent risk which can be unavoidable at times. The darker the skin type the higher the likelihood of developing hypo-pigmentation after tattoo laser fading treatments

Hypo-pigmentation is more difficult to be removed or attenuated than most other types of adverse reactions to laser tattoo fading treatments. This is because the inherent lack of melanin although can improve slightly over time, is permanent and there are not currently known methods to restore the natural melanin production after it has been inhibited by laser burns.

www.voltaicplasma.com   Author: Andreas Russo

While hyperpigmentation, scarring, keloids and certain types of skin texture change can be successfully treated in various ways, hypo-pigmentation can improve slightly over time on its own accord but unfortunately, there are not known aesthetic treatments to reverse it. The most common solution to hypo-pigmentation is tattoo cover-up or permanent make-up.

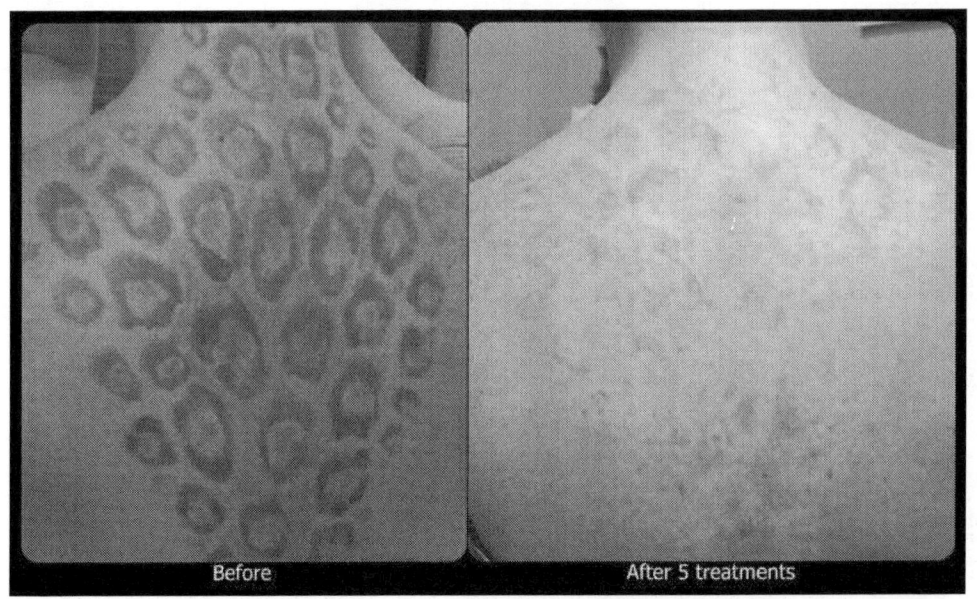

Illustration 249: Hypo-pigmentation and variation in skin tone and texture, in general, is a very common permanent skin reaction to laser tattoo treatments. In the figure above we can see how the brightest colours are still present after 5 laser treatments.

Permanent camouflage makeup is a good solution for those areas rarely exposed to the sunlight. Because exposure to the sun will naturally darken the healthy normal skin, while the hypo-pigmented area will not change in colour, therefore exposure to the sunlight and artificial tanning may accentuate the aesthetic problem even after the use of cover-up tattoos or permanent makeup. Therefore tattooing the hypo-pigmented areas with another colour to blend in the hypo-pigmented area is the most common solution to this adverse reaction.

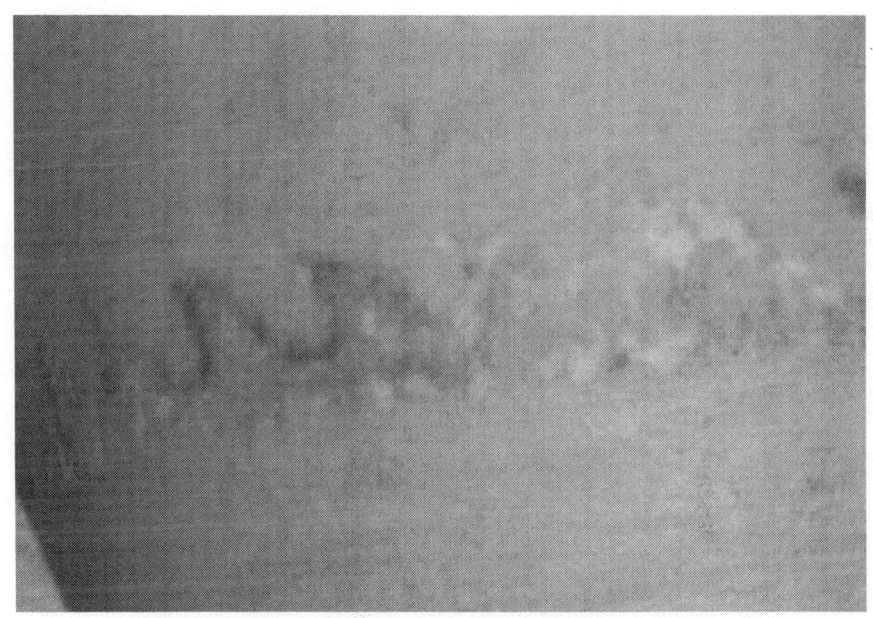

Illustration 250: A further example of hypo-pigmentation. As we can see some pigmentation traces are still present.

Due to the high likelihood of change in skin texture, scarring and hypo-pigmentation many people prefer to only fade the tattoo slightly using a laser. They usually only undergo those treatments that fade the most colours.

28.15 Real Example

The following experience is brought as an example to show the actual results of laser "tattoo removal" treatments. As you will see in these three videos the healing process is accompanied by blistering and it is uncomfortable. In third video the "picture" advertised as safe and more effective than common lasers has caused blistering lasting 5 days and possibly due to the high-intensity treatment, the last session left a certain degree of hypo-pigmentation.

We have chosen these videos because they are a true testimony of what clients go through after the laser removal treatments. As you can see in these videos the immediate and temporary normal reactions are those described previously in this web-page (blistering and discomfort).

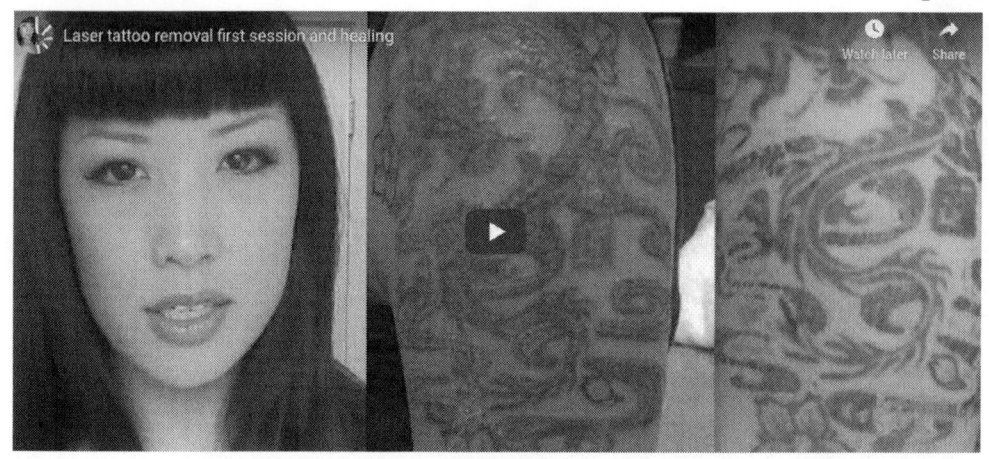

Illustration 251: Click here to watch video

In this video, you can see the real results of a treatment performed with an expensive heavily advertised tattoo fading/"removal" laser the "picture". There are several more published videos on the social media and all show similar experiences. Watch Video on Laser Tattoo Removal First Session

29.0 Electrical Thermabrasion tattoo fading

More and more aesthetic practitioners, aware of the damaging effects caused by repeated exposure to lasers for tattoo removal prefer thermal abrasion with and without osmosis to lasers. This has long been done with devices operating in either elecrofulguration or electrodesssication mode. Electrofulguration is the technique we are going to be focusing on in this section which is also recently referred to as "fibroblast" or plasma tattoo removal.

29.1 Tattoo Removal with Electrical Thermabrasion (Fibroblast) without osmosis.

The first stage to learn when it comes to tattoo removal using electrical arcing is thermabrasion without the use of osmosis. We will look at how osmosis is applied later on in this section.

Electrical arcing tattoo removal without osmosis is applied in those cases where the risks of scarring are increased by the use of osmosis.

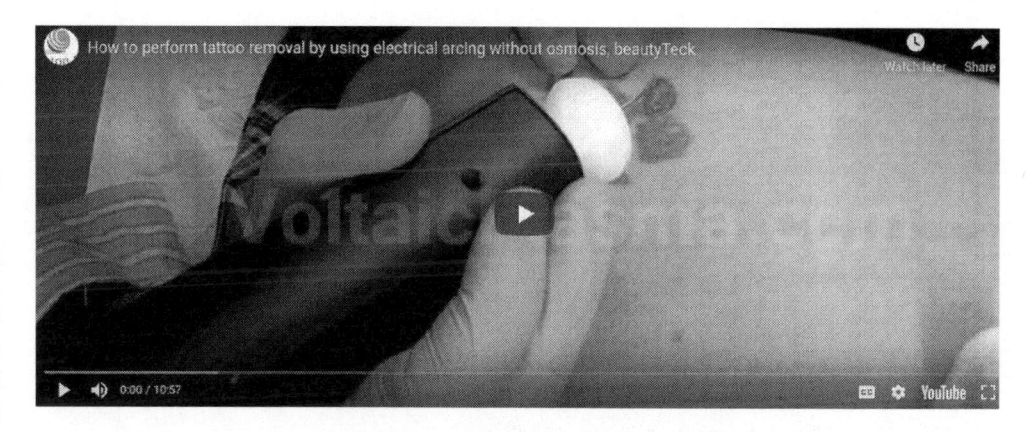

Illustration 252: Watch our video on this topic

Those areas of the body are those parts of the skin subject to continuous stretching and creasing. Like knees, wrists, elbows etc, this is because the continuous creasing and stretching of the skin makes it difficult for the area to heal speedily and therefore more prone to infection and delayed healing. In these cases the use of electrical arcing or electrical thermabrasion on its own may be the best course of action.

However when we use electrical thermabrasion on its own the degree of tattoo fading is rather low after each session. In other words the degree of tattoo fading after each electrical arcing session without osmosis is comparable to that of most Q-Switched lasers for tattoo Removal procedures.

29.2 Plasma or Fibroblast for Tattoo Removal with Osmosis

If performed correctly, electrofulguration, or electrical arcing, provides an effective way to remove tattoos while minimizing the number of sessions required to achieve the desired effects, also minimising the risks of collateral damages or scarring. The risks to the skin are minimized drastically because thermal abrasion with osmosis allows attenuating tattoos, in most cases halving the number of sessions otherwise required with laser treatment.

Although different tattoos present different levels of difficulty in their effective attenuation, depending on the type of ink and instrumentation used to draw it, experience has shown that thermal abrasion with osmosis can remove tattoos within 2 to 4 sessions. If thermal abrasion is applied without osmosis the number of sessions required for tattoo removal increase dramatically and the number of treatments and results can be comparable to those of lasers.

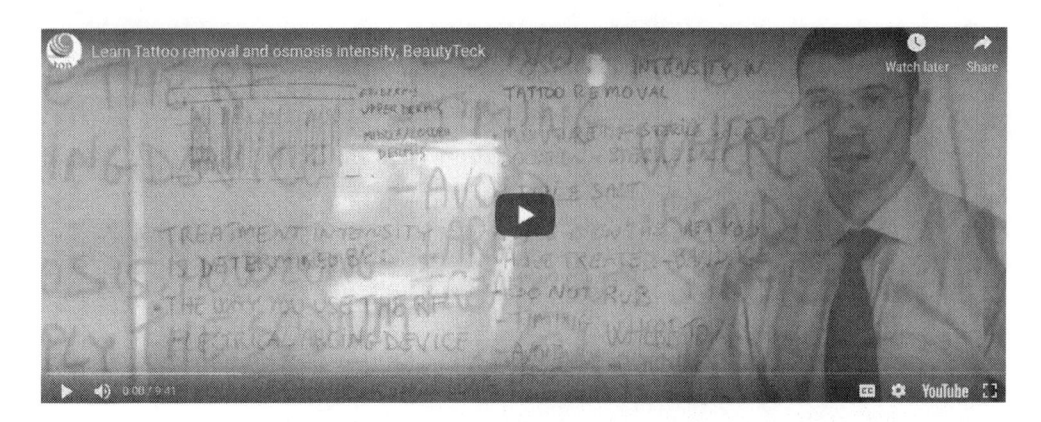

Illustration 253: Watch our video on this topic

Therefore, it has to be noted that there are clinical advantages to using Electrical thermal abrasion with osmosis over laser treatment for tattoo removal. Electrical Thermal abrasion with osmosis is far far more effective and efficient than lasers and it has the following advantages:

- Less potential harm to the client because less sessions are required.
- No collateral damage associated to the repeated use of lasers on the skin.
- The cost of the instruments required for tattoo removal are a fraction of specialized tattoo removal lasers.

Additionally, from a clinical stand point, it is important to try and find any possible way to minimise the number of exposures to burns or to any similar skin abrasions. The more the skin is exposed to laser treatment or any other thermal abrasion techniques the more damage can be caused to the skin. Since fibroblast with Osmosis drastically reduces the number of sessions required to achieve the desired tattoo fading results it is usually one of the best options.

29.3 The importance of Salation or Osmosis when using fibroblasting for tattoo removal.

Salabrasion or salation is one of the first known effective techniques to remove tattoo and it had been around for several hundreds years. Originally Salabrasion was used by literally rubbing the tattoo using salt until the upper part of the dermis become exposed to the sodium chloride.

Modern technology has not made this technique obsolete because it is still more effective than most Q-Switched lasers and inexpensive on top of it. Thermal skin resurfacing before applying salt is key for effectively applying the osmotic effect induced by the sodium chloride.

www.voltaicplasma.com   Author: Andreas Russo

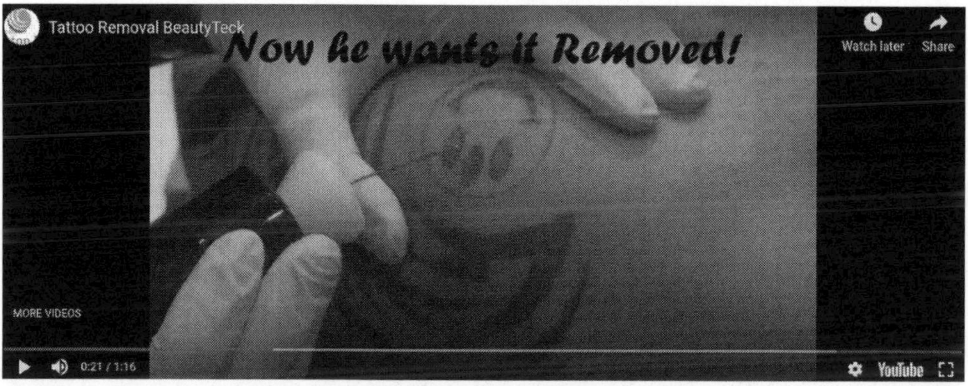

Illustration 254: Watch our video on this topic

When it comes to tattoo removal (or Tattoo fading), the most important part of electrical thermabrasion with osmosis is the osmosis itself. This is the most important ingredient in the recipe of tattoo fading using electrical arcing or Fibroblast. Without osmosis the results would be poor, comparable to those with Q-Switched lasers.

However, whenever mentioning the use of salt for tattoo fading (or tattoo removal) people firstly raise their eyebrows. What do you meal by salt? Yes, we mean sodium Chloride nothing fancy. Too simple and too down to earth to be taken seriously at first, but once you see the results you will take it extremely seriously because it outperforms any expensive Q-Switched lasers' results not by a little but by miles. The results of only one tattoo removal session using electrical arcing coupled with osmosis is often as good as 4 to 5 laser sessions.

The inherent simplicity of osmosis is possibly the reason for this technique, although several times more effective than most expensive Q -Switched lasers, not to be as popular as laser tattoo removal. The first time we saw the results after one session of tattoo removal using electrical arcing with osmosis we were gobsmacked. The results were several times better than with any other laser.

Also, as we will see the use of salt is not as straightforward as the use of lasers alone and you have to time it well. Too long of an application the higher the risks of a scarring, too short the duration the less the tattoo fading.

Like with laser treatment, thermal abrasion causes the colour pigments to be broken down and reabsorbed. However the protocol of thermal abrasion involves also packing the area treated with sodium chloride for a period of half to a full hour after thermal abrasion. The timing of the application of the sodium chloride depends on whether fine salt or a salt paste is used.

Sodium chloride is applied because it causes osmosis. Osmosis draws the broken tattoo pigments to the surface of the skin removing them from the deeper part of the dermis. In other words the osmotic process pulls out as much as the broken pigments as possible so that the more of the unwanted pigments will be trapped in the scab which will subsequently forms during healing. Osmosis therefore facilitates and further speeds up the tattoo discoloration process and hence eventual removal whenever possible (because as we know not all tattoos can be completely removed seamlessly).

In other words tattoo salation has the effect of drawing up the colour pigments towards the surface of the skin. This is why this technique is also referred to as "tattoo osmosis".

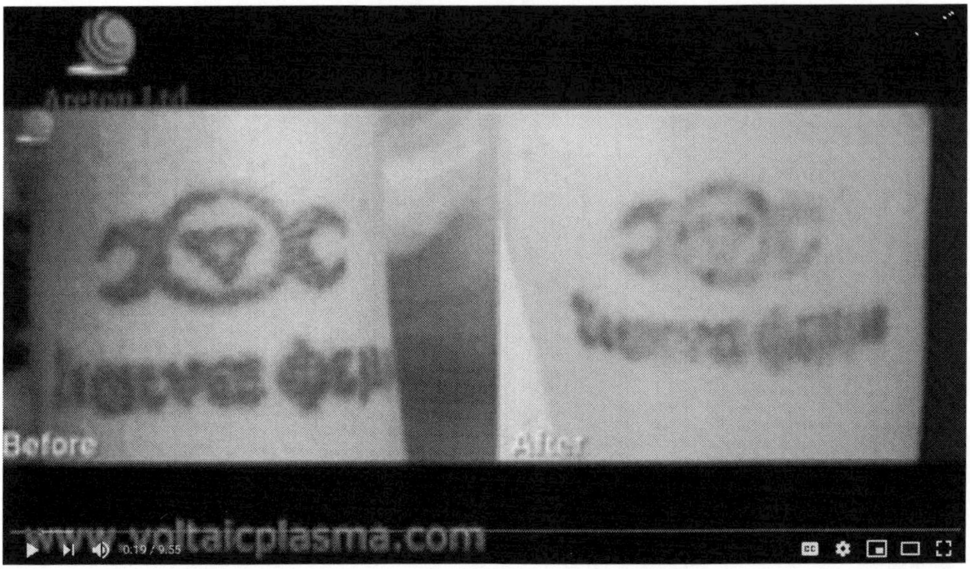

Illustration 255: Watch our video on this topic

Salation or Osmosis has also its degree of treatment intensity. The longer the sodium chloride is left on the exposed tattoo the more the colour pigments are drawn towards the surface, therefore the more the tattoo will fade after each treatment. The intensity of the treatment using sodium chloride on its own is mainly dependent on the duration of the application of the salt on the tattoo itself. Additionally Osmosis can be carried out in two main ways:

1. By applying a dense paste made of sterile saline solution and sterile fine sodium chloride. This has relatively high-intensity results if compared to applying only sterile fine salt. Also the longer the salt is applied on to the tattoo the higher the intensity of the treatment.

2. By applying sterile fine salt on its own. The salt is usually applied on to the tattoo for a predetermined period of time. The duration of the sodium chloride application has a direct impact on the intensity of the treatment. The longer the salt is applied the higher the treatment intensity and the more the osmotic effect on the tattoo pigments, therefore the more the fading of the tattoo after each session.

Keeping the time of application the same the two different osmosis methods have different osmosis intensity. Generally, the sterile sodium chloride paste has a stronger efficacy than fine sterile salt on its own. This is why a sterile paste of sodium chloride is used for permanent make-up removal.

In permanent makeup removal it is not practical to bandage the area treated due to the location of the tattoo, therefore the sterile paste is applied so that the osmotic effect is so strong that the application is only a few minutes and this is enough to achieve the desired result.

29.4 Why using electrical arcing for skin resurfacing before Salabration (or Osmosis)?

Radio frequency or electrical arcing devices have the double function of removing the epidermal layer (necessary for the osmosis to take place) and also heat up and break down the tattoo pigments at the same time. In other words electrical arcing devices have the double effect of not only performing the required skin abrasion necessary for the osmotic effect to take place (once the salt is placed on the tattoo) but it also breaks down part of the tattoo pigments (like lasers do). The latter contributes to speeding up the tattoo fading process.

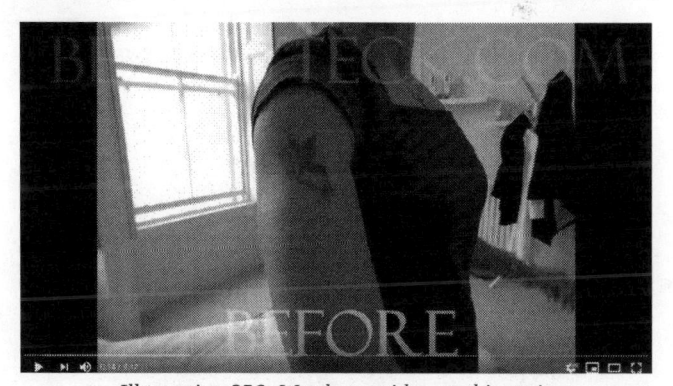

Illustration 256: Watch our video on this topic

Not only Plasma fibroblast devices but also other devices can be used for effective resurfacing before applying salation (or Osmosis). Such as microdermabrasion devices, micro-needling devices injecting the saline salt solution directly into the dermis and any method currently known to expose the upper dermal layer. The upper dermal layer needs to be exposed for the osmosis to be effective. Osmosis on its own is not sufficient in order to remove or fade the tattoo pigments. If the sodium chloride is not in contact with the dermis or at least upper dermis in order to induce an effective osmosis no tattoo fading will take place.

There are several ways to remove the epidermal layer and allow the salt to get in contact with the tattoo pigments. The use of electrical arcing (also referred to as Plasma) and the use of radio frequency devices is one of the best options due to the fact that fibroblasting causes:

1. The dermabrasion necessary to expose the dermis

2. And also it injects heat into the skin at the same time helping break down the tattoo pigments.

This is because the electrical arcing have the double effect of not only abrading the area like microdermabrasion etc, but it also has the effect of breaking down the tattoo pigments by using the heat injected by the electrical arc. Because of this thermal effect the broken pigments will be more easily drawn to the surface by the osmotic effect.

29.5 Intensity of the treatment when using Fibroblasting before osmosis

Usually it is the tattoo removal practitioner the one who decides the degree of ablation and the intensity of the treatment. This is done assessing the client's desires and the aesthetic practitioner's own previous experience. For example, if the client is happy incurring in a higher likelihood of developing a scar but going through fewer treatments then a higher degree of ablation can be carried out.

The intensity of the Electrical thermabrasion is controlled by the depth of the ablation. This in turn is controlled by three factors:

1. The power level of the arc,

2. The sweeping speed of the arc during the spraying operation

3. And of course the number of passes on the area.

The deeper the ablation the more the tattoo will fade after each treatment. This is keeping the intensity of the osmosis the same. Remember that the intensity of the osmosis is dependent on the salt application duration and whether fine salt is applied or the saline paste.

The electrical arcing ablation for tattoo removal or tattoo fading can be carried out at different intensities.

1. The first level of intensity consists in simply removing the epidermis. This is done by setting the specific device at very low power levels to ablate the epidermal layer and then removing the carbon residues with a cotton pad impregnated with non-flammable antiseptic. This is repeated until the carbon residues are removed and the upper dermis is exposed. This alone will suffice to then apply osmosis either by applying sterile salt or a sterile salt paste.

2. The second level of intensity consists not only in removing the epidermal layer as required by the epidermal abrasion, necessary for the osmotic effect to take place, but also break down the tattoo pigments inside the dermal layer where they reside. This can be done in stages by first removing the epidermal layer as described above and then spraying the voltaic arc (fibroblast) into the already exposed upper dermal layer. This has the function of breaking down the tattoo pigments inside the dermis. This technique is called "double pass" this is because the aesthetic practitioner is required to perform two passes on the tattoo in order to apply the osmosis. The first pass is used to remove the epidermis and it exposes the upper dermis. The second pass is used to breakdown the pigments by spraying the electrical arc directly on the dermal layer which is now being exposed. Two passes in total, hence the term "double pass".

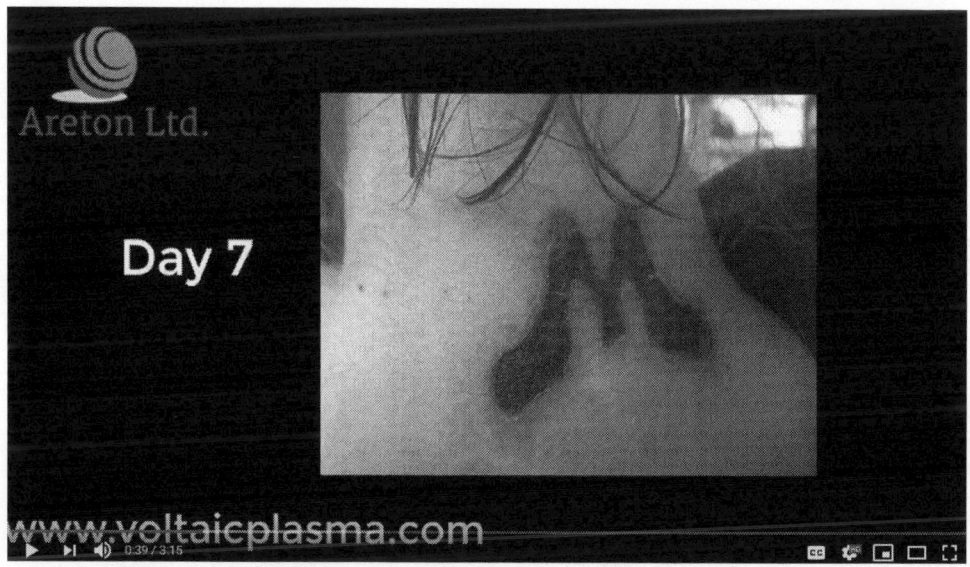

Illustration 257: Watch our video on this topic

Please note that the second intensity level "double pass" can be carried out also by directly increasing the power level of the electrical arcing device to the point where the arc instantly carbonises the epidermal layer and injects the required heat into the dermal layer to break down the tattoo pigments all at the same time.

www.voltaicplasma.com   Author: Andreas Russo

In other words the pigments rooted deeply inside the dermis can be broken down with a single ablation. This is done by setting the device at a relatively high power level and hence the arc has enough power to reach and break down the pigments located in the lower part of the dermis within a single pass.

The tattoo pigments can be also distributed relatively deeply inside the dermis therefore a deeper ablation can be required in order to have an impact on the deeper pigments. In order to do this usually a double pass is performed on the upper dermis. When this is done normally the area treated starts bleeding, this is normal. Please bear in mind that the deeper the ablation the higher the likelihood of permanent adverse effects including scarring.

29.6 Adverse reactions to Tattoo removal by applying electrical thermal abrasion with osmosis

It has been extensively shown that thermal abrasion with osmosis is very effective in removing tattoos without leaving any scars and within only few sessions and in doing so it is more effective than most Q-Switched lasers.

However, scars could develop when:

- thermal abrasion had been carried out to cause extensive damage to the dermis.
- the treated area had become infected.
- the client has a particular predisposition to developing Keloids or hypertrophic scars.

One of the main differences between this type of treatment and laser tattoo removal is that with Electrical Thermabrasion the likelihood of contracting an infection are higher. This is because the treatment will leave an open wound which during the healing process is susceptible to localised inflammatory infections. On the other hand lasers only cause a burn which is not easily susceptible to infections.

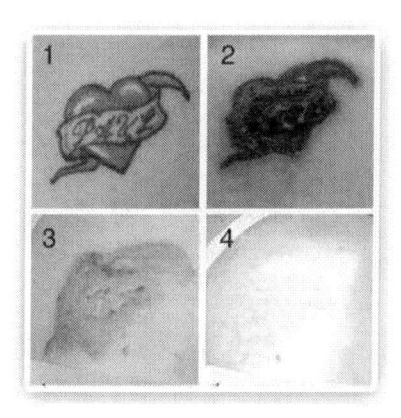

Illustration 258: you can see the characteristic temporary hypertrophic scar formation which will eventually disappear. This is a very common temporary reaction to fibroblast with osmosis.

The main adverse reaction is scarring caused by infections contracted after the tattoo removal procedure during the healing process. Scarring can happen if the treatment has been carried out at too high intensively overall or the treated area has contracted an infection. Although the former eventuality has been rarely reported as being the cause of scarring the latter is more likely to be the leading cause of scarring. This is because a prolonged infection can cause sometimes severe damage to the dermis, hence being the real cause of scarring.

The likelihood of infections are easily minimised by using the appropriate aftercare and keeping the area clean until the scab have formed fully. Once the scabs have formed the likelihood of contracting a localised inflammatory infection is very low because the scab pose an effective barrier to bacteria and avoids infections. The scab must not be removed forcefully by picking it or otherwise. These scabs are usually relatively thick and sometimes contain a relatively large amount of the tattoo colour removed by the procedure.. A Common adverse reaction of osmosis is the formation of a temporary hypertrophic scar. This forms especially if the area has been subject to an infection but it can also form even if an infection has not occurred. Usually, this hypertrofic formation subsides on its own accord over a few weeks.

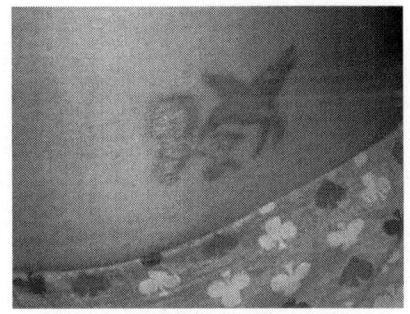

Illustration 259: In this picture, we can see a small hypertrophic formation of the are treated with Electrical arcing and osmosis. In this particular case, the area was on the waist line and an infection had occurred. This small hypertrophic formation disappeared on its own accord.

So far no cases of hypo-pigmentation have been reported after fibroblast with osmosis. As we know hypo-pigmentation is a common adverse reaction to lasers tattoo removal treatments and if it occurs after laser treatments it is permanent.

Hyper-pigmentation is also possible after the use of electrical arcing with osmosis, this is because this treatment involves skin regeneration and skin resurfacing. All skin resurfacing treatments require total sun protection in order to avoid hyper pigmentation. Hence, in order to minimise this likelihood, the client must avoid direct sun exposure while applying sunscreen up to three months after the last treatment like after any other type of plasma aesthetic treatment.

29.7 About the results. How many treatments are required to remove a tattoo?

After Electrical thermabrasion with osmosis the tattoo fades according to the type of tattoo and its location on the body (see kirbey Desai scale). And mainly also depending on the overall intensity of the treatment. Usually the higher the overall intensity of the treatment the more the pigments are drawn from the dermis into the eventual scab. Usually the scab will visibly contain the colours of the tattoo that has been treated. The higher the intensity of the treatment the more the pigments inside the scab. It is not unusual to see scabs containing green, yellow and blue colours after the treatment of multicolour tattoos.

The aesthetic practitioner has double control over the intensity of the overall treatment by varying:

1. the intensity of the electrical thermabrasion treatment and

2. the osmosis intensity.

As we have seen tattoos are all different. The usual rule of the lower the points on the Kirbey desai scale the more quickly the tattoo will be be faded or removed still applies. Always remember that it is sometimes impractical to achieve complete removal of the tattoo without leaving a scar. However all tattoos are often faded more easily than otherwise would with lasers due to the double fading effect of electrical thermabrasion and salation. The average number of treatments required varies between 1 to 3 for an average tattoo.

In general one medium intensity treatment can fade the equivalent amount of 4 Q-Switched tattoo removal laser sessions. In other words on average, 1 treatment with electrical thermabrasion with osmosis is the equivalent of 4 lasers tattoo removal sessions.

29.8 How much of an area can be treated at a time?

Like with laser treatments, also in electrical thermabrasion with osmosis, large tattoos are split into different small areas in order to fade it.

There is no limit to the size of area which can be treated using electrical thermabrasion with osmosis. The wider the area treated the more likely it is to contract an infection due to the extent of the area treated. The larger area treated the more difficult it is to protect the wound against bacterial infections during the healing process.

It is up to the aesthetic practitioner to decide what may be appropriate for each individual case.

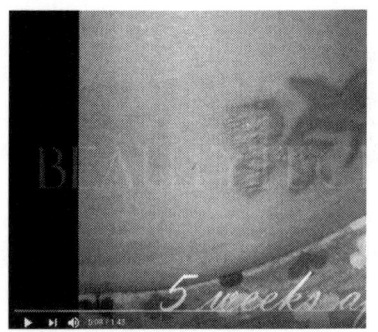

Illustration 260: Watch our video on this topic

www.voltaicplasma.com   Author: Andreas Russo

29.9 Multicolour tattoos

As we know multi colour tattoos are very challenging to be faded with lasers. Some colours cannot be faded by lasers at all.
This is not the case using electrical plasma with osmosis because this type of treatment is colour blind and it is capable to fade all tattoo colours indiscriminately. Since this type of treatment is colour blind it is one of the preferred methods to fade multicolour tattoos. It is not unusual to see scabs literary green or yellow depending on the colours of the original tattoo.

29.10 Tattoo Removal Aftercare

Aftercare after tattoo removal with electrical arcing and osmosis is very important but very simple at the same time.

1. Keep the area clean

2. Do not use any creams on the area

3. Do not use any bandaging on the area treated or any plaster. This is because bandaging or plasters can cause a worm moist environment were bacteria proliferate and hence cause infections and delayed healing.

4. Disinfect periodically up until the area has developed a scab.

Remember that scabs should not be picked and must peel off on their own accord.

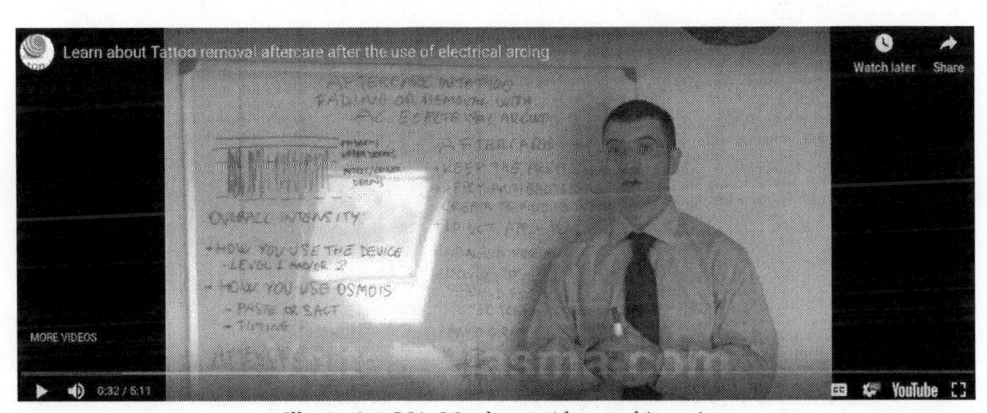

Illustration 261: Watch our video on this topic

www.voltaicplasma.com   Author: Andreas Russo

29.11 Healing time.

The healing time depends on the overall intensity of the treatment. The higher the overall intensity of the treatment the longer the treated area will take in order to recover fully. Usually the scab form within 3 to 4 days from the treatment and falls off on its own accord within 10 days. However, the area may still feel tender to the touch in general up to a few weeks after the scab has fallen off.

Generally the healing time, provided that the area is not infected, occurs within a maximum of 10 days and it is marked by the scabs falling off on their own accord. Watch our video on after care

30.0 Tattoo removal with and without osmosis

Electrical Thermal Abrasion (Fibroblast) with Osmosis

The preferred operational method for this procedure is electro fulguration (also now referred to as "fibroblast") because the ablation requires to be very superficial. If performed correctly, electrofulguration, or electrical arcing, provides an effective way to remove tattoos while minimizing the number of sessions required to achieve the desired effects, also minimising the risks of collateral damages or scarring. The risks to the skin are minimized drastically because thermal abrasion with osmosis allows removing tattoos, in most cases halving the number of sessions otherwise required with laser treatment.

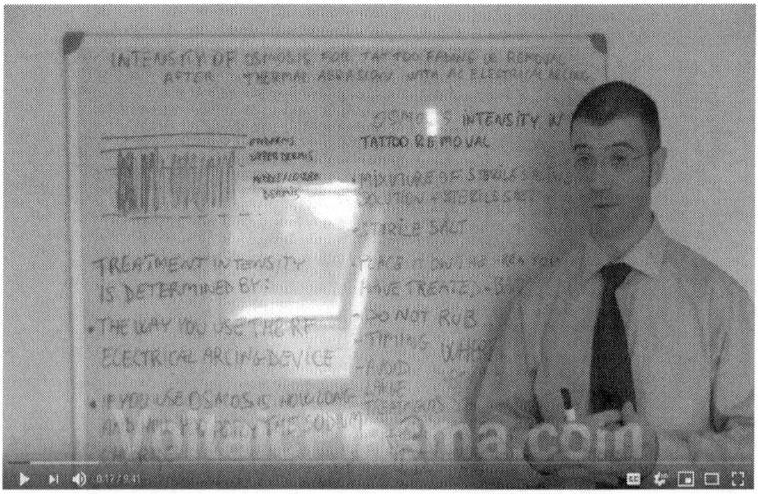

Illustration 262: Watch Our Video on this topic

www.voltaicplasma.com   Author: Andreas Russo

Although different tattoos present different levels of difficulty in their removal, depending on the type of ink and instrumentation used to draw it, experience has shown that thermal abrasion with osmosis can remove tattoos within 3 to 6 sessions, on average, per area treated. If <u>thermal abrasion is applied without osmosis</u> the number of sessions required for tattoo removal increase dramatically and the number of treatments and results can be comparable to those of lasers.

Therefore, it has to be noted that there are clinical advantages of using thermal abrasion with osmosis over laser treatment for tattoo removal. **Thermal abrasion with osmosis is more effective and efficient than lasers and it has the following advantages:**

- Less potential harm to the client because less sessions are required.
- No collateral damage associated to the repeated use of lasers on the skin.
- The cost of the instruments required for tattoo removal are a fraction of specialized tattoo removal lasers.

Why thermal abrasion with osmosis more than halves the number of sessions required compared with conventional laser removal equipment?

Like with laser treatment, thermal abrasion causes the colour pigments to be broken down. However the protocol of thermal abrasion involves also packing the area treated with sodium chloride for a period of half to a full hour after thermal abrasion.

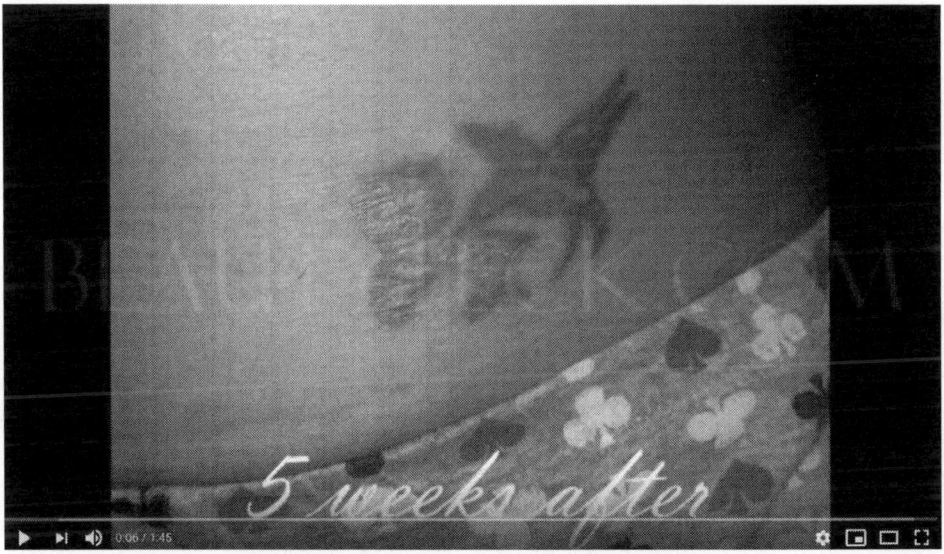

Illustration 263: Click here to watch video

The sodium chloride is applied because it causes osmosis. Osmosis draws the broken tattoo pigments to the surface removing them from the deeper part of the dermis. It therefore facilitates and further speeds up the tattoo discolouration and hence eventual removal.

Additionally, from a clinical stand point, it is important to try and find any possible way to minimise the number of exposures to burns or to any similar skin abrasions. The more the skin is exposed to laser treatment or any other thermal abrasion techniques the more damage is caused to the skin.

Adverse reactions to Tattoo removal by applying electrical thermal abrasion with osmosis

It has been extensively shown that thermal abrasion with osmosis is very effective in removing tattoos without leaving any scars and within only few sessions.

However, scars could develop when:

- Thermal abrasion had been carried out to cause extensive damage to the dermis.
- The treated area had become infected
- The client has a particular predisposition to developing Keloids or hypertrophic scars

Tattoo Removal with Electrical Thermabrasion (Fibroblast) without osmosis.
In those cases where the risks of scarring are increased by the use of osmosis then only thermabrasion should be used.

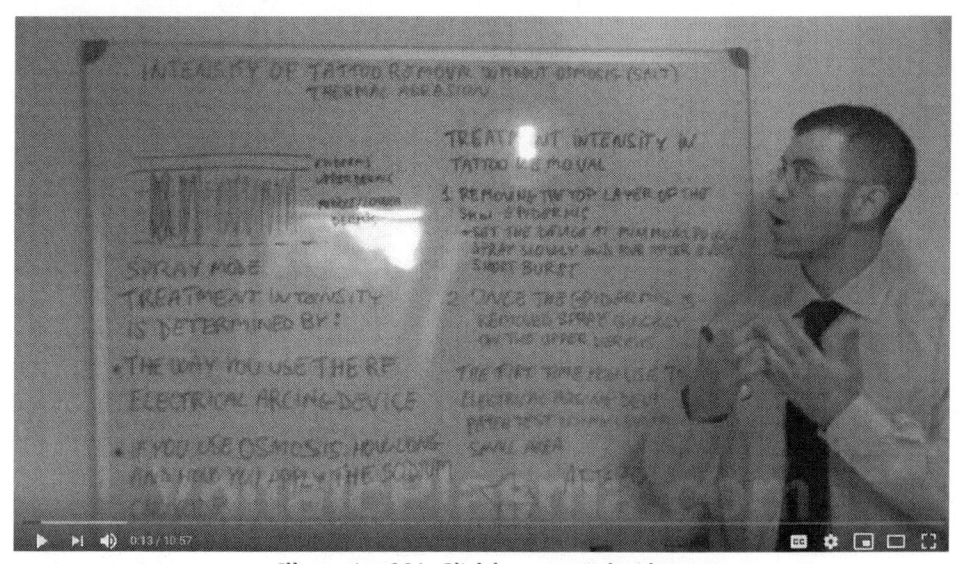

Illustration 264: Click here to watch video

31.0 Permanent make-up removal

This section will only cover eyebrow permanent make-up removal. No tests have been performed on permanent make-up elsewhere on the face. Therefore it is advisable to limit your permanent make up removal treatments to tattooed eyebrows. This type of treatment is generally carried out to correct previous work done by permanent make-up artists.

Permanent make-up removal is much easier than normal tattoo removal. Normally both the equipment and the pigmentation used for permanent make-up are of very high quality. Therefore the removal of permanent make-up is normally much easier than the removal of normal tattoos for a number of reasons:

- high standards of the equipment and pigmentation used to apply the permanent make up in the first place. The better the quality of the work already carried out the easier it becomes to remove the permanent pigmentation.
- the area covered by the permanent make-up is usually very small compared to most other types of tattoos, making permanent make-up removal even easier due to the very small area to treat. From experience, for example, permanent make-up on the eyebrows is removed within one to two sessions if using osmosis.

31.1 Our Electrical Arcing Device Removal Protocol:

- Our device setting: minimum power level.
- Use the spray operation to gently break down the tattoo pigments as shown in the video above. From time to time remove the carbon residues. Remember that this treatment has to be performed so that the ablation is only superficial. If you notice some bleeding this may be the sign that you have already ablated enough by going too deep into the dermis. Remember the ablation has to be very superficial.
- Once you have finished your ablation using the electrical arcing, apply a purpose made paste of sterile fine salt and sterile saline solution. There is no need to apply any occlusion by bandaging or plasters. The paste does not need to be applied on the area for too long. An application between 10 to 20 minutes usually suffices. Please remember that the intensity of the treatment is also very much dependent on the duration of the application of the sterile saline paste. The longer you keep the paste on the area, the more the osmosis intensity and consequently the better the removal results. However please do not exceed the duration of 20 minutes. Once you remove the paste, disinfect the area with a mild antiseptic.

Do not use any bandaging or any plasters to cover the area during healing. The treated area will start scabbing two to three days after the treatment. In the unlikely case the scabbing does not occur within this time-frame, this maybe a sign that ongoing complications are underway (generally infections). If this is the case all efforts have to be made to cure the infection in order to avoid scarring. Any scabs must fall off by themselves and must not be picked.

Repeat the treatment after 8 weeks if required

32.0 Pre Treatment

Here we are going to show you the prerequisites which must be met before undergoing the aesthetic treatments using electrical arcing or aesthetic lasers.

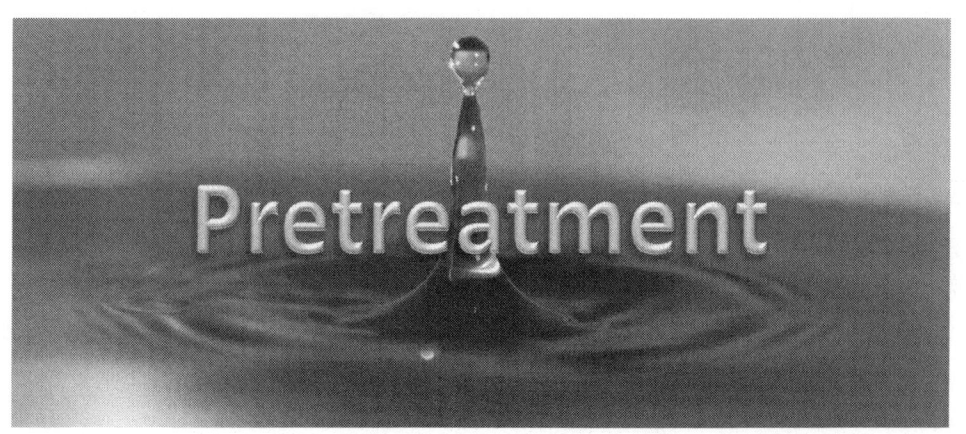

Illustration 265: Pretreatment

32.1 Client's prerequisites to be eligible for the treatment

In order for the client to qualify to undergo the aesthetic treatments using electrical arcing or aesthetic lasers the following prerequisites must be met first:

1) The client must be in good health at the time of the treatment, with no underlining chronic health conditions. If the client displays signs of cold or flue the treatment must be postponed.

2) Those with problems of keloids, skin burns or diabetes should not undergo these aesthetic procedures.

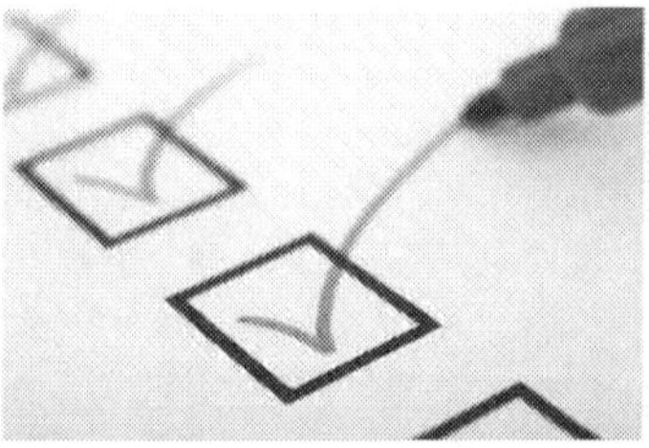

Illustration 266: Eligible for the treatment

3) The area to be treated should not have undergone any previous medical treatment or cosmetic laser treatment. The client must not have taken any medicine for at least 7 days before undergoing the aesthetic treatment.

4) The client must not have undergone any de-pigmentation treatment in the past 3 months.

5) The client should not be waiting for a doctor appointment.

6) The client must not display any tanning at the time of the treatment. This is especially important for tattoo removal or permanent makeup removal.

7) The client must not display herpes simplex and not have had herpes simplex in the past even if dormant at the time of the treatment. In case of clients with herpes simplex, a full antiviral course should be completed before starting the aesthetic treatment.

8) If the client wears a pace-maker avoid treatment with electrical arcing. Consult the pace-maker manufacturer and contact the specific electrical arcing device manufacturer for advice.

32.2 Before applying the numbing product

Before applying the numbing product, if any, remove all makeup from the face thoroughly by using normal makeup removal procedures. Once you have removed all makeup, apply an **appropriate non-flammable antiseptic** on a clean cotton pad and gently rub the area you are going to treat with the electrical arcing device. At that point, you can apply the appropriate numbing product.

32.3 Patch testing

Patch testing should always be performed before starting most aesthetic treatment using AC voltaic arcing. This is because patch testing can demonstrate that, if the after-care is performed correctly, the skin will recover well and there are no adverse effects to the particular aesthetic treatment.

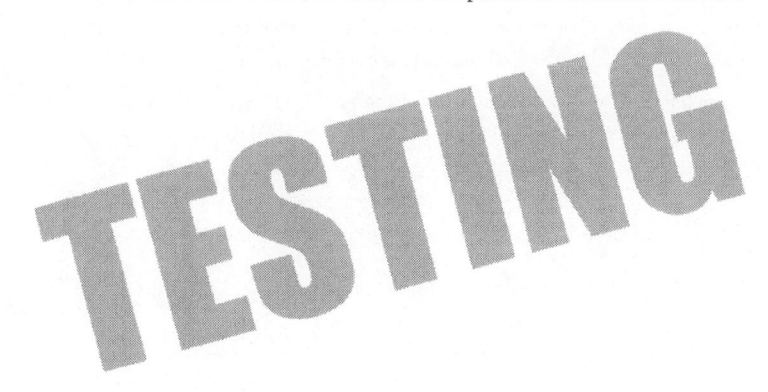

www.voltaicplasma.com   Author: Andreas Russo

However, in case of any benign moles or skin lesions removal, including Xanthelasma, Seborrheic Keratosis, Syringoma etc, patch testing is not strictly required. This is due to the fact that the inherent nature of the treatment does not allow it. Additionally, no aesthetic treatment aiming at removing any benign moles or skin lesion can guarantee scar-free results. The key to patch testing is to carry out, in a small part of the skin, the particular aesthetic procedure **in the same way and using the same treatment intensity you would when you then perform the treatment during the full aesthetic procedure.** For example, if you intend to perform tattoo removal without using osmosis, using an electrical arcing device using a certain equipment configuration, then you only need to carry out the same procedure on a smaller part of the tattoo. In the video below you can see a typical example of a patch test before carrying out a full tattoo removal procedure using electrical arcing with osmosis. The time required for the complete patch testing (including applying sterile Sodium Chloride) is less than 5 minutes.

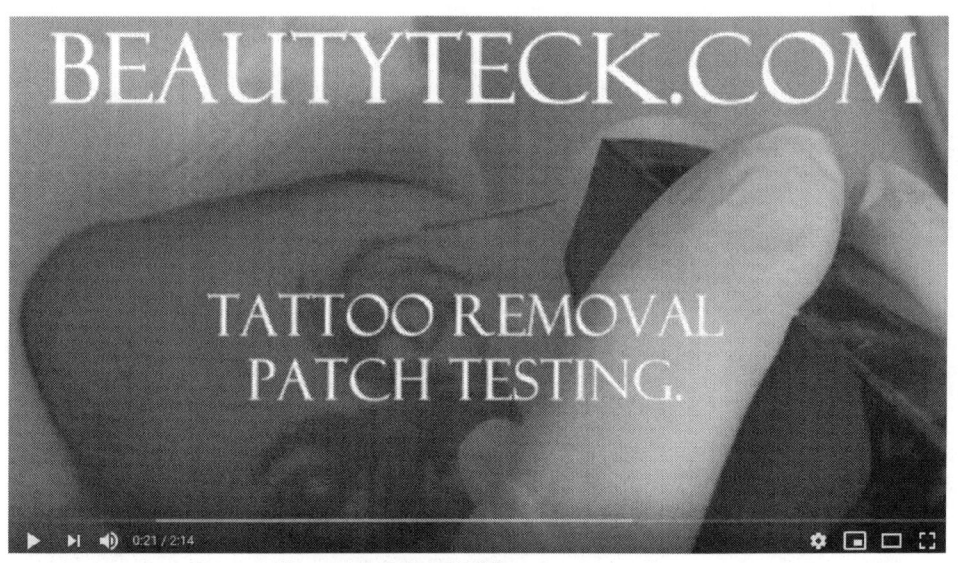

Illustration 267: Click here to watch video

Although the seasoned beauty practitioner can be tempted to carry out full procedures without the use of any patch testing based on one's extensive experience, from time to time any particular client can either overlook the after-care or accidentally contract an infection or some adverse effects could develop. At that point, the experience of the patch test previously carried out provides the peace of mind of knowing that no adverse effects can be attributable to the treatment per se, provided that the treatment is carried out in a similar way as it was carried out during the patch test.

32.4 Use of numbing products before the treatments

It is advisable to numb the area before carrying out any aesthetic treatment using electrical arcing devices for aesthetic applications. This is not always strictly required, however, it is advisable for the client's comfort. Also, because the client is at ease while the area to be treated is numb, the treatment can be carried out speedily and with ease. Not all kinds of numbing solutions are appropriate for all the types of aesthetic treatments possible with electrical arcing. For example, inject-able local anesthetics are purposely avoided in skin tightening as they can interfere with the final results and may lead to adverse reactions. However, electrical arcing has been used for several years for the removal of all sorts of benign skin lesions leading to good results and no direct known cause for concern, even if using inject-able local anesthetics. Please note that, in many countries, only medical practitioners are usually authorised to use inject-able local anesthetics.

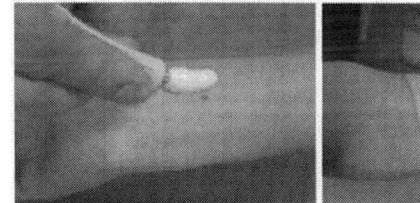

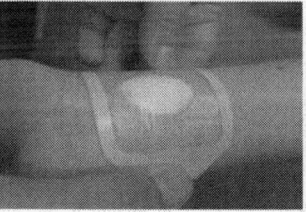

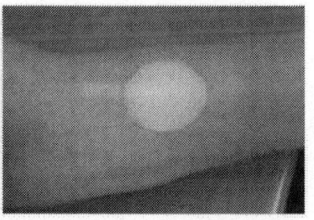

Illustration 268: The three steps to applying correctly most numbing products available on the market without a prescription.

The preferred numbing option is the use of topical products. The advantage of using topical numbing products is that they are suitable for all kind of treatments with electrical arcing including moles and benign skin lesions removal. The main type of numbing topical product available on the market depends on the local legislation. Different professionals are allowed to use different products in each country. (Consult local legislation for further information).

A very common topical numbing product available on the market, in most parts of Europe, including the UK is EMLA. (EMLA is available in 5% formulations from most chemists in the UK).

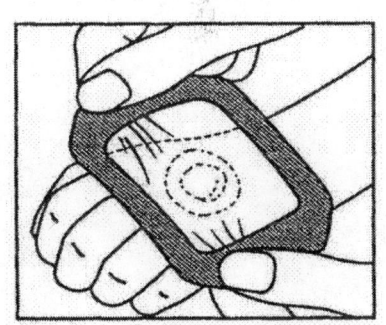

Illustration 269: Occlusion applied to the numbing cream to amplify the numbing effects of the active ingredients in most topical numbing products available without a prescription.

www.voltaicplasma.com   Author: Andreas Russo

This is a product which can be purchased and used without a medical prescription. Because of this, EMLA is also the preferred numbing product used by tattoo artists for tattooing and performing body piercings. EMLA is used by applying the cream on the area you intend to treat (including moles, skin lesions etc) and covering the cream with a normal cling film. The same cling film which can be purchased from any supermarket. The cling film is applied in order to cause an *occlusion effect* which will amplify the effects of the numbing active ingredients in the EMLA numbing cream. The area is then left to rest for approximately 40 to 45 minutes in order to achieve the desired numbing effects.

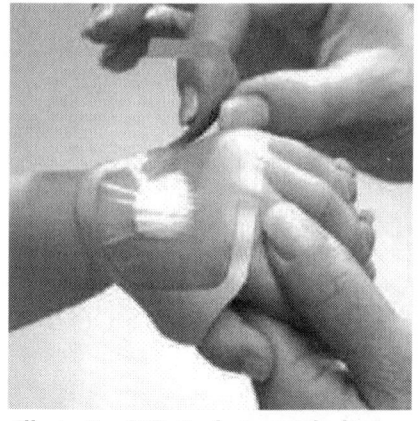

Illustration 270: Occlusion applied using a purpose made patch available from most chemists.

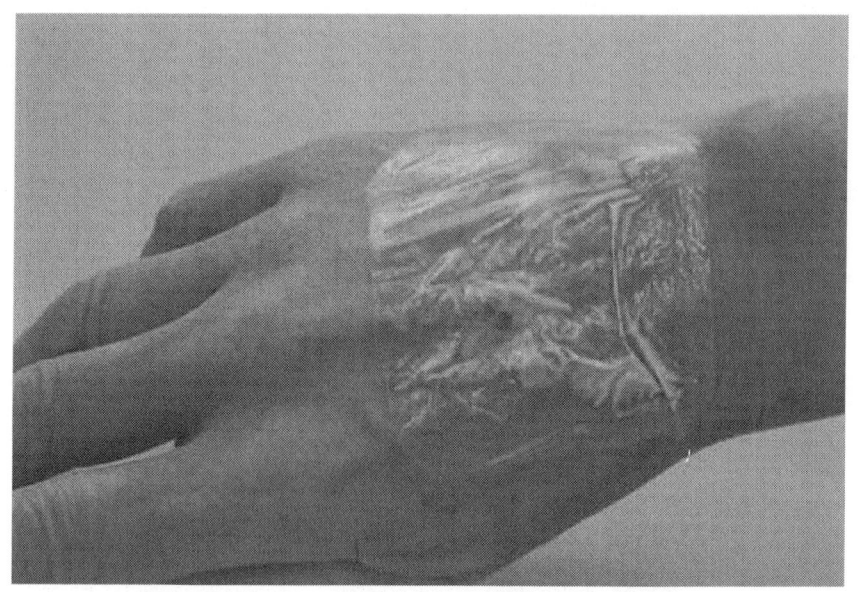

Illustration 271: Occlusion applied on the back of the hand

In our eyelid tightening training videos we can see how, although the aesthetic treatment has started on other parts of the face the product has not been removed from the orbital region because eyelid tightening would be carried out a few minutes later. Unfortunately, although available without prescription form any chemist in the UK, EMLA requires a relative long application time in order to become effective and it is not generally very effective if a cling film is not applied on top of the cream (occlusion). If you attempt to start the aesthetic treatment before the 40 minutes required for the product to become effective, the area may not be numb enough, in order to carry out the aesthetic treatment in ease and comfort. Additionally, the topical effects of the EMLA formulation end within 5 to 10 minutes from the time the cling film is removed and the EMLA residues wiped off. Therefore the window of time while you can perform the aesthetic treatment in comfort is relatively brief.

32.5 Medical topical numbing product

Some Medical practitioners can be authorised to use other numbing products. The formulation that has been extensively and successfully used by medical practitioners who use electrical arcing devices for aesthetic purposes is the following topical custom formulated product: *Formulation active ingredients: Lidocaine 20%, Prilocaine 5%, Tetracaine 5%*. This topical product is either made in a gel or cream formulation. In European countries like Italy and Spain, this is made by most local chemists who also have an internal licensed laboratory to manufacture these types of products. In Europe, this type of topical formulation can only be sold under medical prescription *(therefore under the sole responsibility of the medical practitioner who orders the product)*. Due to current regulations, this is a product which can be used by medical practitioners only or under their direct supervision. The main advantage of using this type of formulation is that the desired numbing effects are achieved almost immediately and are so good that the client will only feel a tickling sensation when the electrical arc is applied. The area where this formulation is applied becomes numb within 5 to 10 minute after the application. Please note that these types of products are not meant to be completely absorbed, therefore all you have to do is applying the cream or gel, on the area you intend to treat and leave the product to work. With this formulation, there will be no need to apply a cling film because the product itself will be strong enough to achieve the desired numbing effects in a relatively short time frame. Additionally, the numbing effects lastlonger than those products available over the counter.

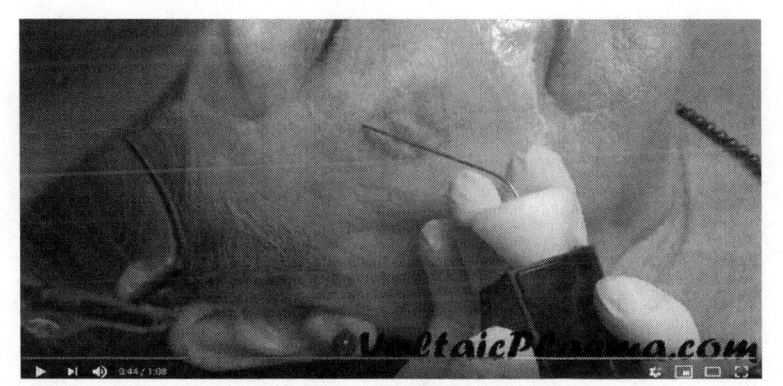

Illustration 272: click here to watch video

In the video above you can see an example of a professional custom made topical numbing product applied on the perioral area in order to numb the skin before a perioral lines attenuation treatment. As you can see occlusion is not necessary.

The numbing effects start within 5 minutes from the application of the cream. The specific treatment you see in the video is atrophic scar attenuation. In any case, whenever you start the treatment on a relatively large area, on a tattoo, for instance, remember to remove the topical anesthetic in small sections. The common mistake made by beginners is to remove all the numbing product all at once. For example, if the topical anesthetic has been placed on both upper eyelids, the untrained beginner usually removes the cream on both eyelids before starting the treatment. The main problem is that the effect of most topical numbing products does not last long (in case of EMLA only 5 to 10 minutes at most). Therefore the effect of the topical anesthetic could start to fade before the end of the treatment making the procedure cumbersome. **For eyelid tightening** *and similar skin tightening procedures, using electrical arcing,* **the use of local injectable anaesthetics must be avoided** *even if the beauty practitioner is authorised to use them.*

So to summarise, the use of appropriate topical numbing products is advisable before any treatment using electrical arcing, while the use of inject-able local anesthetic is not strictly needed and sometimes must be avoided especially for eyelid tightening. Given the fact that topical numbing products are generally easy to use and are sufficient for all types of aesthetic procedures using electrical arcing, the use of inject-able local anesthetics although possible for some treatments are not generally justifiable while using electrical arcing for aesthetic applications.

33.0 Aftercare

In general, aftercare is much more important than the way in which aesthetic treatment is performed.

This does not only apply to equipment that generates electric arcs, but it also applies to lasers, cosmetic peels, and other aesthetic treatments. This is simply because if the area is not kept clean, the likelihood of developing an infection increases.

In this section, you will learn all about the best possible aftercare, the type of antiseptic which are recommended, the optional soothing treatments and warnings.

The Post-treatment to any of the aesthetic treatments described here is very simple:

- Most importantly the area you treated must be kept clean in order to avoid infections until the part has recovered completely (i.e. the scabs have formed and fallen off by themselves or the peeling effect has ended). This occurs within 10 days from the aesthetic treatment. This alone will suffice as after-care.

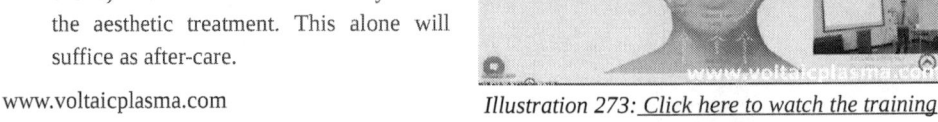

www.voltaicplasma.com

Illustration 273: Click here to watch the training video

- All other aftercare treatments are not strictly required as the body will naturally take care of the healing process.

- It is also important to avoid exposing the treated area directly to the sun for at least 2 to 3 months after the aesthetic procedures. Broad Spectrum Sun Screen must be applied every day on the area treated. Although the likelihood of hyperpigmentation is low cannot be completely eliminated and it is exacerbated by excessive sun exposure too early, even while using total sunscreen. Sunscreen can be applied as soon as any scabs which have formed have fallen on its own accord.

33.1 After Care Main Points

In General after aesthetic treatments using lasers, electrical arcing, or professional cosmetic peels:

1. Keep the area clean and avoid infections until the scabs have formed.

2. If they form, do not pick the scabs and let them fall off by themselves. If the old skin layer is peeling off do not force it off on purpose.

3. Do not apply any make-up (even mineral) until the scabbing or peeling effect has ended and /or any scabs which might have formed have fallen off by themselves.

4. Do not apply any plasters on the treated areas as doing so can delay the natural healing progression and increase the likelihood of undesired effects.

5. Avoid sun exposure and wear broad-spectrum sunblock on the treated area. This has to be done after any scabs which might have formed, have fallen off by themselves. Please note that despite the fact that the appropriate sunblock has been worn direct exposure to intense light sources must be avoided in any case for 3 months after the last treatment.

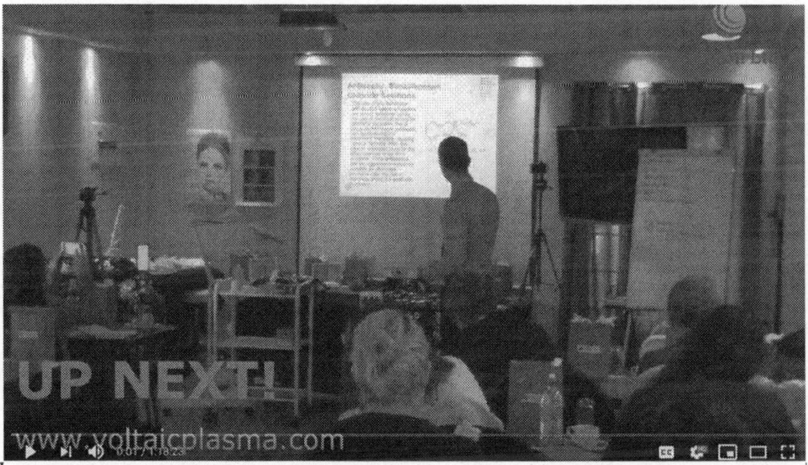

Illustration 274: Click here to watch the training video

33.2 Antiseptic, Benzalkonium Chloride Solutions

The use of any flammable and alcohol-based antiseptics are strictly forbidden during the use of electrical arcing for aesthetic purposes, this is because flammable antiseptic can ignite during the treatment, therefore, causing various hazards. Also, the type of antiseptic used for the after-care has to be fit for purpose. Some antiseptics are too aggressive hence not suitable as after-care products after the use of electrical arcing for aesthetic purposes.

$$n = 8, 10, 12, 14, 16, 18$$

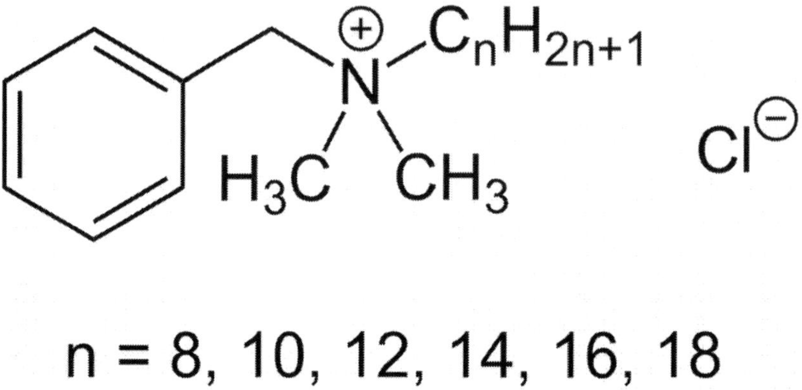

Illustration 275: Antiseptic, Benzalkonium Chloride Solutions

Why is it important to use antiseptics regularly after these treatments? Although the aesthetic treatment has been carried out correctly, and the area is virtually free from a real likelihood of infections at the time of the treatment, the area will be subject to atmospheric agents and in contact with non-sterile garments while recovering. While the client will have to make sure that all unnecessary infection hazards are avoided, some degree of contact with non-sterile objects or garments can sometimes be unavoidable. Therefore the treated area should be cleaned periodically with an appropriate antiseptic

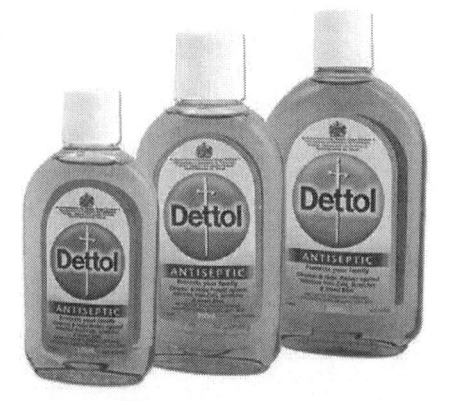

Illustration 276: Dettol

until the scabs will have formed.

Benzalkonium chloride solutions have been shown to be not only effective but leading to the best results if used appropriately. The recommended active ingredient in the antiseptic to be used for these types of aesthetic treatments is Benzalkonium chloride. Antiseptic solutions containing Benzalkonium Chloride are widely available on the market. The concentrations are usually between 0.17% to 0.2%. In the UK these types of antiseptics can be found at any chemist, the most common brand is Dettol Antiseptic Wash 0.198%. This products or equivalent custom solutions should be used to clean the treated area in the morning, early afternoon and evening before going to sleep. No other types of antiseptics should be used. If alcohol-based or other antiseptics are used then there could be some increased likelihood of undesired effects.

Wash the treated area twice a day, in the morning and before bedtime using the Benzalkonium Chloride solution. Increase the number of washes if necessary. Remember to dry very gently without rubbing the area, using a very clean towel (preferably sterile dressing). Do not apply occlusion using plasters of any type (do not bandage the area).

33.3 Optional Soothing Treatment

Apply the appropriate soothing product immediately after you have finished the treatment. Please note that soothing products are most appropriate for upper eyelid tightening. This will minimise the perceived downtime by minimising the swelling.

For all other aesthetic applications of Voltaic Arcing, the use of soothing products is not strictly necessary. After all significant swelling only appears after eyelid tightening and not after other aesthetic treatments possible with electrical arcing. For this reason, the use of soothing products should be avoided in all other aesthetic treatments and be only used after upper eyelid tightening.

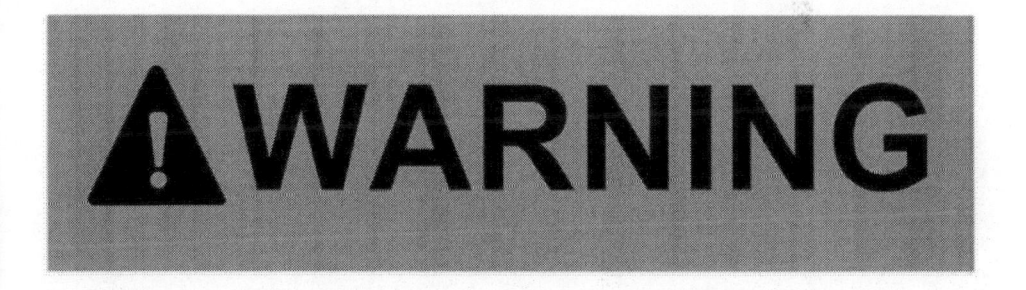

⚠ WARNING

If infections are contracted soon after the treatment they could increase the likelihood of scarring.

1. Picking the scabs can cause scars and/or hypo-pigmentation.

2. The more the client is exposed to sunlight including other artificial light sources (even while wearing Broad Spectrum Sunblock) the higher the risks of hyper-pigmentation.

3. Wearing camouflage make-up or any other type of makeup before the scabs have formed and fallen off, can result in delayed recovery, hypo-pigmentation and red dots where the voltaic spots were applied and increase the risks of infections and hence scarring.

During the recovery period, while the scabbing is still to form, there is a general temptation of using cover up make up, or any makeup to resume the normal day to day activities immediately. This should be avoided.

→ One of the main problems of make-up is the fact that make-up products are not meant to be sterile. Therefore the use of non-sterile products in an area that is still recovering from an aesthetic procedure will increase the likelihood of infections which may eventually result in scarring.

Do NOT apply any plasters to cover the treated area. Do not use antibiotic products as means of preventing infections. The use of antibiotic products as means of prevention is not recommended by the wider scientific community because it can increase future bacterial resistance. Do not use any medicinal products during the aftercare unless prescribed by a medical practitioner.

The use of any type of aftercare bought at the chemist may not always be fit for purpose, and hence increase the likelihood of undesired effects. Therefore if in doubt do not use any drugs, cosmetics healing balms etc that you can buy off the shelf. Make sure the product is fit for purpose.

34.0 Hot and Cold Plasma

Overview of difference between hot plasma and cold plasma.

The definition of hot plasma or cold plasma is dependant on the temperature at the carbonisiation point. In aesthetic treatments and medicine, the carbonisation point is where the electrical arc meets the surface of the skin or the soft tissue dehydrating it quickly into carbon.

When the electrical arc strikes, the temperature at the carbonisation point is proportional to the energy associated with the arc. In turn, the energy associated with the electrical electrical arc is dependant on the dielectric strength of the medium used (normally ambient air). Generally the higher the dielectric strength the higher the energy required to create the electrical arc. In case of most plasma devices for aesthetic applications, the medium used is ambient air. As we know the air normally behaves as an insulator due to its inherent high dielectric strength. Air is generally behaving as an insulator and it takes a relatively high amount of energy to generate an electrical arc in air.

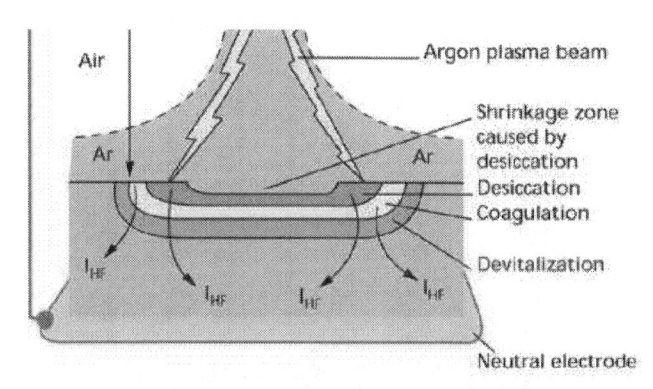

Illustration 277: The desiccation or carbonisation layer is the layer of the skin which experiences the the local highest temperatures. Carbonisation also occurs when using "cold plasma".

This is because the energy required for the arc to take place in a high electric strength material is relatively high. This is why the energy associated to the electrical arc in air has generally high power.

Conversely the lower the dielectric strength the lower the energy associated to the arc. Therefore the energy required to strike the electrical arc is relatively low and hence the low energy allows lower temperatures at the carbonisation point. For this reason one of the most common ways to produce low energy arcs and consequently cold plasma is by using "carrier gasses" with relatively low dielectric strength.

Generally hot plasma is defined as such when electrical arc takes place in air. This is because the temperature of the electrical arc in air (they associated to ddwklaw.com labor lawyer) at the carbonisation point is relatively high. So what is generated by over 90% of devices in the market is hot plasma, because the arc in air and the temperature of the arc is relatively high.

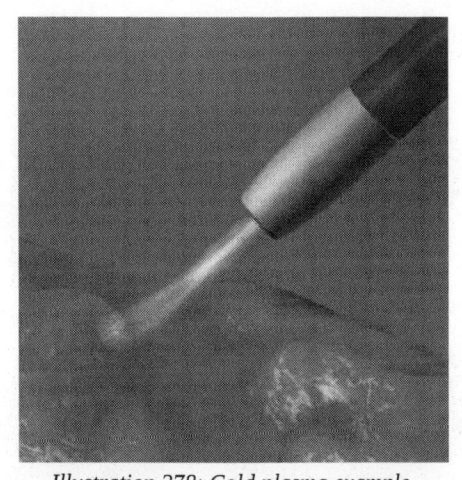

Illustration 278: Cold plasma example, plasma in Argon. The arc is far more stable and looks almost like a flame. The temperature at the point of contact of the arc with the skin is not as high as it is in case of arcing in air because the energy associated with the arc is lower

When the temperature at he carbonisation point is reduced to a certain factor we refer to it as "cold plasma".

www.voltaicplasma.com   Author: Andreas Russo

As we will see the reduction of the temperature at the carbonisation point is possible in various ways.

34.1 What is "hot plasma" ?

"Hot plasma" is that electrical arc generated in atmospheric air. In other words "hot plasma" is electrical arcing which takes place in ambient air without the use of any carrier gasses. It is the same electrical spark you see generated by most devices in the market place. Also because air is made up mostly by nitrogen, some marketers refer to this type of electrical arc as "nitrogen plasma".

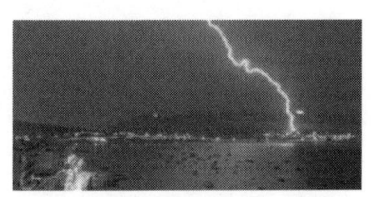

Illustration 279: Lightening is an example of "hot plasma". The energy and temperature at the striking point is so high that it can cause serious damage.

The temperature at the carbonisation point is very high (over 1000 degrees Centigrade).

The high temperature is localised at the carbonisation point and this high temperature occur because the dielectric strength of air is relatively high, hence the air usually behaves as an insulator. In order to generate an electrical arc in air a relatively high amount of energy is required.

In other words, to convert the air from an insulator into a conductor, which is the phenomenon of plasma or electrical arcing, a relatively high amount of energy is required. Hence the electrical plasma in air carries a relatively high amount of energy relative to other types of plasma (like plasma in argon). Therefore the energy associated to plasma in air is relatively high (high energy = high temperatures = high heat transfer).This is the type of plasma we find in most common plasma or electrical arcing devices for medical and aesthetic purposes.

The high temperature at the carbonisation point makes the arc painful during aesthetic procedures (therefore the requirement for numbing products for the treatment).

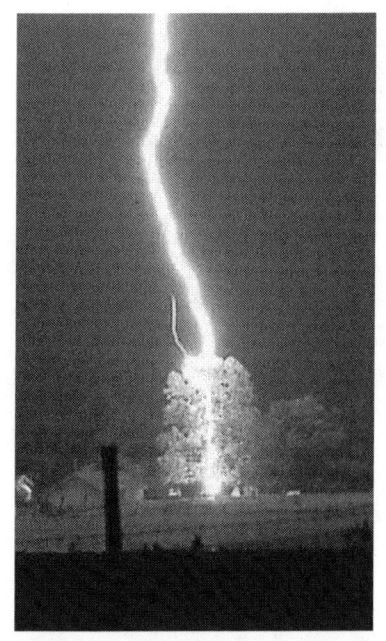

Illustration 280: The temperatures of electrical arcing in air are extremely high. In case of lightening the temperature at the striking point is extremely high. It can set a tree on fire.

www.voltaicplasma.com   Author: Andreas Russo

The heat propagated into the skin is relatively high. At low power intensity the arc is not very easy to sustain.

In hot plasma the amount of heat transferred into the dermal layer is relatively high compared to cold plasma.

To summarise "hot plasma" in aesthetic treatments is:

1. More painful than "cold plasma", this is because the temperature at the carbonisation point is relatively high.
2. The heat transfer to the dermal layer is relatively high.
3. The cross section of the carbonisation point is relatively small.

34.2 What are carrier gasses in Plasma?

Carrier gasses are those gasses which have a dielectric strength lower than air. A lower dielectric strength means that the arc can take place more easily than in air. These gasses require less energy than air to become ionised (become a conductor). This means that the energy associated to the arc is lower, the temperature at the point of contact between the arc and the skin is also lower. These types of gasses are also inert, non flammable and non poisonous.

The most common carrier gas used for this type of application is Argon. This is because:

- Argon is relatively inexpensive ,
- It has a low dielectric strength,
- Inert,
- Non flammable and
- Non poisonous.

For the above reasons Argon has been used for several years in aesthetics and medicine. The advantage of using a carrier gas is that the plasma generated is much more stable, delivers less energy and so, less painful than normal hot plasma.

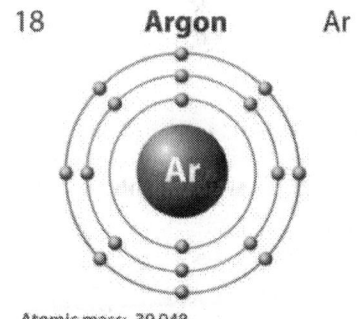

Atomic mass: 39.948
Electron configuration: 2, 8, 8

Illustration 281: Argon

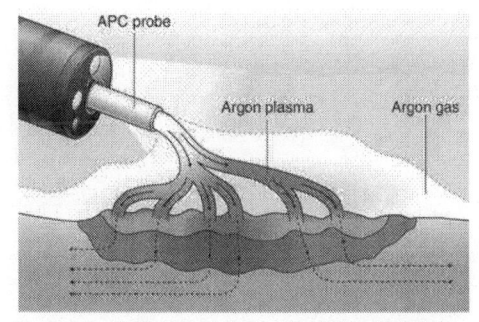

Illustration 282: Argon has a far lower breakdown voltage than air see this link for more information.

www.voltaicplasma.com Author: Andreas Russo

The arc in Argon is easier to sustain and the diameter of the surface contact between the arc and the skin is larger.

34.3 What is "cold plasma"?

As we know "hot plasma" is the electrical arcing in air. Air is normally an insulator (relatively high dielectric strength) therefore the energy required to generate the arc is relatively high. This causes high temperatures at the point of contact between the skin and the electric arc.

In order to stabilise the arc and facilitate the ionisation process (which is another way to refer to as "plasma", electrical sparking etc), Argon or other inert gasses with lower dielectric strength than air are used. This is because lower dielectric strength means lower breakdown voltage and in turn this means that the electrical arc can be generated more easily. The term "cold" is used because, when an inert gas with far lower breakdown voltage than air is used, the temperature at the carbonisation point is much lower. Additionally the arc is much more stable and the diameter of the surface of contact between the arc and the skin is much larger than electrical arc in air ("hot plasma"). This makes the aesthetic treatment less painful and and also allows for some effects not possible with "hot plasma".

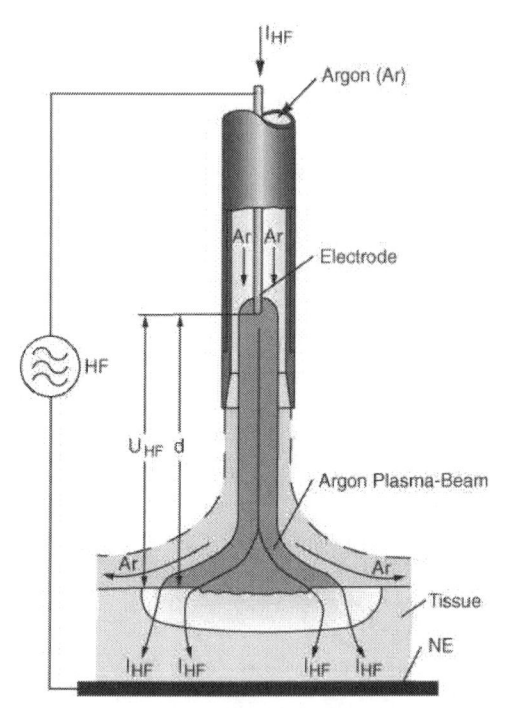

Illustration 283: Cold plasma hand-piece design. Argon is used as carrier gas,

In other words when we use certain carrier gasses with dielectric strength lower than air we have "cold plasma", this is referred to as such because of the lower temperature at the carbonation point. This is because the energy associated with the electrical arc in Argon is much lower than of plasma in air. The temperature is lower because the carrier gasses (or external gasses) used have a lower "breakdown voltage" than air. Because of this, the energy required in order to generate the arc is much lower in this type of electrical arc. In turn since the energy is much lower also the temperature is lower than plasma in air. Hence plasma in Argon is usually referred to as "cold plasma". The lower temperature and lower energy associated to the arc cause less heat transfer into the skin and therefore less pain associated to this type of electrical arc. Also the higher stability of the arc makes this type of electrical arc one of the preferred ways to carry out skin resurfacing using plasma.

www.voltaicplasma.com   Author: Andreas Russo

The main application of "cold plasma" in aesthetics is skin resurfacing. This is because the arc stabilisation allows the user to control the arcing more easily making this type of aesthetic treatment:

- less painful than "hot plasma" (normal arcing in air).
- the diameter of the carbonisation point is larger than that of plasma in air.

35.0 Electrical Arcing and the European New MDD in 2020

35.1 Introduction

Historically there has been a clear distinction between aesthetic and medical applications in Europe, aesthetic applications are those which the person does not require to have done due to medical condition. Aesthetic applications and treatments are aimed at improving the looks of the person.

There is still a clear distinction between aesthetic and medical applications and the new Medical Devices Directive (MDD) which takes place in May 2020 only covers certain types of devices. If they are not part of the new category described by the new legislation they will not be regulated as part of the new MDD starting from May 2020.

As we will see the new legislation will not apply to Plasma devices and even from May 2020 after the new legislation has become effective, any electrical arcing devices which has non medical applications will still the remit of the general safety rules of general devices.

Generally, self certification for any type of devices which are not included in the new MDD covering only lasers IPL, Lasers and all devices which emit High Intensity Electromagnetic Radiations which have some effect on the human body.

In particular here we will:

- ➢ Clarify the operational difference between lasers (or more generally devices emitting High Intensity Electromagnetic Radiation for skin therapy) and plasma devices. We are going to explain how the physics governing the way these devices affect the skin are fundamentally different. This is because the underlining physics of Voltaic plasma, (arcing, electrical sparking etc) is not very well understood by most people in the aesthetic sector and fundamentally different from Electromagnetic remitting Devices . This is why electrical arcing devices are often confused for light emitting devices like lasers.

- Clarify the the purpose of the new European legislation on High Intensity Electromagnetic Radiation devices which is coming into force in May 2020. We will clarify what types of devices the new legislation is intended to cover and the devices that are not intended to cover.

- Demonstrate how plasma devices for aesthetic purposes will still be regulated by the general product safety legislation even after May 2020, because they do not fall in the remit of the new MDD (Medical Devices Directive).

35.2 Plasma or arcing devices for aesthetic purposes and the new european legislation on medical devices

The Annex XVI of the new legislation on medical devices which will come into force in May 2020, states:

"List of groups of products without an intended medical purpose referred to in article 1(2)
5.High intensity electromagnetic radiation (e.g. infra-red, visible light and ultra-violet) emitting equipment intended for use on the human body, including coherent and non-coherent sources, monochromatic and broad spectrum, such as lasers and intense pulsed light equipment, for skin resurfacing, tattoo or hair removal or other skin treatment."

Above we only quoted the part of the new legislation which would appear to be applicable to this type of aesthetic devices, we ignore all the other points of Annex XVI as they are clearly not applicable. To read the full publication please click here.
In order to understand the new legislation properly we have to first understand the basic physics of electromagnetic radiations so that we can interpret this legislation correctly.

36.0 The principle of exclusion in legislation

The principle of legislative exclusion means that if the specific legislation does not appear to cover explicitly a certain sector or type of product, that sector or product will not be the remit of that legislation. In this case by default a more general legislation will apply. Hence, like in this case, if the new legislation does not apply to plasma devices then the more general product safety legislation will apply instead, as of before May 2020.

36.1 Why the word "High Intensity"? Because all objects radiate electromagnetic radiations.

As we can see the new text refers to High Intensity Electromagnetic Radiation Emitting Equipment. The "High Intensity" is a crucial definition. This is because all devices and object radiate (or emit) "Electromagnetic Radiations".

It is a well known fact in physics that any object which has a temperature of above the absolute zero (0 Degrees Kelvin or -274 Degrees centigrade) emits electromagnetic radiations. This is a verifiable fact and common knowledge in science. Additionally this is how infrared cameras (or thermal cameras) capture the image of objects and also measure their temperature. These devices (thermal cameras) directly capture the Electromagnetic radiation emitted by any object and they do not require any external light of any kind to capture the images.

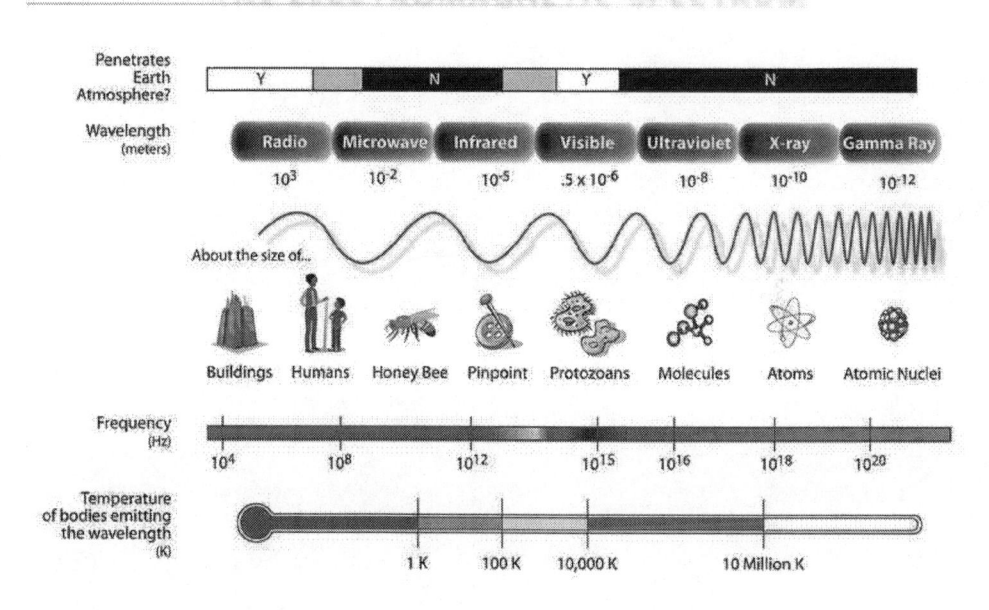

Illustration 284: The Electromagnetic Spectrum

Whereas other conventional cameras capture the light reflected by the object and hence require an external light source to be able to see the objects. For more information about Thermal

www.voltaicplasma.com　　　　　　　　　　　　　　　　　　Author: Andreas Russo

Cameras and how objects always radiate Electromagnetic energy please refer to the following video (watch Video on the relevant page of VoltaicPlasma.com). **All devices, like any other object, emit electromagnetic radiation due to their temperature and more.**

Any screen or LED light emits electromagnetic radiation (light). These emissions although visible do not have any significant effect onto the human body other than the visibility of the light itself.

As seen above all objects radiate electromagnetic energy and therefore also all devices emit electromagnetic radiations irrespective of the way they are designed or manufactured.

As we will see, besides the electromagnetic emissions related to the temperature of the object itself, different devices emit different intensities and levels of electromagnetic emissions.

The total electromagnetic emissions of a device are due to:

1. the object's own temperature. All devices heat up due to their normal operation and reach a certain temperature. At any given temperature the object radiates a certain electromagnetic emission at a certain frequency and intensity, which becomes visible only to infrared cameras/thermal cameras but not the human eye. Of course this type of electromagnetic radiation is of low intensity and has no effect on the human body.

Illustration 285: Led Screen Device

2. The device's user interface, (like the screen, touch screen, displays, led lights in the controls) and its own mode of operation produce additional electromagnetic emissions. This type of electromagnetic radiations is of very low intensity, sometimes visible to the human eye but has no detrimental effect on the human body. or eyes.

3. Purposeful High Intensity Electromagnetic radiations. Only these types of radiations can cause any significant heat transfer into the human body (and skin). These high intensity electromagnetic emissions can be harmful to the human eye, hence appropriate eye-wear protection must be used for health and safety. This is the case for IPLs, Lasers and High Intensity LED Light Therapy devices. These are devices designed in a way to emit high intensity electromagnetic emissions which have a clear effect which are of so high intensity that produce significant heat transfer into the body. In all these cases exposure to this high intensity emissions are clearly felt by the human body.

Generally, almost all devices for skin therapy are part of case 1 and 2 described above. Most devices have either a user interface emitting light (electromagnetic radiation) and all of them operate at a temperature above 0 Degrees Kelvin. Because of the low intensity of the Electromagnetic emissions these devices although all emit electromagnetic radiations they will not be remit of the new category, even if they are intended to treat the body.

www.voltaicplasma.com   Author: Andreas Russo

Only the last type of radiations emitted by devices intended to treat the body will be remit of the new category and hence regulated by the new MDD (Medical Devices Directive).

37. 0 Why does the legislation refer to as "High Intensity Electromagnetic Radiation" (HIER) and not only "Electromagnetic Radiation" ?

Up until May 2020 devices which have no clear medical remit are not covered by the MDD (Medical Devices Directive). Only certain devices clearly defined by the new legislation will be covered by the MDD (Medical Devices Directive) after May 2020.

As we have seen, all devices and objects emit electromagnetic radiations. Without the term "High Intensity" all devices would have fallen into the new category by default. In other words because all devices do emit electromagnetic radiation, the term "High intensity Electromagnetic Radiation (HIER) is to be interpreted as the type of radiation which has some intended or tangible effects onto the skin.

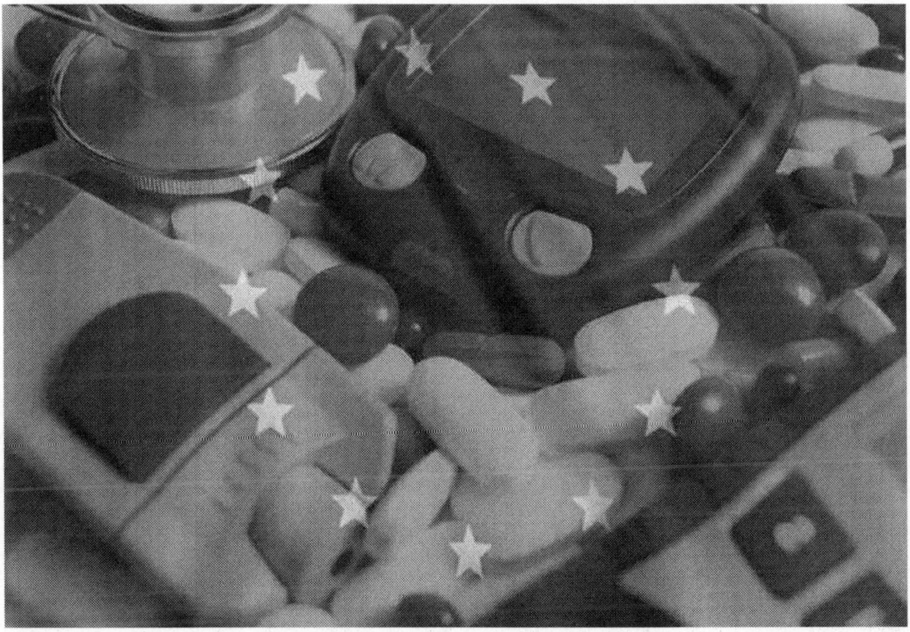

Illustration 286: Medical Devices Directive

It is clear that the new legislation do not include all Electromagnetic Emitting Devices, otherwise all devices would have been included in the new category. If the legislator wanted to include all devices for skin therapy then the new text of law would have not chosen the wording "High Intensity" and more specifically it would have included all devices for skin treatment.

The legislator intended to purposefully single out only those devices that emit such "high intensity" electromagnetic radiations, the emissions of which do cause a significant heat transfer into the skin, which is then resulting in skin resurfacing, tattoo removal and other aesthetic skin treatments.

In other words, the main reason for the legislator to place the wording "High Intensity" before the term "Electromagnetic Radiation" is to include only certain types of devices within the new MDD (Medical Devices Directive) remit . These are those devices which emit high enough electromagnetic emissions which will cause enough heat transfer into the skin in order to achieve the aesthetic treatments desired.

This does not mean that all devices which transfer heat into the body or skin by other means are included within the new category. If a device transfers heat into the skin in a different way other than using light to do so, it will not be included in the new category and old more general legislation will still apply as after May 2020. Only those devices which use light (or High Intensity Electromagnetic Radiations) to cause the heat transfer into the skin for the purposes outlined in the new legislation will be regulated by the new MDD (Medical Devices Directive). But all other equipment although they all emit light or electromagnetic emission will be unaffected by the new legislation.

Clearly, devices (although emitting light) that transfer heat by means other than electromagnetic radiations and are intended for skin treatments including tattoo removal etc will not require MDD regulation.

37.1 are High Intensity Electromagnetic Radiation (HIER) devices as defined by the new legislation?

So we have seen that all devices emit Electromagnetic radiation. Therefore what types of devices does the new legislation refer to?

High Intensity Electromagnetic Emitting equipment are all devices which are designed in order to emit such a high intensity radiation which in and of itself (the Electromagnetic radiation) has a noticeable effect into the human skin.

The new legislation does not set set any physical parameters as the intensity of the electromagnetic radiation. Since the new legislation mentions the wording "High Intensity" only, and it does neither provide any specific quantitative limits nor thresholds in intensity or frequency of the electromagnetic radiation itself, how can we practically recognise such HIER devices?
The two examples (lasers and IPLs) mentioned by the legislation itself can come to help.

1. Lasers. As we know it is actually the very coherent light produced by the laser that causes the effect on to the skin.

www.voltaicplasma.com   Author: Andreas Russo

2. The new legislation also refers to IPL (Intense Pulsed Light) devices. These devices are an example of the light source generating equipment, whose light is of such high intensity and has a tangible effect on the skin and human body. This is because the light emitted is broad spectrum and incoherent and the light emitted has such high intensity that it has an appreciable and significant effect on the skin.

All these HIER devices do require protective eye-wear for their operation. This is because even indirect exposure of the eyes to this High Intensity Electromagnetic Radiation can cause damage to the eyesight which could be also permanent in some cases and this is an health and safety requirement.

So HIER Devices are those which the Intensity Of the Electromagnetic Radiation is of so "High Intensity" that the radiation itself has a significant effect on the skin and protective eye-wear is required to be used during their normal operation.

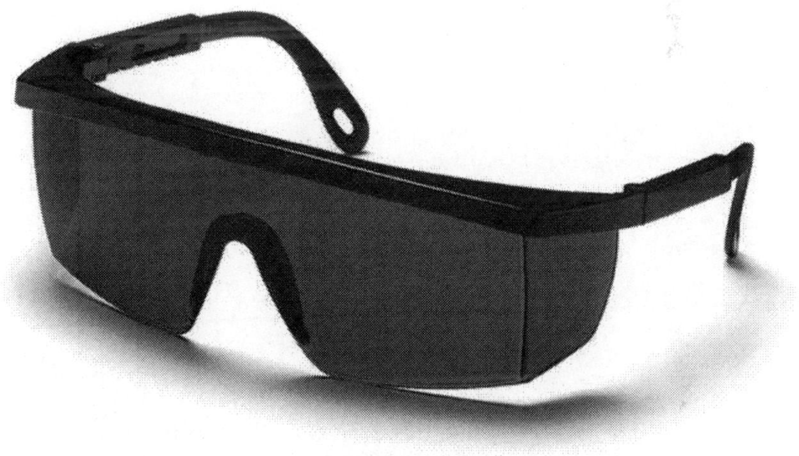

Illustration 287: Protective eye-wear to be worn during the normal use of HIER Devices. This is because direct and sometimes indirect exposure to HIER can be harmful to the eyes.

37.2 Plasma (or Electrical Arcing) Devices for aesthetic purposes are not equipment emitting High Intensity Electromagnetic Radiation

The new legislation is intended to cover only those devices emitting high intensity electromagnetic radiations which have some effect on to the skin.

The intensity of the light emitted by arcing or plasma devices is very low. These broadband low intensity electromagnetic emissions of the electrical arc, although visible to the eye (like the light emitted by most users interfaces) cannot be felt by the human body. This light has no effect whatsoever on the skin or the human body. Generally the emissions intensity is so low, that plasma is generally adopted in several different industries without the use of any protective eye-ware, like in case of lasers.

The most powerful electrical arcs known are lightening. Even the light emitted by lightening has no effect on the human body and it can be observed by the naked eye without any hazards to the vision. Also, the light associated to such powerful arcs does not affect the human body (like heat transfer etc). It has to be borne in mind that it is not the light emitted by the lightening that makes it dangerous, but the power associated to its electric discharge. Obviously the power associated to most voltaic arcing devices is thousands of times lower than those of lightening.

The physics behind heat transmission using plasma are very different than those of HIER, The way heat is transmitted during arcing is the same as that of radio frequency devices, "electrolysis" etc (which is by means of electric discharge or using electricity).

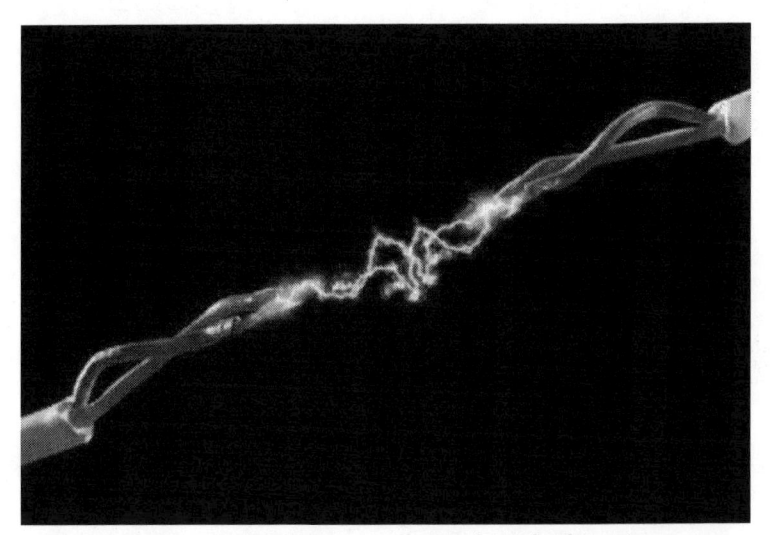

Illustration 288: Electrical Arcing or Electrical Spark. The arcing process produces a very low light source with has no effect on the human body. The light emitted can be observed by the naked eye without risk to the vision. This is due to the very low intensity of the electromagnetic emissions of electrical sparking.

Plasma (or electrical arcing) devices for aesthetic purposes, emit low intensity electromagnetic radiations (which are of lower intensity than most user interface screens).

The new legislation is intended to cover only those devices emitting high intensity electromagnetic radiations which has some effect on to the skin.

www.voltaicplasma.com   Author: Andreas Russo

2. The new legislation also refers to IPL (Intense Pulsed Light) devices. These devices are an example of the light source generating equipment, whose light is of such high intensity and has a tangible effect on the skin and human body. This is because the light emitted is broad spectrum and incoherent and the light emitted has such high intensity that it has an appreciable and significant effect on the skin.

All these HIER devices do require protective eye-wear for their operation. This is because even indirect exposure of the eyes to this High Intensity Electromagnetic Radiation can cause damage to the eyesight which could be also permanent in some cases and this is an health and safety requirement.

So HIER Devices are those which the Intensity Of the Electromagnetic Radiation is of so "High Intensity" that the radiation itself has a significant effect on the skin and protective eye-wear is required to be used during their normal operation.

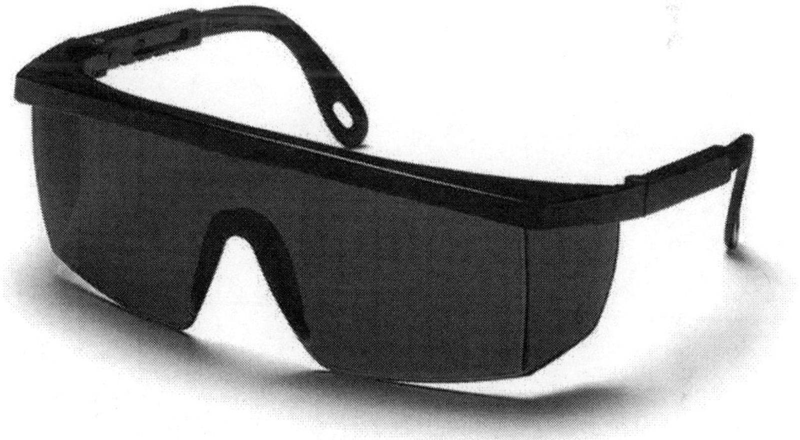

Illustration 287: Protective eye-wear to be worn during the normal use of HIER Devices. This is because direct and sometimes indirect exposure to HIER can be harmful to the eyes.

37.2 Plasma (or Electrical Arcing) Devices for aesthetic purposes are not equipment emitting High Intensity Electromagnetic Radiation

The new legislation is intended to cover only those devices emitting high intensity electromagnetic radiations which have some effect on to the skin.

www.voltaicplasma.com   Author: Andreas Russo

The intensity of the light emitted by arcing or plasma devices is very low. These broadband low intensity electromagnetic emissions of the electrical arc, although visible to the eye (like the light emitted by most users interfaces) cannot be felt by the human body. This light has no effect whatsoever on the skin or the human body. Generally the emissions intensity is so low, that plasma is generally adopted in several different industries without the use of any protective eye-ware, like in case of lasers.

The most powerful electrical arcs known are lightening. Even the light emitted by lightening has no effect on the human body and it can be observed by the naked eye without any hazards to the vision. Also, the light associated to such powerful arcs does not affect the human body (like heat transfer etc). It has to be borne in mind that it is not the light emitted by the lightening that makes it dangerous, but the power associated to its electric discharge. Obviously the power associated to most voltaic arcing devices is thousands of times lower than those of lightening.

The physics behind heat transmission using plasma are very different than those of HIER, The way heat is transmitted during arcing is the same as that of radio frequency devices, "electrolysis" etc (which is by means of electric discharge or using electricity).

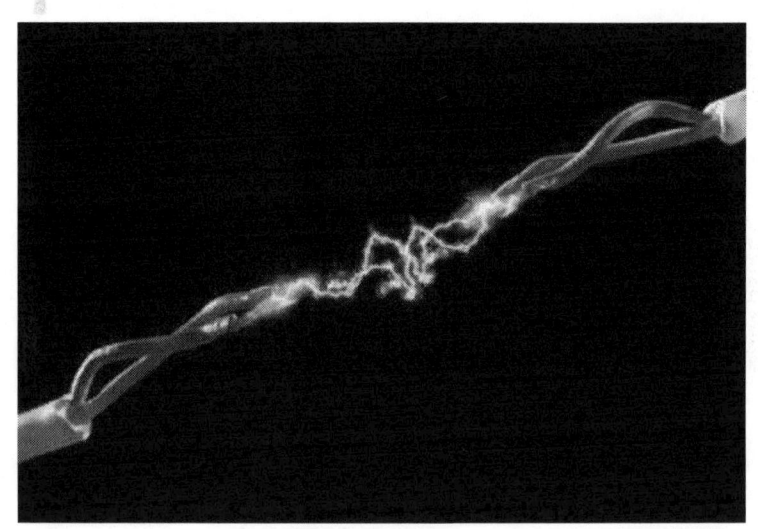

Illustration 288: Electrical Arcing or Electrical Spark. The arcing process produces a very low light source with has no effect on the human body. The light emitted can be observed by the naked eye without risk to the vision. This is due to the very low intensity of the electromagnetic emissions of electrical sparking.

Plasma (or electrical arcing) devices for aesthetic purposes, emit low intensity electromagnetic radiations (which are of lower intensity than most user interface screens).

The new legislation is intended to cover only those devices emitting high intensity electromagnetic radiations which has some effect on to the skin.

www.voltaicplasma.com   Author: Andreas Russo

The intensity of the light emitted by arcing or plasma devices is very low. These broadband low intensity electromagnetic emissions of the electrical arc, although visible to the eye (like the light emitted by most users interfaces) cannot be felt by the human body. This light has no effect whatsoever on the skin or the human body. Generally the emissions intensity is so low, that plasma is generally adopted in several different industries without the use of any protective eye-ware, like in case of lasers .

The most powerful electrical arcs known are lightening. Even the light emitted by lightening has no effect on the human body and it can be observed by the naked eye without any hazards to the vision. Also, the light associated to such powerful arcs does not affect the human body (like heat transfer etc). It has to be borne in mind that it is not the light emitted by the lightening that makes it dangerous, but the power associated to its electric discharge. Obviously the power associated to most voltaic arcing devices is thousands times lower than those of lightening.

The physics behind heat transmission using plasma are very different than those of HIER, The way heat is transmitted during arcing is the same as that of radio frequency devices, "electrolysis" etc (which is by means of electric discharge or using electricity).

Plasma (or electrical arcing) devices for aesthetic purposes, emit low intensity electromagnetic radiations (which are of lower intensity than most user interface screens).

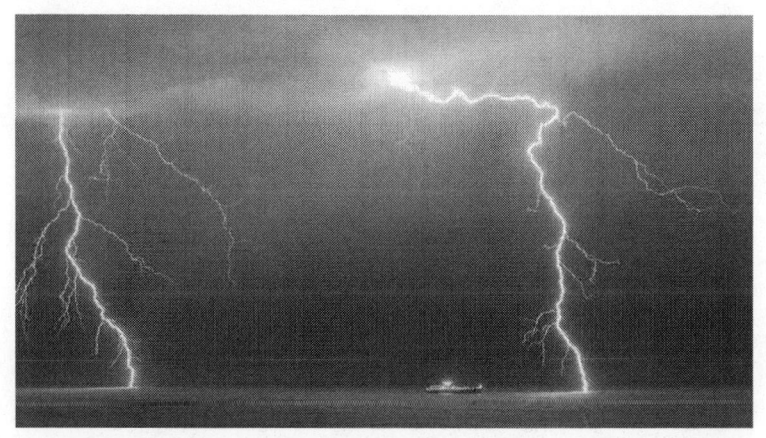

Illustration 289: Lightning is the most powerful arc in nature. The light emitted by this high power phenomenon has no effect on the human body, even when the electrical discharges are this powerful.

Plasma is used in all industries, including manufacturing and assembly lines as well as medicine and aesthetics. In no instances protective eye-ware is required.

www.voltaicplasma.com   Author: Andreas Russo

This is because the broad spectrum electromagnetic energy (light) emitted by the electric spark is of such low intensity that is not dangerous and it can be observed directly by the human naked eye without any hazards.

Also as we know there are more potent sparks in nature than those used in aesthetic by electrical arcing devices, these are Lightening. No one has ever been blinded or affected by the light produced in lightening. No one has ever issued a warning to wear protective eye-ware during a thunderstorm. This is clear simply because the light emitted by the potent electrical spark (lightening) is of very low intensity and does not cause any harm on the human body. To be clear the danger posed by lightening is not due to the light itself, but the power of the electrical discharge itself.

Therefore if the light emitted by a lightening (the highest intensity electrical arc known in nature) can be observed by the naked eye at any distance and has no effect on the human body then the electromagnetic radiations of those small arcs emitted by devices used in aesthetic applications are extremely low.

Also trying to compare the luminescence of the electrical arcs used in aesthetics and those of a mobile phone screen it is easily found that the light intensity of the mobile device screen is several times higher than that of the electrical arc.

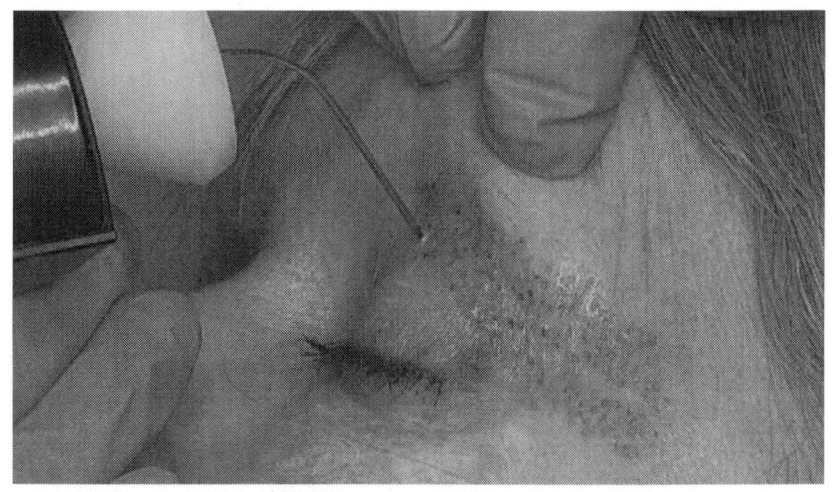

Illustration 290: Electrical discharge in air during a routine aesthetic treatment. The light emitted by the electrical arc has very low intensity. No protective eye-wear is used by the user and the subject undergoing the treatment. This is because the light emitted by the arc has so low intensity that it can be observed by the naked eye without incurring into any health and safety hazards.

To summarise we have seen that:

1. Electrical arcing devices emit low intensity electromagnetic radiations. These radiations are incoherent and of broad spectrum like those radiated by most other user interfaces like LED screen and touch screens. However the light emitted by plasma devices is of lower intensity than that of a mobile phone screen and most other user interfaces.

2. The light emitted by the electrical discharge has neither effect on the skin nor the human body. It is the electrical discharge (and not the light emitted by the electrical discharge) which causes the heat propagation into the skin. This aplies to any type of arcing in air and carrier gasses.

3. The light emitted by the electrical arcing for aesthetic purposes has very low intensity and it has clearly neither any effect on the human body nor the skin.

For all the reasons above plasma devices for aesthetic purposes are **not** High Intensity Electromagnetic Emitting devices and therefore they are not part of the new legislation's remit. As a consequence the MDD (Medical Devices Directive) will not apply to plasma devices also after the new legislation will come into force in May 2020.

Annex I

In this annex you can watch an online seminar where the difference between HIER and Plasma device was explained in detail. To download the relative power point presentation please CLICK HERE

www.voltaicplasma.com					Author: Andreas Russo

Made in the USA
San Bernardino, CA
12 May 2020